AF429424

Introduction to Pharmaceutical Analysis

Introduction to Pharmaceutical Analysis

Dr. Hemant R. Badwaik

Dr. Shiv Shankar Shukla

Dr. D.K. Tripathi

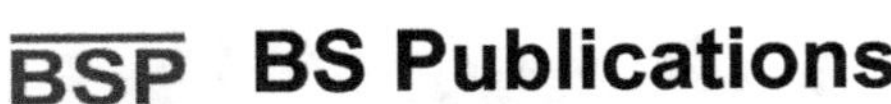

BS Publications

A unit of **BSP Books Pvt. Ltd.**

4-4-309/316, Giriraj Lane, Sultan Bazar,

Hyderabad - 500 095 - T.S.

Introduction to Pharmaceutical Analysis
by *Dr. Hemant R. Badwaik, Dr. Shiv Shankar Shukla and Dr. D. K. Tripathi*

Published by:

BSP **BS Publications**

A unit of **BSP Books Pvt., Ltd.**

4-4-309/316, Giriraj Lane, Sultan Bazar,
Hyderabad - 500 095, T.S.
Phone : 040 - 23445688, 23445600
e-mail : info@bspbooks.net
Website : www.bspbooks.net

ISBN: 978-93-89354-19-5

PREFACE

The content of the book has been prepared as per the syllabus of Pharmaceutical Analysis, recommended by the Pharmacy Council of India for 1st semester, Bachelor in Pharmacy course. Each and every topic of the syllabus has been covered and discussed adequately. There are eleven chapters which cover entire syllabus for the subject.

The book contains two appendixes, in which most of the test solutions and common volumetric solutions have been discussed in terms of their concentration, preparation. Standardization methods of volumetric solutions have also been included there in. The precautions to be taken for preparing or storing have been mentioned in respective places.

Sufficient care has been taken during preparation of the content in terms of language, so that the students can easily understand.

However, the authors would be thankful for any kind of suggestion given for further development of the book as well as for the benefit of the students.

-Authors

ACKNOWLEDGEMENT

The authors are thankful to the Pharmacy Council of India for providing a uniform syllabus for all subjects of Bachelor in Pharmacy course. In fact, this has long been awaited and ultimately has been done. Hence, we again thank the Council and its members.

The author, Dr. D.K. Tripathi expresses his sincere gratitude to the management, Santosh Rungta Group of Institutions, in particular to Sri Santosh Rungta the Chairman, Dr. Saurav Rungta, the Director (Tech) and Sri Sonal Rungta, the Director (F&A) for extending cooperation for preparing the book. Thanks to the colleagues of Dr. Tripathi working Rungta College of Pharmaceutical Sciences & Research, Bhilai for their support extended as and when required. Particularly Dr. Ajazuddin, Dr. Amit Alexander, Shri. Ayushmaan Roy, and Sri. Gyanesh Sahu.

Finally, for the cooperation extended by the members of the family, Dr. Tripathi remains thankful to them.

-Authors

CONTENTS

CHAPTER 1: DEFINITION AND SCOPE

CHAPTER 2: ERRORS

CHAPTER 3: ACID-BASE TITRATION

CHAPTER 7: GRAVIMETRY

CHAPTER 8: REDOX TITRATIONS

CHAPTER 9: CONDUCTOMETRY

Definition and Scope

Pharmaceutical manufacturing industries are supposed to conduct both qualitative and quantitative analysis to assure that the raw materials used meet the desired specifications and to ensure the quality of the final product.

Analysis plays a very important role during the development and manufacturing of a pharmaceutical product. The market, as well as regulatory authority, demands evidence-based data regarding qualitative as well as quantitative measurement of a drug. This is required to make a formulation of definite strength to ensure the desired dose and safe therapeutic activity. Analysis conducted in pharmaceutical industries or laboratory on drugs or on their products is named Pharmaceutical analysis.

Various types of solutions are used in the analysis. For example; test solution, reagent solution, stock solution, dilute solution, volumetric or standard solution, etc. Each type of solution has got separate applications and importance.

LEARNING OBJECTIVES

After studying the chapter the students familiarize themselves with the following concepts:

- ✓ Different Techniques of Analysis
- ✓ Methods of Expressing Concentration
- ✓ Primary and Secondary Standards
- ✓ Preparation and standardization of various molar and normal solutions- Oxalic acid, sodium hydroxide, hydrochloric acid, sodium thiosulphate, sulphuric acid, potassium permanganate, and ceric ammonium sulphate

1.1 DIFFERENT TECHNIQUES OF ANALYSIS

A sample is analyzed primarily for two purposes – identification and determination of content. Accordingly, the techniques of analysis are classified into two categories – qualitative and quantitative.

Qualitative tests are generally conducted to detect whether the desired compound or substance is present in the sample or not. Hence, this type of tests is for identification of the compound in the sample or for the limit test.

Quantitative tests are done to quantify or determine the amount of a particular compound or substance present in a sample. These techniques are based on (1) the quantitative measurement of the amount of the reagent added to complete the reaction or measurement of the amount of the reaction product, (2) measuring the characteristic movement of a substance in a specific medium under controlled conditions, (3) measurement of electrical properties of the compound, (4) measurement of some spectroscopic properties of the compound.

Therefore, the techniques used in the pharmaceutical analysis can be classified into four types;

1. Chemical methods:
   - Volumetric or titrimetric method
   - Gravimetric method
   - Gasometric method
2. Electrical methods:
   - Potentiometry
   - Conductometry
   - Polarography
   - Voltammetry
   - Amperometry
3. Instrumental method
4. Biological or microbiological method

(i)   Chemical methods

Volumetric or titrimetric method: In this method, a definite amount of sample is dissolved in water or in a suitable solvent and titrated with a titrant of known concentration using a suitable indicator till the end point is reached. The volume of titrant required is used to calculate the amount of the active substance present in the sample is calculated. This may be neutralization, complexometric, precipitation, oxidation-reduction, or nonaqueous titration.

Gravimetric methods: In this method, the substance to be determined is converted into an insoluble compound (precipitate) in the purest form. The precipitate is separated, washed, dried, and then weighed. The method is a time consuming one. In the electro-gravimetric method, the sample is electrolyzed over the electrode and the compound deposited is weighed after drying.

In thermogravimetry (TG) the changein weight is recorded, in differential thermal analysis (DTA) the difference in temperature between the sample and an inert reference substance is observed. While in differential scanning calorimetry (DSC) the energy required to establish a zero-temperature difference between the sample and reference substances measured.

Gasometric analysis: It refers to the measurement of the volume of gas evolved or absorbed in a chemical reaction. The gases analyzed in this method are CO_2, N_2O, N_2, cyclopropane, amyl nitrate, ethylene, helium, etc.

(ii) Electrical methods

In these methods, the electric current, voltage or resistance is measured with respect to the concentration of the same species present in the solution. This type of methods includes

Potentiometry: In this method, the electrical potential of an electrode in equilibrium with an ion is measured.

Conductometry: This method involves the measurement of electrical conductivity of an electrode with reference to a reference electrode.

Polarography, Voltammetry, and Amperometry: In these methods, electrical current at a microelectrode is measured.

(iii) Instrumental methods

In these methods, some physical properties of the compound or a substance are measured. When a very small quantity of the compound or substance is present in a sample, these methods are used. These methods are very selective, sensitive, accurate and simple. Any change in the properties such as absorbance, specific rotation, refractive index, migration difference, and charge to mass ratio of the compound or substance can be measured very quickly.

Spectroscopic methods include ultraviolet, visible, infrared, atomic absorption, x-ray, and nuclear magnetic resonance spectroscopy. These methods of analysis measure the amount of radiant energy of a particular wavelength either absorbed, scattered or emitted by the sample.

Emission spectroscopic method involves heating or electrical treatment of the sample to excite the atoms in the sample so that these emit the energy and measure the intensity of this energy. This method includes flame photometry, fluorometry, etc. While in absorption spectroscopy the amount of radiation absorbed by the sample being studied. For example, UV and visible spectroscopy, IR, NMR, AAS, etc. can be used for this purpose.

Chromatographic technique and Electrophoretic methods are based on the separation of the compounds in a mixture. The methods are used to identify the compounds of mixtures. The chromatographic techniques involve TLC, HPTLC, HPLC, GC, etc.

In Mass spectrometry, the material is vaporized using a high vacuum and the vapor is bombarded by a high energy electron beam. The molecules in vapor state fragment and produce ions of varying sizes. These ions are differentiated by accelerating them in the electrical field and then these are deflected in a magnetic field. Each type of ion produces a peak in the mass spectrum.

(iv)   Biological and microbiological methods

Biological methods are used to determine or measure the potency of a drug or its derivative when there is no suitable physical or chemical method. Such methods of analysis are called bio-assays.

Microbiological methods are used to determine the potency of antibiotics or anti-microbial agents. The inhibition of growth of bacteria by the sample is compared with that by a standard antibiotic. These methods include cup and disc, or turbidimetric.

1.2 METHODS OF EXPRESSING CONCENTRATION

The concentration of a solution means how much solute is present in a definite amount (mass or volume) of solvent or solution. It can be expressed in various ways. For example, percentage, normality, molarity, molality, mole fraction. Since a liquid can be measured by volume or mass, the percentage concentration may be weight/weight, weight/volume, volume/ volume or volume/weight.

Percentage concentration (w/w)

It refers to a number of grams of solute present in 100g of the solution according to the metric system.

That is,

$$\% \, (w/w) = \frac{\text{Mass of solute}}{\text{Mass of solution}} \times 100$$

Sometimes, the quantity of the solute or solution is expressed in volume along with the density of the solute or solution. In such a case, the mass of the solute/solution is calculated prior to the calculation of percent (w/w). This is illustrated through an example below.

Example 1: A solution of sodium chloride contains 5g of sodium chloride in 250g of solution. Find out the concentration (w/w) of the solution.

Solution: Percent concentration $(w/w) = \dfrac{5g}{250g} \times 100 = \mathbf{2}$

Example 2: 125g of a solution contains 25mL of glycerin. The density of glycerin is 1.285g/mL. Calculate the concentration of the solution in %w/w.

Solution: Density of glycerin = 1.285g/mL, Volume of glycerin present in 125g of solution = 25mL

Mass of glycerin present in 125g of solution = density × volume = 1.285g/mL × 25mL = 32.125g

So, the percent concentration (w/w) of glycerin = $\dfrac{32.125g}{125g} \times 100 = \mathbf{25.7}$

Example 3: 400mL of a solution contains 320.5g of sucrose. Density of the solution is 1.255g/mL. Calculate the concentration of the solution in %w/w.

Solution: Density of the solution = 1.255g/mL,

Volume of the solution = 400mL

Mass of the solution = density × volume = 1.255g/mL × 400mL = 502.0g

Mass of the sucrose present in 502g of solution = 320.5g

So, the percent concentration (w/w) of the solution = $\dfrac{320.5g}{502g} \times 100 = \mathbf{63.84}$

Percentage concentration (w/v)

According to metric system it refers to number of grams of solute present in 100mL of solution.

That is,

$$\% \,(w/v) = \dfrac{\text{Mass of solute}}{\text{Volume of solution}} \times 100$$

Sometimes, the quantity of the solute or solution is expressed in grams along with the density of the solute or solution. In such a case, the volume of the solute/solution is calculated prior to the calculation of percent (w/v). This is illustrated through an example below.

Example 4: 500g of sucrose is dissolved in water to prepare 600mL of syrup. Find out the concentration of the syrup.

Solution: Volume of the syrup = 600mL,

Mass of the solute = 500g

Concentration of the syrup, $\% \,(w/v) = \dfrac{\text{Mass of solute}}{\text{Volume of solution}} \times 100 = \dfrac{500g}{600mL} \times 100 =$ **83.33**

Example 5: To prepare150 mL of 10%w/v solution of hydrochloric acid how many milliliters of HCl of 98.5%w/v would be required?

Solution: Concentration of HCl = 98.5%w/v;

Required amount of HCl = 10g

Volume of HCl $=10g = \dfrac{100mL}{98.5g} \times 10g = \mathbf{10.15mL}$

Percentage concentration (v/v)

According to the metric system, it refers to a number of milliliters of solute present in 100mL of solution.

That is,

$$\% \,(v/v) = \dfrac{\text{Volume of solute}}{\text{Volume of solution}} \times 100$$

Sometimes, the quantity of the solute or solution is expressed in grams along with the density of the solute or solution. In such a case, the mass of the solute/solution is converted into volume prior to the calculation of percent (v/v). This is illustrated through an example below.

Example 6: The concentration of a solution of sorbitol liquid is expressed as 15%w/v. If the density of the sorbitol liquid is 1.287g/mL; calculate the volume of sorbitol liquid required to make 900mL of the solution.

Solution: Density of sorbitol liquid = 1.287g/mL;

Volume of solution = 900mL

Concentration of the solution = 15%w/v = 15g in 100mL

For 900mL solution the amount of sorbitol liquid would be required $= \dfrac{15g}{100mL} \times 900mL = 135g$

Volume of 135g of sorbitol liquid $= \dfrac{Mass}{Density} = \dfrac{135g}{1.287g/mL} = \mathbf{104.9mL}$

Normality

Normality of a solution is defined as the number of gram-equivalents of a solute present in one litre of the solution. In other words, number of milli gram-equivalents in one mL.

Thus,

$$\text{Normality} = \frac{\text{Number of gramequivalents}}{\text{Number of litres}} = \frac{\text{Number of milligramequivalents}}{\text{Number of millilitres(mL)}}$$

To define normality the term *equivalent weight* is used. However, the value of equivalent weight varies with the type of chemical reaction, and it is difficult to give a clear and universal definition of the term. It is found that the same compound can have different equivalent weights in different chemical reactions.

The definition of the term, equivalent weight, with respect to the type of chemical reaction is being explained below.

Equivalent weight

Neutralization reactions:

The equivalent weight of an acid refers to the amount of the acid containing a one-gram atom of replaceable hydrogen, i.e., 1.0078g (1.008g) *of hydrogen.* The replaceable hydrogen in an acid is alternatively called as basicity of an acid. The number of replaceable hydrogens in monobasic acid such as hydrochloric acid, acetic acid, Hydrobromic acid, hydroiodic acid is one. Dibasic acid such as sulphuric acid contains two and tribasic acid such as phosphoric acid contains three replaceable hydrogens. Thus, the equivalent weight of monobasic acid is its molecular weight, that of a dibasic acid is ½ of its molecular weight and that of a tribasic acid is 1/3 of its molecular weight.

The equivalent weight of a base is the weight of it containing one replaceable hydroxyl group, 17.008g of an ionizable hydroxyl group (17.008g of hydroxyl are equivalent to 1.008g of hydrogen).

In other words, the equivalent weight of monoacidic base sodium hydroxide, potassium hydroxide is their molecular weight. The equivalent weight of diacidic base such as calcium hydroxide, barium hydroxide, strontium hydroxide is ½ of their molecular weight.

Salts of strong bases and weak acids such as sodium carbonate or sodium acetate hydrolyzes in water and the resulting solution is alkaline. Each molecule of such salt reacts with two molecules of hydrochloric acid; hence, the equivalent weight of such salt is ½ of the molecular weight.

$$\text{Equivalent weight} = \frac{\text{Molecular weight}}{\text{Acidity}} \quad \text{(for base)}$$

$$\text{Equivalent weight} = \frac{\text{Molecular weight}}{\text{Basicity}} \quad \text{(for acid)}$$

Example 7: The molecular weights of sulphuric acid, hydrochloric acid, acetic acid, and oxalic acid dihydrate are 98, 36.5, 60, and 106 respectively. Calculate their equivalent weights.

Solution: For acid, the equivalent weight $= \dfrac{\text{Molecular weight}}{\text{Basicity}}$

Basicity of sulphuric acid, hydrochloric acid, acetic acid, and oxalic acid dihydrate are 2, 1, 1, 2 respectively.

Hence, equivalent weight of sulphuric acid $= \dfrac{98}{2} = \textbf{49}$

$$\text{Equivalent weight of hydrochloric acid} = \frac{36.5}{1} = \textbf{36.5}$$

$$\text{Equivalent weight of acetic acid} = \frac{60}{1} = \textbf{60}$$

Similarly, equivalent weight of oxalic acid dihydrate $= \dfrac{106}{2} = \textbf{53}$

Note: Since oxalic acid is stable with two molecules of water of crystallization its equivalent weight should be calculated including its water of crystallization $[(COOH)_2, 2H_2O]$.

Normality can also be defined as;

$$\text{Normality} = \frac{\text{Number of gram\,--\,equivalents}}{\text{Number of litres}}$$

$$= \frac{\text{Number of milligram\,--\,equivalents}}{\text{Number of millilitres (mL)}}$$

So, number of milligram-equivalents = Normality × Number of milliliters (mL)

Say, two substances X and Y are dissolved in sufficient water to make standard solutions having strength Sx and Sy respectively. If two solutions are reacted and Vx mL of X is found exactly equivalent to Vy mL of Y (that is Vx mL neutralizes completely Vy mL);

Then, Vx mL × Sx (Normality of the solution of X) = Vy mL × Sy (Normality of the solution of Y)

Example 8: Calculate the volume of 0.5N hydrochloric acid to be required to precipitate 0.45g of silver nitrate completely.

Solution: The reaction is $AgNO_3 + HCl = AgCl + HNO_3$

Equivalent weight of $AgNO_3$ being 169.89g; 1N solution of it contains 169.89g per lt.

In other words, 169.89g of $AgNO_3$ per litre makes 1N solution

Then, 0.45g of $AgNO_3$ per litre makes $\dfrac{0.45g}{169.89g} = 0.002648N$

Say, the volume of $AgNO_3$ solution required = 1000 mL

Given that, the strength of hydrochloric acid solution = 0.5N

Volume of hydrochloric acid solution consumed = V mL

Then, V mL × 0.5N = 0.002648N × 1000mL

$$V = \frac{0.002648N \times 1000mL}{0.5N} = \mathbf{5.296mL}$$

Example 9: How many milliliters of 0.125N solution A need to be diluted to prepare 500mL of 0.1N of solution?

Solution: Say, V mL of 0.125N solution A would be diluted.

Given that, the strength of solution A = 0.125N

The strength of the required solution = 0.1N

Volume of required solution = 500mL

Then, V mL × 0.125N = 500mL × 0.1N

So, $\qquad V = \dfrac{500mL \times 0.1N}{0.125N} = \mathbf{400mL}$

Complex formation and precipitation reaction

The equivalent weight of the substances take part in these reactions is the amount which contains or reacts with 1gm atom of a universal cation, M^+. In other words, *the equivalent of a substance in these reactions is the amount equivalent to* 1.008g *of hydrogen*. Thus, in case of a cation, the equivalent weight would be its atomic weight divided by its valency and the equivalent weight of the substance is its weight that reacts with one equivalent of the cation.

In a precipitation reaction, the equivalent weight of salt is its gm molecular weight divided by total valency of the reacting ion. Hence, the equivalent weight of silver nitrate in the titration of chloride ion would be the molecular weight of it (silver nitrate).

In case of complex formation reaction, the equivalent weight is calculated with the help of the ionic equation of the reaction. For example, the equivalent weight of potassium cyanide in the titration with silver ions would be 2 moles (2 × 65.118).

$$2CN^- + Ag^+ \leftrightarrow [Ag(CN)_2]^-$$

Similarly, zinc is titrated with potassium ferrocyanide. According to the ionic equation as shown below the equivalent weight of potassium ferrocyanide is one-third of its formula weight.

$$3Zn^{2+} + 2K_4Fe(CN)_6 \rightarrow 6K^+ + K_2Zn_3[Fe(CN)_6]_2$$

Oxidation-reduction reaction

The equivalent weight of an oxidizing or reducing substance (reagent) is commonly defined as the weight of the substance which contains or reacts with 1.008g of available hydrogen or 8.000g of available oxygen.

The term 'available' means 'the amount actually being utilized in the oxidation or reduction'. By writing the hypothetical equation for the reaction the amount of available oxygen can be known. An example is given below,

$$2KMnO_4 => K_2O + 2MnO + 5O \quad \text{(in acidic medium)}$$

The equation shows that in acidic medium two molecules of $KMnO_4$ release 5 atoms of available oxygen.

In an actual oxidation-reduction reaction (redox reaction) electrons are transferred from the reducing agent to the oxidizing agent. Thus, oxidation is a process in which loss of one or more electrons by atoms or ions takes place while reduction is a process in which gain of one or more electrons by a reducing atom or ion takes place.

Method of calculating the equivalent weight on the basis of oxidation number has been described in Chapter 7 (Red-ox titration).

Molality

The molality of a solution is defined as the number of moles of a substance present in one kg of solvent.

$$\text{Molality or molal concentration } (m) = \frac{\text{No of moles of solute}}{\text{kg of solvent}}$$

Molarity

Molarity of a solution is defined as the number of moles of a substance present in one litre of solution. One mole is the amount of a substance that contains one gram molecular weight of that substance. In case of an element, it refers to its atomic/molecular weight, in case of a molecule it refers to the sum of the atomic weights of constituting elements, in case of a radical the same is true. For example;

One mole of hydrogen = 2 × its atomic weight = 2 × 1 = 2g, (hydrogen is diatomic; its molecular formula is H_2).

One mole of carbon = 1 × 12.01 = 12.01g ≈ 12g

One mole of SO_4^{2+} = 1 × S + 4 × O = 1 × 32.06 + 4 × 16 = 32.06 + 64 = 96.06g

One mole of Na_2CO_3 = 2 × 23 + 1 × 12 + 3 × 16 = 46 + 12 + 48 = 106g

One molar solution means one gram molecular weight of a substance is present in 1000mL of solution. Thus,

$$\text{Molarity or molar concentration } M = \frac{\text{No of moles of solute}}{\text{Liter of solutions}}$$

For example, 2g of Na_2CO_3 is dissolved in sufficient water to produce 50mL of solution. molecular weight of Na_2CO_3 and valency is 2; $50 \text{ mL} = \frac{50\text{mL}}{1000} = 0.05\text{lt}$.

The molarity of the solution $= \frac{2\text{g}}{50\text{mL}} = \frac{2\text{g}}{0.05\text{lt}} = 40\text{M}$

1.3   PRIMARY AND SECONDARY STANDARDS

Primary standards

If a substance is available in a pure and stable state, a solution of definite concentration (normality/molarity) can be prepared. This is done by accurate weighing the calculated amount of the substance, dissolving in a solvent to prepare a definite volume of the solution. Such a substance is called a *primary standard.*

The standard solution is a solution of known concentration used for titrating another solution to find out the concentration of the solution titrated.

Thus, the concentration of such standard solution, used in various titrations, is called the *strength* of the solution. This is illustrated through an example below.

Example 10:   In a titration 24.65mL of 1.0053M solution of potassium dihydrogen phthalate was consumed by 25mL of sodium hydroxide solution. Find out the strength of the sodium hydroxide solution.

Solution: Volume of potassium dihydrogen phthalate solution consumed (V) = 24.65mL

Volume of sodium hydroxide solution (V_1) = 25.00mL

Strength of potassium dihydrogen phthalate solution (S) = 1.0052M

Strength of sodium hydroxide solution (S_1) = ?

According to the rule of neutralization, $V \times S = V_1 \times S_1$

So, the strength of the sodium hydroxide solution, $S_1 = \dfrac{V \times S}{V_1} = \dfrac{24.65 \times 1.0052 \text{ M}}{25} =$ **0.9911M**

Example 11: 20.00mL of ferrous sulphate solution reacts completely with 25.50mL of 0.15N potassium permanganate solution. Calculate the strength of ferrous sulphate solution in terms of molarity.

Solution: In this reaction, ferrous sulphate acts as reducing agent and its normal solution contain 1 mol per lt or 151.90g per lt.

Say, the strength of ferrous sulphate solution is S

Given that the volume of ferrous sulphate solution consumed = 20.00mL

The volume of potassium permanganate solution = 25.50mL

The strength of potassium permanganate solution = 0.15N

Then, $S \times 20.00 = 25.50\text{mL} \times 0.15\text{N}$

So, $$S = \frac{25.50\text{mL} \times 0.15\text{N}}{20.00\text{mL}} = 0.191\text{N}$$

Since the concentration of ferrous sulphate in its normal and moral solution is the same, the strength of ferrous sulphate solution would be **0.191M**.

Properties of a primary standard:

To become a primary standard, a substance should possess the following properties;

1. It should be easily obtained, purified, dried (preferably at around 105°C), and preserve in a pure state for a reasonable period of time. (Hydrated substances cannot fulfill this criterion because without partial decomposition their surface moisture cannot be removed completely.)

2. During weighing a substance is exposed to air. So, it must be stable in the presence of air. That is, it should not oxidize or absorb moisture (hygroscopic). It should not be affected by carbon dioxide too. The composition of the substance must remain unchanged during storage.

3. The substance should not contain impurities more than 0.02%. The impurities should be qualitatively and quantitatively measurable by using a sensitive method.

4. It should have a high equivalent weight; so that it can be weighed accurately. The precision in weighing is usually $0.1 - 0.2$ mg. However, for an accuracy of 1 in 1000, at least 200 mg should be weighed.

5. The substance should be readily soluble in water or in another solvent under the normal conditions.

6. The reaction between the standard solution and the substance being titrated should be stoichiometric and instantaneous. There should be a negligible error in titration and should be easily determined.

Practically it is very difficult to get a substance which can be used as an ideal primary standard. It is necessary to compromise between the ideal properties. Different substances are used as the primary standard in specific titration. For example, sodium carbonate, borax, potassium hydrogen phthalate, succinic acid, etc., are used as the primary standard in acid-base titrations. The primary standards used with respect to the type of titration are mentioned in Table 1.1 below.

Table 1.1: List of substances used as the primary standard

Type of titration	Substances used as Primary standards
Acid-base	Potassium hydrogen phthalate $KH(C_8H_4O_4)$ Sodium carbonate $[Na_2CO_3]$ Borax $[Na_2B_4O_7]$ Thallous carbonate $[Tl_2CO_3]$ (poisonous) Potassium bi-iodate $[KH(IO_3)_2]$

Table 1.1: *Contd...*

	Succinic acid [$H_2(C_4H_4O_4)$]
	Benzoic acid [$H(C_7H_5O_2$]
	Adipic acid [$H_2(C_6H_8O_4)$]
	Furoic acid [$H(C_5H_3O_3)$]
	Hydrochloric acid [HCl] (constant boiling)
Complexometric	Silver nitrate [$AgNO_3$]
	Sodium chloride [$NaCl$]
	Potassium chloride [KCl]
	Disodium ethyl enediaminetetra-acetate dihydrate and anhydrous
	Soluble salts of various metals such as Zinc, Magnesium, Copper, and spectroscopically pure manganese depending on the reaction
Precipitation	Silver [Ag]
	Silver nitrate [$AgNO_3$]
	Sodium chloride [$NaCl$]
	Potassium chloride [KCl]
	Potassium bromide (obtained from potassium bromate)
Oxidation-reduction	Potassium dichromate [$K_2Cr_2O_7$]
	Potassium bromate [$KBrO_3$]
	Potassium iodate [KIO_3]
	Potassium bi-iodate [$KH(IO_3)_2$]
	Iodine [I_2]
	Sodium oxalate [$Na_2C_2O_4$]
	Arsenious oxide [As_2O_3]
	Electrolytic or pure iron

Usually, hydrated salts are not used as primary standard; because these cannot be dried efficiently. The salts such as borax [$Na_2B_4O_7, 10H_2O$], oxalic acid [$H_2C_2O_4, 2H_2O$], copper sulphate [$CuSO_4, 5H_2O$] do not effloresce. Experimentally, these have been found satisfactory as a secondary standard.

In general, the standard solution (*titrant*) is added from a burette. Addition of standard solution or titrant is continued till the reaction is complete. The substance being titrated is called *titrate* and the process is called *titration*. The point at which the reaction becomes complete is called *endpoint* or *equivalencepoint*. The completion of the titration is detected by the change of color of a substance added in the form of solution to the titration mixture. Such a substance is called an *indicator*.

Secondary standards

The name itself tells that this is a standard which comes second. That's why the name is secondary. In laboratories,the secondary standard is used to prepare reagents, kits or to produce quality control material for other labs. The primary standard is used as the primary calibrator or primary reference material. A secondary standard is used for the purpose of calibration of control material for analysis of the unknown concentration of a substance. So principally, secondary standard serves the purpose of external quality control. This makes it essential that the secondary standard must first be standardized against the primary standard. There are other points to remember. For preparing the standard solutions distilled water must be used.

Similarly, before using the chemicals it is necessary to check the date of manufacture, expiry date, date of receipt of chemical, whether the conditions for its transport was followed or not, whether the seal tampers, etc. Solutions of these substances are routinely used in laboratories of institutes and industries also. The secondary standard substances possess many of the properties of primary standards, but not all. These substances are not available as purest and stable form. For example, sodium hydroxide and potassium hydroxide are commonly used as standards. These are extremely hygroscopic, are not obtained as purest form, contain some amount of carbonates. Exact results cannot be obtained in the presence of carbonate. Hence, these substances are used as a secondary standard. Certain important properties of secondary standards are given below;

- It has less purity than the primary standard
- Less stable and more reactive
- Their solutions remain stable for a long time
- Standardized against a primary standard

The best and common example is anhydrous sodium hydroxide (NaOH) and potassium hydroxide (KOH). It is extremely hygroscopic. As soon as the bottle is opened, sodium hydroxide starts absorbing moisture from the atmosphere and within a short time it becomes moist.

Another example is potassium permanganate ($KMnO_4$) very often used as a secondary standard. It is a good oxidizing agent or in other words, it is reactive hence, less stable. Due to its reactivity, it is oxidized to manganese oxide (MnO_2) which contaminates the $KMnO_4$. For this reason, it is unsuitable for being a primary standard. But it can be used very well as a secondary standard.

1.4 PREPARATION AND STANDARDIZATION OF VARIOUS MOLAR AND NORMAL SOLUTIONS

Preparation of various molar and normal solutions

These are primarily standard solutions because their concentrations in terms of normality or molarity have to be measured and maintained. The solution may be of a primary standard or secondary standard substance.

A solution of definite strength can be prepared by accurately weighing the substance, dissolving in an appropriate solvent, usually water to make up a definite volume. This is done when the substance is available in a pure and stable state, and if it neither absorbs nor releases moisture. The solution is prepared in a volumetric flask.

When a solution of exact strength such as 0.1 N or 0.1 M is required, the solution can be prepared as follows;

Initially, a slightly concentrated solution is prepared. After determining the actual strength of the solution, a measured volume of the solvent is added to the standardized solution and mixed thoroughly. The solution thus prepared possesses the exact strength. This is explained through the following example. Say, 500mL of the 0.1M solution of NaOH is to be prepared. According to the molecular weight, 2g is to be dissolved in water to make 500mL. Now, 2.2g of NaOH is taken and 500mL of its solution is prepared, standardized against potassium hydrogen phthalate. Say, the actual strength is 1.127(0.1)M or 0.1127M and during titration 53.00mL of alkali solution is consumed. Then the balance amount of alkali solution becomes $500 - 53 = 447$ mL.

So,$\qquad 0.1M \times V \text{ mL} = 0.1127M \times 447 \text{ mL}$

Or,$\qquad V = \dfrac{0.1M \times 447mL}{0.1127M} = 503.769mL \approx 503.80 \text{ mL}$

Thus, 503.80 mL $-$ 447.00 mL $= 56.8$ mL of water should be added to 447mL of alkali solution and mixed thoroughly to obtain the exact strength of 0.1M.

Note that the extra volume of water must be accurately measured.

When substances such as most alkali hydroxides, some inorganic acids, etc. are not available in a pure and stable state, their solutions nearest to the required strength are prepared. These solutions are standardized with appropriate primary standard solutions to find out their actual strength. This type of substance is called a secondary standard.

Preparation of molar solutions

The one molar solution is prepared by dissolving one gram molecular weight of a substance in sufficient solvent, usually water, to make 1000mL of the solution.

Preparation of normal solutions

Normal solution

Normal solutions solutionthat contains 1 g. the equivalent weight of a substance per litre of solution. It is expressed as N. The strength of a solution can be N, N/2 (0.5N), N/5 (0.2N), N/10 (0.1N), N/50 (0.02N), N/100 (0.01N), etc.

For example, equivalent weight of NaOH $= \dfrac{40}{1} = 40$; similarly, equivalent weight of $Na_2CO_3 = \dfrac{106}{2} = 53$

Thus, when 40g of NaOH present in one litre it makes 1N solution and 1N solution of Na_2CO_3 means 53g of Na_2CO_3 is present in one litre of solution.

If the substance is available in pure form, a solution of particular strength (normality/molarity) can be easily prepared by weighing the required amount accurately and dissolving in the solvent, usually distilled water to make the required volume.

If the substance can absorb some moisture (unbound moisture), the substance should be dried in a hot air oven or under vacuum drier and cooled in a desiccator, thereafter it is used.

1. Preparation and standardization of 0.1M Oxalic acid

The molecular formula of oxalic acid is $(COOH)_2, 2H_2O$ and its molecular weight is 126.068. Hence, 1M solution of oxalic acid shall contain 126.068g per litre. A.R. oxalic acid has been widely used as standard. Since the water content of oxalic acid is uncertain, it is not really recommended to use as a primary standard. Only it is used by elementary students. It should be stored or preserved in well-closed container in a desiccator over an appropriate deliquescent such as sodium bromide.

Preparation of 0.1M Oxalic acid

To prepare 250mL of the 0.1M solution of oxalic acid $\dfrac{126.068}{4}$ g = 31.517g would be required.

> Weigh accurately 31.517of oxalic acid, transfer into a clean 250mL volumetric flask.
> Dissolve in freshly prepared distilled water and make up the volume.

Standardization of 0.1M Oxalic acid against 0.1M potassium permanganate

> Pipette out accurately 25.00mL of oxalic acid solution in a 250mL clean conical flask, add 100mL of freshly prepared distilled water.
> Add 6mL of concentrated sulphuric acid slowly, mix; if necessary heat the solution to 70°C.
> Rinse a 50mL clean burette with 0.1M potassium permanganate solution, fill the burette with 0.1M potassium permanganate solution, open the stopcock and drain the solution to remove air bubble from the jet completely.
> Refill the burette with 0.1M potassium permanganate solution; adjust the meniscus at zero marks of the burette.
> Titrate the hot solution (temperature should be within 65° – 70°C) of oxalic acid slowly with 0.1M potassium permanganate solution until a pale pink color appears which persists for at least 30 seconds. Note the volume of 0.1M potassium permanganate solution consumed (titer value).
> Repeat the determination twice and take the average of the titer values for calculation.

Calculation

Say, the volumes of 0.1M potassium permanganate solution consumed are 24.90mL, 24.90mL and 24.95mL. The average volume, $V = \dfrac{24.90+24.90+24.95}{3}$ mL = 24.92mL

Strength of 0.1M potassium permanganate solution, S = 1.0006

The volume of oxalic acid solution titrated, $V_1 = 25.00$ mL

The strength of 0.1M oxalic acid solution, $S_1 = \dfrac{24.92 \times 1.0006}{25.00} = 0.9974$

Or, the strength of oxalic acid solution is 0.09974M

2. Preparation and standardization of 0.1M Sodium hydroxide

The molecular formula of sodium hydroxide is NaOH; it is most commonly used as a standard alkali because it is very cheap. However, potassium hydroxide and barium hydroxides are also used as standard alkali. All these alkalis are the strong base. But, none of these is available in the purest form. Sodium and potassium hydroxides are very hygroscopic and mostly contain a certain amount of carbonate along with water. Hence, none of these can be used as a primary standard, because the exact result would not be obtained with due to the presence of carbonate. A.R. Sodium hydroxide contains 1 - 2% sodium carbonate and commercially available sodium hydroxide which is prepared from metallic sodium contain less than 1% of sodium carbonate. Due to extreme hygroscopicity, it is not chosen as the primary standard.

The molecular weight of sodium hydroxide, NaOH is 40. Thus, one-liter solution of 1M NaOH will contain 40g of it. Since it is a monoacidic base, its equivalent weight is also 40. Hence, one-liter solution of 1N NaOH will contain 40g of it. It is available in the form of sticks, flakes, or pellets.

Since sodium hydroxide contains extra moisture 10 − 15% more of the calculated quantity should be taken. That is in place of 40g one should take 48 − 50g for making 1lt of 1N/1M solution.

Preparation of 0.1M Sodium hydroxide solution

Take a clean and dry weighing bottle of 15mL capacity, weigh it. Transfer about 2.2g of A.R. NaOH as quickly as possible, close the bottle with lid and weigh the weighing bottle accurately and transfer the content into a clean 500mL volumetric flask. Weigh the empty bottle. The difference in two weights provides the amount of sodium hydroxide taken. Dissolve in freshly distilled water. Shake well and make up the volume up to the mark.

Sodium hydroxide solution can be standardized against various substances such as standard hydrochloric acid, potassium hydrogen phthalate, benzoic acid, succinic acid, adipic acid, potassium bi-iodate, oxalic acid, potassium bi-tartrate, etc. Among these substances, potassium hydrogen phthalate is widely used.

Preparation of 0.1M potassium hydrogen phthalate

A.R. potassium hydrogen phthalate, $HK(C_8H_4O_4)$, is available with a purity of 99.9%. As such it is not hygroscopic. If it is not properly stored, it may contain some moisture. It is to be dried at 120°C for 2 hrs and cooled in a desiccator before use. The molecular weight of potassium hydrogen phthalate is 204.22. Since it has one replaceable hydrogen atom, its equivalent weight would be 204.22. Thus, one litre of the 1M solution will contain 204.22g of potassium hydrogen phthalate and the 0.1M solution will contain 20.422g of potassium hydrogen phthalate per litre.

Standardization of 0.1M Sodium hydroxide against potassium hydrogen phthalate

➢ Take about 2.05g of potassium hydrogen phthalate in a clean and dry weighing bottle, weigh accurately (x)g.

- Transfer the content of the bottle into a clean 100mL volumetric flask, weigh the empty bottle accurately (y)g. The difference between the two weights (i.e., $[x - y]$) would be the amount of potassium hydrogen phthalate taken.
- Rinse the inner walls and add $60 - 70$mL of freshly prepared hot water to the flask, dissolve potassium hydrogen phthalate.
- After complete dissolution adds freshly distilled up to the mark, shake well.
- Pipette out 25.00mL of the potassium hydrogen phthalate solution into a 250mL clean conical flask, add few drops of phenolphthalein solution.
- Rinse a 50mL clean burette thrice with sodium hydroxide solution, fill the burette with sodium hydroxide solution, open the stopcock and drain some solution to remove air bubble completely and to fill the jet with an alkali solution.
- Refill the burette with alkali solution up to the zero marks, titrate potassium hydrogen phthalate solution till a pink color is noticed. Note the titer value.
- Repeat the titration twice more and note the titer values, take the average of the three values for calculation of the strength of the sodium hydroxide solution.

Calculation

Say, the volume of potassium hydrogen phthalate solution $(V_1) = 25.00$mL

Say, the amount of potassium hydrogen phthalate taken, $x - y = 2.0498$g

$$\text{Strength of 0.1M solution of potassium hydrogen phthalate } (S_1) = \frac{\text{Practical weight}}{\text{Theoretical weight}}$$

$$= \frac{2.0498\text{g}}{2.0422\text{g}} = 1.0037$$

$$\text{Volume of sodium hydroxide solution consumed } (V) = \frac{24.95 + 24.95 + 25.00}{3} = 24.97\text{mL}$$

$$V \times S = V_1 \times S_1$$

$$\text{The strength of 0.1M solution of sodium hydroxide } (S) = \frac{25.00\text{mL} \times 1.0037}{24.97\text{mL}} = \mathbf{1.0049}$$

Preparation and Standardization of 0.1N Sodium hydroxide against potassium hydrogen phthalate Same procedure as described above for preparation and standardization of 0.1N Sodium hydroxide against potassium hydrogen phthalate shall be followed.

3. Preparation and standardization of 0.1N hydrochloric acid

Concentrated hydrochloric acid is about $10.5 - 12$ N if it is stored properly and not opened frequently. If this concentrated acid is diluted appropriately with freshly distilled water, a standard solution of desired strength can be prepared. Usually concentrated hydrochloric acid contains vapor of hydrogen chloride. When the bottle is opened the vapor goes out and the acid loses its concentration with time. To avoid this volatility and hygroscopicity, and to maintain the concentration constant, constant-boiling-point HCl can be used. In fact, the constant-boiling-point HCl can be prepared with regular concentrated HCl.

In practice, normal or molar solution of HCl is prepared by diluting regular concentrated HCl. The strength of concentrated HCl available is 10.5 N – 12N. To prepare 1N HCl 90.00mL of concentrated HCl is diluted with freshly prepared distilled water to make 1000mL.

Preparation of 0.1N HCl: The solution of 0.1N HCl is prepared by diluting 9.00mL of concentrated HCl to 1000mL with freshly distilled water.

Standardization

(A) Standardization against anhydrous sodium carbonate

For this purpose, A.R. sodium carbonate having 99.9% purity is used. This may contain little moisture. So, it needs to be dried at 260 – 270°C for 30 min and cooled in a desiccator before use. If it is dried at a temperature above 270°C, sodium carbonate may lose carbon dioxide. The equivalent weight of Na_2CO_3 is 106/2 = 53. Hence, to make a 1N solution of Na_2CO_3 53g of it should be contained in 1 L of solution.

To prepare 0.1N solution 5.3 g of Na_2CO_3 should be present in one litre of solution. Here only 100mL of 0.1N solution shall be prepared; so, 0.53g of Na_2CO_3 shall be dissolved in water to make 100mL.

Preparation of 0.1N solution of sodium carbonate

Weigh accurately about 0.53g of A.R. sodium carbonate (dried) taken in a weighing bottle and transfer into a 100mL volumetric flask, weigh the empty bottle.

The difference in two weights provides the exact amount of sodium carbonate transferred. Dissolve the sodium carbonate in sufficient freshly prepared distilled water, make up the volume with water, and shake well.

Procedure

- Pipette out 25.00mL of sodium carbonate solution and take it in a clean 250mL conical flask, add 2 - 3 drops of methyl orange indicator solution to the alkali solution.
- Take a clean 50mL burette; rinse it thrice with an acid solution; then fill the burette with alkali solution above the zero marks.
- Open the stopcock of the burette, drain the acid to ensure complete removal of air bubble from the jet and filling of the jet with the acid, close the stopcock.
- Refill the burette with the acid slightly above the zero marks; adjust the meniscus of the acid at zero marks.
- Titrate the alkali solution with the acid and rotate the flask so that reaction is completed; continue the titration till the color of the solution becomes faint yellow.
- Wash the walls of the conical flask with fresh water, mix and add the acid dropwise with constant swirling.
- Continue the addition of acid dropwise till the color of the solution changes to orange or light pink.
- Note the volume of acid required for titration (titer value).
- Repeat the process twice more and take the average titer value for calculation.

Calculation of strength of 0.1N HCl solution

Say, the average titer value is 24.75mL (V_1, volume of acid required),

Amount of Na_2CO_3 to be taken (theoretical weight) = 0.53g for 100mL of 0.1N solution

Weight of Na_2CO_3 taken =0.5297g

$$\text{Strength of 0.1N solution of } Na_2CO_3 \,(S) = \frac{\text{Practical weight}}{\text{Theoretical weight}} = \frac{0.5297g}{0.53g} = 0.9994$$

Volume of Na_2CO_3 solution = V mL

Say, strength of acid solution = S_1

According to law of mass action, $V_1 \times S_1 = V \times S$

$$24.75mL \times S_1 = 25mL \times 0.9994$$

So, the strength of 0.1N HCl solution, $S_1 = \dfrac{25mL \times 0.9994}{24.75mL} = 1.009$

In other words, the strength of acid = **0.1009N**

Standardization against borax

Borax is tetraborate decahydrate ($Na_2B_4O_7, 10H_2O$) is a primary standard. The advantages of borax are;

- Its equivalent weight (190.72) is more than that of Na_2CO_3 (53), the extent of error will be less since more amount of borax is to be weighed.
- It can be easily and economically purified by recrystallization from water,
- Drying for making anhydrous is not required,
- It is practically non-hygroscopic, and
- By using methyl red indicator, a sharp endpoint can be observed. Methyl red is not affected by boric acid, a very weak acid.

$$B_4O_7^{2-} + 2H^+ + 5H_2O \leftrightarrow 4H_3BO_4$$

Procedure

The equivalent weight of borax is 190.72; hence to prepare a 1N solution of it 190.72g should be dissolved in water to make 1000mL.

Hence, to make 1000mL of 0.1N solution 19.072g of borax would be required and $\dfrac{19.072 \times 25}{1000}$ g = 0.4768g would be required for 25mL of 0.1N solution.

- ➢ Weigh accurately 0.48g of A.R. borax and transfer into a clean 250mL conical flask, dissolve in 50 – 60mL of freshly prepared distilled water, add few drops of methyl red solution.
- ➢ Take a clean 50mL burette; rinse it thrice with an acid solution; then fill the burette with alkali solution above the zero marks.

> Open the stopcock of the burette, drain the acid to ensure complete removal of air bubble from the jet and filling of the jet with the acid, close the stopcock.
> Refill the burette with the acid slightly above the zero marks; adjust the meniscus of the acid at zero marks.
> Titrate the borax solution with the acid and rotate the flask so that reaction is completed; continue the titration till about 24mL of the acid is consumed.
> Wash the walls of the conical flask with fresh water, mix and add the acid dropwise with constant swirling.
> Continue the addition of acid dropwise until the pink color is observed.
> Note the volume of acid required for titration (titer value).
> Repeat the process twice more and take the average titer value for calculation.

Calculation of strength of 0.1N HCl solution

Strength of borax solution: Amount of borax to be taken = 0.4768g (Theoretical weight)

Say, the amount of borax taken (1) 0.4729g, (2) 0.4770g, and (3) 0.4765g

Strength of borax solution,

$$S = \quad 1. \quad \frac{\text{Practical weight}}{\text{Theoretical weight}} = \frac{0.4729g}{0.4768g} = 0.9918$$

$$2. \quad \frac{\text{Practical weight}}{\text{Theoretical weight}} = \frac{0.4770g}{0.4768g} = 1.0004$$

$$3. \quad \frac{\text{Practical weight}}{\text{Theoretical weight}} = \frac{0.4765g}{0.4768g} = 0.9994$$

Volume of borax solution, V = 25.00mL

Say, the Volume of HCl solution consumed, V_1 in three titrations are 25.00mL, 24.95mL, and 25.00mL

If the strength of HCl solution is S; then $SV = S_1V_1$

$$1. \quad S_1 = \frac{S \times V}{V_1} = \frac{25.00\text{mL} \times 0.9918}{25.00\text{mL}} = 0.9918$$

$$2. \quad S_1 = \frac{S \times V}{V_1} = \frac{25.00\text{mL} \times 1.0004}{24.95\text{mL}} = 1.0024$$

$$3. \quad S_1 = \frac{S \times V}{V_1} = \frac{25.00\text{mL} \times 0.9994}{25.00\text{mL}} = 0.9994$$

The average strength of 0.1N HCl solution is $\dfrac{0.9918 + 1.0024 + 0.9994}{3} = \mathbf{0.9978}$

In other words, the strength of HCl solution is 0.09978N

Preparation and standardization of 0.1M hydrochloric acid

The molarity and normality of hydrochloric acid are same, since basicity of it is unity (one). Hence, for preparation of 0.1M HCl solution 9.00mL is diluted to 1000mL with freshly distilled water (free from dissolved CO_2).

Preparation of 0.1M Sodium carbonate

The molecular weight of sodium carbonate (Na_2CO_3) being 106, 1M solution of it contains106g of Na_2CO_3. For 0.1M solution, 10.6g of Na_2CO_3 should be dissolved in sufficient water to make 1000mL or 1.06g of Na_2CO_3 in 100mL of solution.

The method of preparation and standardization would remain the same as mentioned for preparation and standardization of 0.1N HCl solution.

Calculation of strength of 0.1M HCl solution

Say, the average titer value is 24.95mL (V_1, volume of acid required),

Amount of Na_2CO_3 to be taken (theoretical weight) = 1.06g for 100mL of 0.1N solution

Weight of Na_2CO_3 taken =1.0608g

$$\text{Strength of 0.1N solution of } Na_2CO_3 \text{ (S)} = \frac{\text{Practical weight}}{\text{Theoretical weight}} = \frac{1.0608g}{1.06g} = 1.0007$$

Volume of Na_2CO_3 solution, V = 25.00mL

Say, strength of acid solution = S_1

According to law of mass action, $V_1 \times S_1 = V \times S$

$$24.95mL \times S_1 = 25.00mL \times 1.0007$$

$$\text{So, strength of 0.1N HCl, } S_1 = \frac{25mL \times 1.0007}{24.95mL} = 1.0027$$

In other words, the strength of acid = **0.1003N**

Preparation of 0.1M Borax

The molecular weight of borax is 381.44; hence, 1M solution of borax 381.44g shall be present in 1000mL of solution. To prepare 1000mL of 0.1M solution 38.144g of borax should be dissolved in sufficient water to make 1000mL and 100mL of the 0.1M solution will contain 3.8144g of borax. 25mL of 0.1M solution shall contain 0.9536g of borax.

Standardization

The method of titration shall be the same as followed in case of standardization of 0.1N solution of HCl.

Calculation of strength of 0.1M HCl solution

Strength of borax solution: Amount of borax to be taken = 0.9536g (Theoretical weight)

Say, the amount of borax taken (1) 0.9565g, (2) 0.9537g, and (3) 0.9542g

Strength of borax solution,

$$S = \quad 1. \quad \frac{\text{Practical weight}}{\text{Theoretical weight}} = \frac{0.9565g}{0.9536g} = 1.003$$

$$2. \quad \frac{\text{Practical weight}}{\text{Theoretical weight}} = \frac{0.9537g}{0.9536g} = 1.0001$$

$$3. \quad \frac{\text{Practical weight}}{\text{Theoretical weight}} = \frac{0.9542g}{0.9536g} = 1.0006$$

Volume of borax solution, $V = 25.00\text{mL}$

Say, the Volume of HCl solution consumed, V_1 in three titrations are 25.00mL, 24.95mL, and 25.00mL

If the strength of HCl solution is S; then $SV = S_1V_1$

1. $S_1 = \dfrac{S \times V}{V_1} = \dfrac{25.00\text{mL} \times 1.003}{25.00\text{mL}} = 1.003$

2. $S_1 = \dfrac{S \times V}{V_1} = \dfrac{25.00\text{mL} \times 1.0001}{24.95\text{mL}} = 1.0001$

3. $S_1 = \dfrac{S \times V}{V_1} = \dfrac{25.00\text{mL} \times 1.0006}{25.00\text{mL}} = 1.0006$

The average strength of 0.1M HCl solution is $\dfrac{1.003 + 1.0001 + 1.0006}{3} = 1.0012$

4. Preparation and standardization of 0.1M Sodium thiosulphate

Preparation of 0.1M Sodium thiosulphate

Sodium thiosulphate ($Na_2S_2O_3$, $5H_2O$) is readily available as a pure state. It is a reducing agent. But, it is efflorescent in nature. Due to this, its water content may vary. As a result, it is not used as a primary standard. The half-cell reaction is

$$2S_2O_3^{2-} \leftrightarrow S_4O_6^{2-} + 2e$$

The molecular weight of $Na_2S_2O_3$ is 158.11 and that of $Na_2S_2O_3$, $5H_2O$ is 248.18 and its valency is 2. Hence, 1M solution of $Na_2S_2O_3$, $5H_2O$ contains 248.18g per litre. The valency of $Na_2S_2O_3$, $5H_2O$ being 2; its equivalent weight would be $\dfrac{248.18}{2} = 124.09$. Thus, 1N solution of sodium thiosulphate contains 124.09g per litre.

Sodium thiosulphate solution has certain stability problems, such as

- The water used to prepare the solution should be freshly prepared or conductivity water, because dissolved carbon dioxide accelerates the decomposition of sodium thiosulphate.
  $$S_2O_3^{2-} + H^+ \rightarrow HSO_3^- + S$$
- Microbial contamination (e.g., Thiobacillusthioparas) can facilitate the decomposition of sodium thiosulphate if the solution is kept for some time.
- Sodium thiosulphate is photosensitive. Light accelerates the decomposition of sodium thiosulphate.

Thus, sodium thiosulphate solution should be prepared with freshly prepared distilled water and per one litre of the solution either 3 drops of chloroform or 10mg of mercuric iodide should be added.

- ➤ If the pH of the solution is kept within 9 to 10, the decomposition activity of the bacteria is negligible.
- ➤ If 0.1g of sodium carbonate is added to each litre of solution, the pH of the solution becomes alkaline (9 – 10).
- ➤ Borax should not be added, because it can accelerate the decomposition.
  - $S_2O_3^{2-} + 2O_2 + H_2O \leftrightarrow 2SO_4^{2-} + 2H^+$

➢ Sodium thiosulphate solution should be stored in an amber color bottle to protect it from sunlight.

Procedure

For making 1 L of 0.1M solution weigh 25g of sodium thiosulphate, A.R. ($Na_2S_2O_3$, $5H_2O$) and transfer it into a 1 L volumetric flask. Dissolve the sodium thiosulphate insufficient amount of freshly distilled water. Once it goes into solution, make up the volume with freshly distilled water. If the solution is stored for more than a few days, add 0.1g of sodium carbonate, A.R. Shake well to dissolve the sodium carbonate. Store the solution in an amber color bottle.

Standardization of 0.1M Sodium thiosulphate

(a) With the 0.1M solution of potassium iodate

The purity of A.R. potassium iodate is 99.9%, it is dried at 120°C. Potassium iodate reacts with potassium iodide and molecular iodine is formed;

$$IO_3^- + 5I^- + 6H^+ = 3I_2 + 3H_2O$$

Sodium thiosulphate solution can be standardized with various substances such as potassium iodate, potassium bromate, potassium dichromate, pure copper, pure iodine, a standard solution of iodine, potassium permanganate, and with ceric sulphate. Here, few shall be described.

Preparation and standardization of 0.1N Sodium thiosulphate

Preparation of 0.1N Sodium thiosulphate

Dissolve about 26g of sodium thiosulphate and 0.2g of sodium carbonate in 1000mL of freshly prepared distilled water. Shake well.

Standardization of 0.1N Sodium thiosulphate

As mentioned above standardization of sodium thiosulphate solution with potassium iodate solution, potassium dichromate solution and with standard iodine solution are discussed below.

With 0.1N potassium iodate (KIO_3) solution

The purity of potassium iodate A.R. grade is not less than 99.9%, it can be dried at 120°C without any stability problem. The molecular weight of KIO_3 is 214.001g/mol and equivalent weight is $1/6^{th}$ of its molecular weight as an oxidizing agent. That is, its 1N solution contains 35.67g per litre of solution and 0.1N solution should contain 3.567g per litre of solution.

Dry about 0.5g of KIO_3 at 110°C for 2 hrs and then put in a desiccator to cool to room temperature.

➢ Weigh accurately about 0.145g of dried KIO_3 transfer carefully into a 250mL iodine flask.

➢ Add 25mL of freshly boiled and cooled distilled water and dissolve the potassium iodate.

➢ Add 2g of pure potassium iodide (iodate free) and dissolve.

➢ Add 5mL of 2N H_2SO_4 solution.

- ➢ Stopper the flask.
- ➢ Rinse thrice a clean 50mL burette with 0.1N sodium thiosulphate solution.
- ➢ Fill the burette with 0.1N sodium thiosulphate solution up to the zero marks.
- ➢ Titrate the liberated iodine with 0.1N sodium thiosulphate solution with constant stirring until a pale-yellow color is produced.
- ➢ Wash the inner walls of the flask with about 150mL of freshly boiled and cooled distilled water.
- ➢ Add 2mL of starch solution, the blue color is produced.
- ➢ Continue the titration with 0.1N sodium thiosulphate solution until the solution becomes colorless. The endpoint is sharp. Note the volume of 0.1N sodium thiosulphate solution consumed (titer value).
- ➢ Repeat the titration twice more and take the average titer value (V) for calculation.

Calculation

Theoretical weight of KIO_3 = 0.14268g

Say, the amount of KIO_3 taken (average) = 0.1427g

Strength of 0.1N KIO_3 solution (S_1) = $\dfrac{\text{Practical weight}}{\text{Theoretical weight}}$ = $\dfrac{0.1427g}{0.14268g}$ = 1.0001

Volume of 0.1N KIO_3 solution (V_1) = 40mL

Say, average volume of 0.1N sodium thiosulphate solution consumed (V) = 39.83mL

Strength of 0.1N sodium thiosulphate solution, $S = \dfrac{40mL \times 1.0001}{39.83mL}$ = 1.00436 ≈ **1.0044**

With 0.1N potassium dichromate solution

The molecular weight of potassium dichromate, $K_2Cr_2O_7$ is 294.22g/mol. In acidic medium potassium dichromate is reduced by the acid. According to the equation given below, its equivalent weight would be 1/6th of the molecular weight; that is, 49.037g.

$$Cr_2O_7^{2-} + 6I^- + 14H^+ = 2Cr^{3+} + 3I_2 + 7H_2O$$

There are certain errors related to this reaction;

- The HI (from excess of iodide and acid) is readily oxidized by air, particularly in the presence of chromic salt.

- The reaction is not instantaneous. Thus, a current of carbon dioxide should be passed through the reaction flask before and during titration. However, there is an alternative and simple way to pass carbon dioxide. To the acid solution, some amount of sodium bicarbonate is added and the flask is kept closed as much as possible; so that the reaction between $NaHCO_3$ and acid can produce CO_2 which can pass through the reaction.

Preparation of 0.1N potassium dichromate solution

A.R. grade potassium dichromate has a purity of 99.9%. Take 5 – 6g of potassium dichromate crystals, crush it in glass mortar to make powder, transfer the powders into a weighing bottle, dry at about 145°C for 60min, close the weighing bottle and keep it in a desiccator to cool to room temperature.

- Weigh accurately about 2.45g of dried potassium dichromate.
- Transfer the material carefully into a 500mL clean volumetric flask, to avoid loss during transfer using a glass funnel.
- Rinse the funnel and inner walls of the flask with freshly prepared distilled water, remove the funnel, and close the flask tightly.
- Shake the flask to dissolve the material.
- Add sufficient water to make up the volume.
- Mix thoroughly.

Take 500mL clean glass-stoppered flask (iodine flask), pour 100mL of freshly boiled and cooled distilled water.

- Add 3g of pure potassium iodide (iodate free) and 2g of pure sodium bicarbonate; rotate the flask to dissolve the solids.
- Add slowly 6mL of concentrated HCl, rotate the flask to mix the contents thoroughly.
- Measure 25.00mL of 0.1N potassium dichromate solution accurately and transfer into the flask, stopper the flask tightly and keep it in the dark for 5min to complete the reaction.
- Rinse the flask with the distilled water.
- Rinse a 50mL clean burette with the 0.1N sodium thiosulphate solution thrice.
- Fill the burette with 0.1N sodium thiosulphate solution up to the zero marks.
- Titrate the 0.1N potassium dichromate solution with 0.1N sodium thiosulphate solution until a yellowish green color is produced.
- Add 2mL of starch solution to the content in the flask, blue color is produced.
- Note the volume of 0.1N sodium thiosulphate solution consumed (titer value, V').
- Continue titration till the blue color turns to light green color. The endpoint is sharp.
- Carryout a blank determination with 25mL of distilled water in place of 0.1N potassium dichromate solution.
- Note the volume of 0.1N sodium thiosulphate solution consumed (v).
- Subtract the v from V', this gives the volume of 0.1N sodium thiosulphate solution consumed by 25.00mL of 0.1N potassium dichromate solution (V)
- Repeat the determination twice more using 25.00mL of 0.1N potassium dichromate solution at each time. Take the average of three titer values for calculation.

Calculation

Theoretical weight of potassium dichromate = 2.4517g

Say, the amount of potassium dichromate taken = 2.4525g

$$\text{Strength of 0.1N potassium dichromate solution} = \frac{\text{Practical weight}}{\text{Theoretical weight}} = \frac{2.4525\text{g}}{2.4517\text{g}}$$

= 1.0003

The volume of 0.1N potassium dichromate solution taken, V_1 = 25.00mL

Say, the average volume of 0.1N sodium thiosulphate solution consumed (V) = 24.93mL

$$\text{The strength of 0.1N sodium thiosulphate solution} = \frac{25.00\text{mL} \times 1.0003}{24.93\text{mL}} = \mathbf{1.0031}$$

With 0.1N iodine solution

Preparation of 0.1N iodine solution

Solubilization of iodine in water has two problems:

- Iodine is almost insoluble in water. Its solubility in water is 0.0335g in 100mL of water.
- Despite this poor solubility, iodine volatilizes, and the vapor of iodine exists over the solution.

Both of these problems can be solved by dissolving iodine in a solution of potassium iodide. The solubility of iodine increases with increase in the concentration of potassium iodide. This is due to the formation of the tri-iodide ion as shown below;

$$I_2 + I^- \leftrightarrow I_3^-$$

The solution thus produced allows much less iodine to vaporize and remain in the vapor state. Hence, the loss of iodine is much less. Maybe in a very lesser amount, some amount of iodine is lost from its solution if the solution is kept open or in lightly sealed condition. Following precautions should be taken while storing an iodine solution;

- The solution of iodine should be stored in amber colored, airtight bottle.
- Iodine interacts with rubber. So, iodine solution should never be kept in contact with a rubber material.
- Potassium iodide used to prepare the iodine solution should be free from iodate.
- The solution of iodine should be kept away from light.

Iodine solution can be standardized against pure arsenious oxide, pure barium thiosulphate monohydrate, or with sodium thiosulphate solution.

Procedure

- ➢ Transfer about 14g of iodine into a 1000mL volumetric flask.
- ➢ Add a solution of 36g of potassium iodide in 100mL of freshly prepared distilled water.
- ➢ Dissolve the iodine in potassium iodide solution.
- ➢ Add 3 drops of concentrated hydrochloric acid and mix thoroughly.
- ➢ Dilute the solution to 1000mL with freshly prepared distilled water.
- ➢ Stopper the flask and mix thoroughly.

Standardization of 0.1N iodine solution

The purity of A.R. arsenious oxide or arsenic trioxide (As_2O_3) may be not less than 99.9%. Its molecular weight is 197.84g/mol. Arsenious oxide has been used as a favored primary standard for iodine solutions since long. Because of its poisonous effect, even the use of small amounts of arsenic-containing compounds is avoided. Barium thiosulfate monohydrate and anhydrous sodium thiosulfate have been favored as alternative standards. Perhaps the most convenient method of determining the concentration of an iodine solution is the titration of aliquots with a sodium thiosulfate solution that has been standardized against pure potassium iodate. Instructions for this method follow. The reaction between arsenious oxide and iodine is,

$$H_3AsO_3 + I_2 + H_2O \leftrightarrow H_3AsO_4 + 2H^+ + 2I^-$$
$$H_3AsO_3 + I_3^- + H_2O \leftrightarrow H_3AsO_4 + 2H^+ + 3I^-$$

The reaction proceeds towards right quantitatively if the HI produced in the reaction is removed immediately after formation. For this reason, sodium bicarbonate ($NaHCO_3$) not sodium carbonate (Na_2CO_3) or sodium hydroxide (NaOH) is added to the reaction mixture. Sodium carbonate (Na_2CO_3) or sodium hydroxide (NaOH) reacts with iodine and forms iodide, hypo-iodide, and iodate.

➤ Weigh accurately about 130mg of pure arsenious oxide (arsenic trioxide).
➤ Transfer it into a 250mL iodine flask, add 20mL of 1N NaOH solution,
➤ Dissolve by warming, if necessary.
➤ Dilute the solution with 40mL of water.
➤ Add 2 drops of methyl orange T.S.
➤ Add diluted HCl dropwise until the yellow color is changed to pink.
➤ Add 2g of sodium bicarbonate and 50mL of water.
➤ Add 3mL of starch T.S.
➤ Titrate the solution with an iodine solution from a burette until a permanent blue color is produced.
➤ Note the volume of iodine solution consumed.
➤ Repeat the process twice more and take the average titer value for calculation.

Calculation

Say, the weight of arsenious oxide taken (practical weight) = 0.1303g

The weight of arsenious oxide to be taken (theoretical weight) = 0.12365g for 25mL

The strength of arsenious oxide solution $= \dfrac{\text{practical weight}}{\text{theoretical weight}} = \dfrac{0.1303g}{0.12365g} = 1.054$

Say, the strength of iodine solution = S and volume of iodine solution required = 25.05mL

Now, S × 25.05mL = 1.054 × 25mL

$$S = \frac{1.054 \times 25mL}{25.05mL} = \textbf{1.052N}$$

5. Preparation and standardization of 0.1N Sulphuric acid

Preparation

The molecular weight of sulphuric acid is 98.08 and its basicity is 2. Hence, the equivalent weight of sulphuric acid is $\dfrac{98.08}{2} = 49.04g$. The 1N solution of sulphuric acid contains 49g in 1000mL. Say, the density of sulphuric acid used is 1.834g/mL.

Then, the volume of 49.04g of sulphuric acid $= \dfrac{49.04\text{g}}{1.834\text{g/mL}} = 26.74\text{mL}.$ $[\rho = \dfrac{m}{v}]$

- Measure 27.00mL of concentrated sulphuric acid.
- Take a clean and washed 1000mL volumetric flask.
- Pour 800mL of distilled water, cool it in an ice bath.
- Transfer the acid gradually into the volumetric flask with constant swirling.
- Once the acid is transferred completely, allow the solution to cool to room temperature.
- Make up the volume with water and stopper the flask, mix thoroughly.

Standardization

As mentioned earlier anhydrous sodium carbonate is used for standardization of hydrochloric acid or sulphuric acid. The process of standardization is given below.

- ➤ Take about 2g of anhydrous sodium carbonate A.R. into a clean dry weighing bottle, dry it in a hot air oven at about 105°C for 2 hrs.
- ➤ Close the bottle with its lid, transfer the bottle into a desiccator.
- ➤ Weigh accurately about 1.10g of anhydrous sodium carbonate.
- ➤ Transfer the weighed anhydrous sodium carbonate into a 250mL of the conical flask.
- ➤ Add 50mL of distilled water and dissolve.
- ➤ Add 2 drops of methyl red T.S.
- ➤ Titrate the solution with sulphuric solution from a burette until pink color is produced.
- ➤ Boil the solution and titrate with the sulphuric acid solution until the faint pink color produced does not fade away.
- ➤ Note the volume of sulphuric acid solution consumed.
- ➤ Repeat the process twice more and take the average titer value for calculation.

Calculation

Say, the weight of sodium carbonate taken (average practical weight) = 1.0655g

The weight of sodium carbonate to be taken (theoretical weight) = 1.0599g for 20mL

Strength of sodium carbonate solution $= \dfrac{1.0655\text{g}}{1.0599\text{g}} = 1.0053\text{N}$

Say, the average volume of sulphuric acid solution consumed = 20.03mL and the strength of sulphuric acid solution = S

Then, S × 20.03mL = 1.0053N × 20.00mL

So, S $= \dfrac{1.0053\text{N} \times 20.00\text{mL}}{20.03\text{m}} = \mathbf{1.0038N}$

Preparation and standardization of 0.1M Sulphuric acid

Preparation

The molecular weight of sulphuric acid is 98.08. One molar solution contains 98.08g of sulphuric acid.

Its density should be 1.84g/mL. since the purity of concentrated sulphuric acid varies from 95 - 98%, its density is less than the theoretical value. To prepare one litre of 1M solution of sulphuric acid 57mL of concentrated sulphuric acid is diluted to 1000mL with distilled water. The method is similar to that described above. Thus, to prepare one litre of 0.1M solution of sulphuric acid 5.7mL of concentrated sulphuric acid is diluted to 1000mL with distilled water.

Standardization

Follow the method described earlier for 0.1N Sulphuric acid.

6. Preparation and standardization of 0.1M Potassium permanganate

The molecular weight of potassium permanganate is 158.034. The 1M solution contains 158.034g of potassium permanganate per liter. So, the 0.1M solution contains 15.8034g of potassium permanganate per litre. Potassium permanganate, $KMnO_4$ is not a primary standard. It is very difficult to obtain Potassium permanganate in the purest form.

- It contains free manganese dioxide as a common impurity that catalyzes auto-decomposition of potassium permanganate on standing. The decomposition reaction is

$$4MnO_4^- + 2H_2O \rightarrow 4MnO_2 + 3O_2 + 4OH^-$$

- Potassium permanganate is inherently unstable in the presence of manganese ion, Mn^{2+}

$$2MnO_4^- + 3Mn^{2+} + 2H_2O \rightarrow 5MnO_2 + 4H^+$$

- Potassium permanganate is reduced on contact with organic material such as rubber; hence its solution should not be kept in contact with such materials.
- In acidic medium, the decomposition reaction is slow; while in the neutral medium the reaction is relatively faster.
- When exposed to bright sunlight it and even its pure solution decompose slowly.
- The bottle should be rinsed with dichromate-sulphuric acid and then washed thoroughly with distilled water. The bottle is then used to preserve potassium permanganate solution.

Preparation of 0.1M Potassium permanganate
- Weigh 7.9g of A.R. potassium permanganate on a watch glass, transfer it to a 1000mL beaker,
- Add 500mL of distilled water, cover the beaker with a beaker-cover,
- Boil for 15 – 30 min, allow to cool to room temperature,
- Filter the solution through a funnel plugged with purified glass wool or through a sintered glass crucible,

- Collect the filtrate in a container which has been cleaned with the chromic acid mixture and subsequently washed with distilled water,
- Store the filtered solution in clean, amber color glass bottle fitted with stopper, keep the bottle in dark or under diffuse light.

Standardization of 0.1M Potassium permanganate against arsenious oxide

- Take about 1g of arsenious oxide in a weighing bottle, dry it at $105° - 110°C$ for 2hrs and keep it in a desiccator at room temperature to cool.
- Weigh accurately 0.25g of arsenious oxide accurately from the weighing bottle, transfer to a 500mL clean conical flask.
- Weigh the weighing after the transfer of arsenious oxide, the difference between the two weights shall be the weight of arsenious oxide taken.
- Add 10mL of 20% sodium hydroxide solution and mix.
- Allow standing for $8 - 10$ min with occasional stirring.
- When the arsenious oxide is completely dissolved add 100mL of water, 10mL of concentrated HCl, and 1mL of 0.0025M iodine-monochloride (ICl) solution.
- Titrate the solution with potassium permanganate solution until a faint pink color appears and persists for at least 30 seconds.
- If the color disappears within 30 sec, add potassium permanganate solution dropwise; once the first drop disappears add next. Continue till the faint pink color persists for 30 secs.
- Note the volume of potassium permanganate solution consumed.
- Repeat the same for two more determinations. Take the average value for calculation of the strength of potassium permanganate solution.

Calculation

The molecular weight of arsenious oxide is 197.82. The 1M solution of arsenious oxide will contain 197.82g per litre. Or, 0.1M solution of arsenious oxide will contain 19.782g per litre (0.019782g/mL).

For 50mL of 0.1M solution $50 × 0.019782g = 0.9891g$ of arsenious oxide should be taken (theoretical weight)

Say, the weight of arsenious oxide taken = 0.9902g (average of three weights of three determinations)

So, the strength of 0.1M solution of arsenious oxide, $S_1 = \dfrac{\text{Practical weight}}{\text{Theoretical weight}} = \dfrac{0.9901g}{0.9891g} = 1.0010$

Volume of arsenious oxide solution, $V_1 = 50.00mL$

Volume of potassium permanganate solution consumed, $V = 49.90mL$

Strength of potassium permanganate solution = S

$$S \times V = S_1 \times V_1$$

$$S = \frac{S_1 \times V_1}{V} = \frac{50 \times 1.001}{49.90} = 1.0030$$

Preparation of 0.1N Potassium permanganate

The molecular weight of potassium permanganate is 158.034g. The equivalent weight of potassium permanganate depends on the acidity of the medium. The valency state of Mn in $KMnO_4$ is +7 which gains 5 electrons in acidic medium. Hence, the equivalent weight of $KMnO_4 = \frac{158.034}{5} = 31.6068$g. When the pH of the medium is alkaline or neutral $KMnO_4$ gains 3 electrons; hence, its equivalent weight in the alkaline or neutral medium is $\frac{158.034}{3} = 52.678$g. Usually, 0.1N solution of potassium permanganate is prepared by dissolving 15.8034g in sufficient water to prepare one liter.

Standardization of 0.1N Potassium permanganate against arsenious oxide

Arsenious oxide oxidizes rapidly and stoichiometrically at room temperature in presence of trace amount of iodine. Iodine works as a catalyst. Compounds containing iodine reduce and form iodine when added to arsenious acid (H_3AsO_3). Permanganate oxidizes iodine rapidly to all. The iodine-monochloride then oxidizes arsenious acid and itself reduces to iodine (I_2).

$$5I_2 + 2MnO_4^- + 10Cl^- + 16H^+ = 10ICl + 2Mn^{2+} + 8H_2O$$

$$10ICl + 5H_3AsO_3 + 5H_2O = 5I_2 + 5H_3AsO_4 + 10H^+ + 10Cl^-$$

One molecule of arsenious oxide consumes two atoms of oxygen as indicated below;

$$As_2O_3 + 2O = As_2O_5$$

Thus, the above equation manifests that the equivalent weight of arsenious oxide is $\frac{1}{4}$ th of its molecular weight; that is the equivalent weight $= \frac{1 \times 197.82}{4} = 49.455$g. In other words, 1N solution of arsenious oxide will contain 49.455g per litre. Or, 0.1N solution of arsenious oxide will contain 4.9455g per litre or 0.0049455g/mL.

For 50mL of 0.1N solution 50 × 0.0049455g = 0.247275g of arsenious oxide should be taken (theoretical weight).

Say, the weight of arsenious oxide taken = 0.2499g (average of three weights of three determinations)

So, the strength of 0.1N solution of arsenious oxide, $S_1 = \frac{\text{Practical weight}}{\text{Theoretical weight}} = \frac{0.2499g}{0.2473g} = 1.0105$

Volume of arsenious oxide solution, $V_1 = 50.00$mL

Volume of potassium permanganate solution consumed, $V = 49.90$mL

Strength of potassium permanganate solution = S

$$S \times V = S_1 \times V_1$$

$$S = \frac{S_1 \times V_1}{V} = \frac{50 \times 1.0105}{49.90} = 1.0125$$

Standardization of 0.1N Potassium permanganate against sodium oxalate

The molecular weight of sodium oxalate, $Na_2C_2O_4$ is 134 and valency is 2. So, its equivalent weight is $\frac{134}{2}$ = 67g. To prepare a 1N solution of sodium oxalate, 67g should be present in one litre. Thus, a 0.1N solution contains 6.7g of sodium oxalate per litre of solution.

Take about 1g of sodium oxalate in a weighing bottle, dry it in a hot air oven at 110°C for about 2 hrs, cool it to room temperature in a desiccator.

- Weigh accurately 0.67g of sodium oxalate from the weighing bottle, transfer it into a 100mL volumetric flask and dissolve it in freshly prepared distilled water.
- Pipette out exactly 25.00mL of sodium oxalate solution into a 250mL conical flask, add 100ml of distilled water, then add slowly 6ml of concentrated sulphuric acid, if required heat to about 70°C.
- Rinse a 50mL clean burette with potassium permanganate solution, fill, then open the stopcock to remove some potassium permanganate solution; once the jet is completely filled with potassium permanganate solution and air is completely removed, refill the burette up to the zero mark.
- Titrate the hot sodium oxalate slowly with potassium permanganate solution with constant stirring until a pale pink color is produced and persists for at least 15 seconds. Note the volume of potassium permanganate solution consumed (titer value).
- Repeat the determinations twice more; make the average of three titer values and use for calculation.

Note that till end of the titration the temperature of the solution must remain within 60° – 65°C.

Calculation

Say, the amount of sodium oxalate taken = 0.6704g for 250mL solution

Theoretical weight of sodium oxalate to be taken = 0.6700g for 250mL of 0.1N solution

The strength of 0.1N solution of sodium oxalate, $S_1 = \dfrac{\text{Practical weight}}{\text{Theoretical weight}}$

$$= \frac{0.6704g}{0.6700g} = 1.0006$$

The volume of sodium oxalate solution used, $V_1 = 25mL$

Say, the average volume of potassium permanganate solution consumed,

$$V = \frac{25.05 + 25.00 + 25.00}{3}$$

$$= 25.02 \text{mL}$$

$$V \times S = V_1 \times S_1$$

The strength of 0.1N potassium permanganate solution, $S = \dfrac{25.00 \times 1.0006}{25.02} = 0.9998$

In other words the strength of potassium permanganate solution = 0.09998N

7. Preparation and standardization of 0.1N Ceric Ammonium Sulphate solution

Preparation

The molecular weight of ceric ammonium sulphate, $(NH_4^-)_4[Ce(SO_4)_4],2H_2O$ is 632.57. Its equivalent weight is also 632.57. Hence, 1N or 1M solution of ceric ammonium sulphate contains 632.57g per lt.

➢ Weigh about 66g of ceric ammonium sulphate and transfer it into a clean 500mL conical flask, add a mixture of 30mL concentrated sulphuric acid and 500mL of distilled water and heat gently to dissolve the ceric ammonium sulphate completely.

➢ Allow the solution to cool to room temperature.

➢ Transfer the solution into a clean 1000mL volumetric flask, dilute to 1000mL with distilled water, stopper the flask tightly and shake well.

Standardization

➢ Weigh accurately about 0.1g of dried arsenic trioxide, transfer it into a 500mL conical flask.

➢ Wash thoroughly the inner walls of the flask with 100mL of distilled water.

➢ Add 300mL of dilute sulphuric acid, 0.15mL of osmic acid and 0.1mL of ferroin T.S. (indicator).

➢ Take a 50mL clean burette, rinse with ceric ammonium sulphate solution and then fill.

➢ Adjust the meniscus at zero mark of the burette.

➢ Titrate arsenic trioxide solution with ceric ammonium sulphate solution until the pink color of the solution changes to pale blue or yellowish green color.

➢ Repeat the titration twice and take the average titer value for calculation of the strength of the ceric ammonium sulphate solution.

Calculation

Each mL of 0.1N ceric ammonium sulphate solution ≈ 4.946mg ≈ 0.004946g of arsenic trioxide

Gram-equivalent wt of arsenic trioxide = 49.46g; that is 0.1N solution of it contains 4.946g/lt

Say, the amount of arsenic trioxide taken = 0.1076g for making 1000mL solution and average titer value is 20.05mL.

Say, the average titer value = 20.05mL; in other words, 20.05mL of ceric ammonium sulphate solution is consumed by 0.1076g of arsenic trioxide.

0.004946g of arsenic trioxide $\approx$ 1mL of 0.1N ceric ammonium sulphate solution

So, 0.1076g of arsenic trioxide $\approx \dfrac{1 \times 0.1076g}{0.004946g} = 21.75mL$ of 0.1N ceric ammonium sulphate solution

Say, the strength of ceric ammonium sulphate solution = xN

Then, x N × 20.05mL = 0.1N × 21.75mL

Or, the strength of ceric ammonium sulphate solution, $x = \dfrac{0.1N \times 21.75mL}{20.05mL} = \mathbf{0.1085N}$

Preparation and standardization of 0.1M Ceric Ammonium Sulphate solution

Since the gram-molecular weight and gram-equivalent weight of ceric ammonium sulphate are same, 632.57g, the method of preparation and standardization of 0.1M ceric ammonium sulphate solution is same.

Determination of strength of a primary standard solution

The strength of a primary standard solution is not calculated through titration, it is calculated on the basis of the exact amount dissolved in the solution. Hence, proper care must be taken to achieve accurate strength. The accuracy in the strength of the solution depends on;

> Accuracy in weighing,
> Transferring the material into the flask,
> Dissolving, and
> Making up the volume.

The strength of a solution of the primary standard can be calculated as;

$$\text{Strength of a solution of primary standard} = \frac{\text{Practical weight}}{\text{Theoretical weight}}$$

Example 12: A molar solution of sodium carbonate should contain 165.012g of Na_2CO_3 in one litre of its solution. If a litre of solution contains 164.625g of Na_2CO_3, what would be the strength of the solution?

Solution: Sodium carbonate is a primary standard.

$$\text{The strength of the solution} = \frac{\text{Practical weight}}{\text{Theoretical weight}} = \frac{164.625}{165.012} = \mathbf{0.9976\ M}$$

Example 13: A normal solution of sodium carbonate should contain 82.506g of Na_2CO_3 in one litre of its solution. If 250 mL of 1N solution is to be prepared, calculate the amount of Na_2CO_3 required.

Solution: 1 litre = 1000mL of the solution contains 82.506g of sodium carbonate

250mL of the solution should contain $\dfrac{82.506g}{1000mL} \times 250mL = \textbf{20.6265g}$ of sodium carbonate

Example 14: In a neutralization reaction 25.00 mL of the 0.1N hydrochloric acid solution is completely neutralized by 12.50 mL of sodium hydroxide solution. Find out the strength of the sodium hydroxide solution.

Solution: Given that, $V_{HCl} = 25.00$ mL, $V_{NaOH} = 12.50$ mL

$S_{HCl} = 0.1N$, $S_{NaOH} = ?$

It is known that $S \times V = S_1 \times V_1$

Hence, $V_{HCl} \times S_{HCl} = V_{NaOH} \times S_{NaOH}$

Or, 25.00 mL $\times 0.1N = 12.50$ mL $\times S_{NaOH}$

Or, $S_{NaOH} = \dfrac{25.00mL \times 0.1N}{12.50mL} = \textbf{0.2N}$

Determination of strength of a secondary standard solution

Depending on the chemical property a solution of the secondary standard is standardized. For example, sodium hydroxide solution is standardized using a standard solution of hydrochloric acid or potassium hydrogen phthalate solution. Potassium permanganate solution is standardized against a standard solution of sodium oxalate. A perchloric acid solution is standardized against potassium hydrogen phthalate. Iodine solution is standardized against a standard solution of sodium thiosulphate or arsenic trioxide. Few are described below.

Standardization of 0.1N solution of sodium hydroxide

Dry about 11g of potassium hydrogen phthalate in powder form at 105°C for 3 hrs, cool it in a desiccator.

Weigh accurately about 10.21g and transfer it into a 50mL clean volumetric flask. Add 40mL of freshly prepared distilled water, dissolve. If necessary, warm it to complete dissolution. Allow to cool to room temperature and make up the volume, mix thoroughly. Pipette out accurately 20mL of potassium hydrogen phthalate solution and transfer into a clean 250mL conical flask. Add 2 drops of phenolphthalein solution T.S. and titrate with sodium hydroxide filled in a burette till a permanent pink color is produced. Repeat the titration and take the average titer value for calculation of the strength of sodium hydroxide solution.

Calculation

Say, the weight of potassium hydrogen phthalate taken (practical weight) = 10.225g

The strength of potassium hydrogen phthalate solution $= \dfrac{\text{practical weight}}{\text{theoretical weight}}$

$= \dfrac{10.225g}{10.21g} = 1.0015N$

Say, the average titer value (volume of NaOH solution consumed) = 20.05mL

Then, the strength of NaOH solution $= \dfrac{20 \text{ mL} \times 1.0015N}{20.05mL} = \textbf{0.9990N}$

Standardization of 0.1N solution of potassium permanganate

Dry about 1g of sodium oxalate in powder form at $110^\circ C$ until a constant weight is obtained, cool it in a desiccator. Weigh accurately about 200mg of dried sodium oxalate and transfer it into a 500mL conical flask. Dissolve the sodium oxalate in 250mL of freshly prepared distilled water; add 7mL of sulphuric acid. Heat the mixture to about $70^\circ C$ and then titrate slowly with potassium permanganate solution from a burette with constant stirring until a pale pink color which persists for at least 15 sec, is produced. The temperature of the titration mixture should not fall below $60^\circ C$. Each mL of 0.1N potassium permanganate solution is equivalent to 6.700mg of sodium oxalate. Repeat the titration twice and take the average titer value to calculate the strength of the potassium permanganate solution.

Calculation

Say, the average titer value = 29.03mL and the amount of sodium oxalate taken = 198.98mg

Each 6.700mg of sodium oxalate $\approx$ 1mL of 0.1N potassium permanganate solution.

198.98mg of sodium oxalate $\approx \dfrac{1\text{mL of } 0.1\text{N} \times 198.98\text{mg}}{6.700\text{mg}} = 29.70\text{mL}$ of 0.1N potassium permanganate solution

If the strength of 0.1N potassium permanganate solution is x(N)

Then, x(N) $\times$ 29.03mL = 0.1N $\times$ 29.70mL

The strength of 0.1N potassium permanganate solution is;

$$x = \frac{0.1\text{N} \times 29.70\text{mL}}{29.03\text{mL}} = \mathbf{0.1023(N)}$$

A. MULTIPLE CHOICE QUESTIONS

1. A sample contains 10ppm of iron, this is the result of
    (a) Qualitative test
    (b) Quantitative test
    (c) General test
    (d) None of the above

2. A sample contains sulphate, this is the result of
    (a) Qualitative test
    (b) Quantitative test
    (c) General test
    (d) None of the above

3. Qualitative tests are generally conducted to
    (a) Detect whether the desired compound or substance is present in the sample
    (b) Detect whether the desired compound or substance is not present in the sample
    (c) Identify the presence of the compound
    (d) All of the above

4. Chemical methods of analysis include
    (a) Gasometric analysis
    (b) Polarographic analysis
    (c) Voltametric analysis
    (d) Amperometric analysis

5. Electrical method of analysis include
   - (a) Gasometric method
   - (b) Potentiometric method
   - (c) UV-spectrophotometric method
   - (d) All of the above

6. Conductometry is a
   - (a) Chemical method of analysis
   - (b) Electrical method of analysis
   - (c) Instrumental method of analysis
   - (d) None of the above

7. Titrimetry is a
   - (a) Chemical method of analysis
   - (b) Electrical method of analysis
   - (b) Instrumental method of analysis
   - (d) None of the above

8. A microelectrode is required for
   - (a) Polarography
   - (b) Voltametry
   - (c) Amperometry
   - (d) All of the above

9. Ingasometry method which gas is used?
   - (a) CO_2
   - (b) NO
   - (c) O_2
   - (d) H_2

10. Absorption spectroscopy include
    - (a) TLC
    - (b) IR
    - (c) HPTLC
    - (d) None of the above

11. Number of gram-equivalents of a solute present in one liter of the solution is called as
    - (a) Molality
    - (b) Molarity
    - (c) Normality
    - (d) None of the above

12. Sodium hydroxide solution should be standardized against
    - (a) Potassium dihydrogen phthalate solution
    - (b) Potassium permanganate solution
    - (c) Sodium oxalate solution
    - (d) None of the above

13. Solution whose strength is measured, is called
    - (a) Reagent solution
    - (b) Volumetric solution
    - (c) Test solution
    - (d) Indicator solution

14. Which of the following is a primary standard?
    - (a) Oxalic acid
    - (b) Sulphuric acid
    - (c) Acetic acid
    - (d) None of the above

15. Which of the following is used to express concentration?
    - (a) %w/v
    - (b) N
    - (c) M
    - (d) All of the above

16. Sulphuric acid volumetric solution can be standardized with
    - (a) Sodium sulphate
    - (b) Potassium sulphate
    - (c) Sodium hydroxide
    - (d) Potassium permanganate

17. Sodium thiosulphate volumetric solution can be standardized with
    (a) Potassium dichromate
    (b) Potassium permanganate
    (c) Oxalic acid
    (d) Hydrochloric acid
18. Silver nitrate is used as primary standard in
    (a) Complexometric titration
    (b) Potentiometric titration
    (c) Acid-base titration
    (d) None of the above
19. Number of moles present in 1lt of solution, the concentration of the solution is expressed as
    (a) Molality
    (b) Molarity
    (c) Normality
    (d) None of the above
20. Which of the following is secondary standard?
    (a) Sodium carbonate
    (b) Potassium dihydrogen phthalate
    (c) Sodium hydroxide
    (d) Silver nitrate

B. SHORT QUESTIONS

1. Name the types of solutions used in analysis.
2. Name the methods used for the analysis of various substances.
3. What are the methods used in the chemical analysis?
4. What are the electrical methods of analysis?
5. Name the instruments used in chromatographic analysis.
6. Define the term used to express the concentration of sodium hydroxide solution T.S.
7. Define the term used to express the concentration of dilute alcohol.
8. How many grams of sodium carbonate would be required to prepare 0.1M solution?
9. How can you express the concentration of a powder mix?
10. Define the term 'Equivalent weight'.
11. What is molarity?
12. Define the term 'Molality'
13. What is 'mole fraction'?
14. Define the term 'Normality'.
15. What is a 'Primary standard'?
16. What is 'Secondary standard'?
17. How can you prepare 1 L of 10%v/v solution of hydrochloric acid?
18. Calculate the equivalent weight of potassium permanganate.
19. What is a neutralization reaction?
20. Mention how precipitation reaction takes place.
21. What are the properties of secondary standards?
22. What are the factors influencing the accuracy of a primary standard solution?

C. LONG QUESTIONS

1. Explain briefly volumetric analysis using a suitable example.
2. Classify the techniques of analysis.
3. What is the utility of different types of analysis in the pharmacy?
4. Mention the desired characteristics of the primary standard.
5. Explain why sodium hydroxide is not considered as a primary standard.
6. Distinguish between molarity and molality with example.
7. Describe briefly how you can prepare decinormal solution of potassium permanganate.
8. Describe the method of preparation of 500 mL of 0.01N Sulphuric acid.
9. Explain the principle of gravimetric analysis.
10. Write down the properties of primary standards.
11. Describe the method of preparation and standardization of 0.1M solution of oxalic acid.
12. Write down the names of two substances used as primary standards with respect to various types of analysis.
13. Describe the method of preparation and standardization of 0.1N Sodium hydroxide solution.
14. Describe the method of preparation and standardization of 0.1N Hydrochloric acid using anhydrous sodium carbonate as a primary standard.
15. What do you mean by Complex formation and precipitation reaction? Mention a suitable example.
16. What do you mean by the oxidation-reduction reaction? Mention a suitable example.
17. Describe the method of preparation and standardization of 0.1M Sodium thiosulphate against KIO_3.
18. Describe the method of preparation and standardization of 0.1N potassium permanganate against sodium oxalate.
19. Describe the method of Preparation and standardization of 0.1M Ceric Ammonium Sulphate solution.
20. Describe the method of Preparation and standardization of 0.1N Ceric Ammonium Sulphate solution.

CHAPTER 2

Errors

During a chemical analysis, one analyzes a quantity with full effort and greatest care so that the instrument and method used can produce an exact result. In practice, the difference between the results of successive determinations is found. The difference in the results may be small or large. The average of the results is accepted or reported as the most probable. However, this average or reported result may not be equal to the true result. The reliability of the experimental result depends on the magnitude of the difference between the true value and observed/experimental value (average value). There are some factors that affect the reliability of the result. Therefore, it is necessary to understand these factors.

LEARNING OBJECTIVES

After studying the chapter the students familiarize themselves with the following concepts:
- ✓ Sources of errors
- ✓ Types of errors
- ✓ Methods of minimizing errors
- ✓ Accuracy
- ✓ Precision and significant figure

The difference between the true value and the observed or measured value is called *absolute error*. The absolute error indicates the accuracy of the measurement or determination. Thus, accuracy indicates how close the observed value to the true value is. In other words, the *accuracy increases with a decrease in absolute error*. The ratio of absolute error to the true value is called *relative error* $\left(\dfrac{\text{Absolute error}}{\text{True value}}\right)$. It is usually expressed in terms of percentage or parts per thousand. There are some situations where true value cannot be obtained experimentally. For example, the molecular weight of a pure substance is the sum of the atomic weights of constituent atoms. It is assumed that the atomic weights have been determined by expert analysts using established methods and with utmost care. The results are considered as the most reliable and the accuracy is much higher accuracy than ordinary experimentations. If several analysts determine the same compound present in the same sample by using different methods, the most probable value (average value) can be calculated from their results. However, the establishment of most probable value requires the application of statistics and the concept of *precision*.

The closeness between a series of results is measured by calculating their *mean deviation*. This is determined by calculating the arithmetical mean of the results and then, calculating the deviation of each individual result from the mean. Finally, the sum of the deviations, regardless of the sign, is divided by the number of measurements. The *relative mean deviation* is the ratio of mean deviation with mean. This can also be expressed in terms of percent or parts per thousand. This is illustrated with an example below.

Example 1: The percentages of drug content in a tablet were found to 67.43, 67.75, 67.50, 67.49, 67.70, and 67.72. Calculate the mean deviation and relative mean deviation.

Drug content (%)	Deviation
67.43	- 0.17
67.75	0.15
67.50	- 0.10
67.49	- 0.11
67.70	0.10
67.72	0.12
Total = 405.59	0.75

$$\text{Mean} = \frac{405.59}{6} \qquad\qquad \text{Mean deviation} = \frac{0.75}{6}$$

$$= 67.598 \qquad\qquad\qquad\qquad = 0.125$$

$$\approx 67.60$$

$$\text{Relative mean deviation} = \frac{0.125}{67.60} \times 100 = 0.185\% = 1.85 \text{ parts per thousand}$$

2.1 SOURCES OF ERRORS

There are two major sources of errors

Reading Error

In most of the direct measurements whether it is reading a scale, tape, a ruler, caliper, stopwatch, analog voltmeter, etc. or a digital display system such as digital multimeter or digital clock there may an error either in reading or in the device. The uncertainties may be caused by the limitations of our measuring equipment (instrumental error) and/or our own limitations (personal error) at the time of measurement. For example, our reaction time while starting or stopping a stopwatch leads to personal error. This does not refer to any mistakes may be made while taking the measurements. Errors for both the reasons are considered as personal error. In fact, it refers to the uncertainty inherent to the instrument and personal ability to minimize this uncertainty. The precision of the experiment can be affected by a reading error. The uncertainty associated with the reading of the scale and the need to interpolate between scale markings is relatively easy to estimate. Let us consider the millimeter (mm) marking on a scale is the smallest marking and a person with a normal vision can read the marking to the nearest millimeter at best. Therefore, in this case, a reasonable estimate of the uncertainty would be $\Delta l = \pm 0.5$ mm which is half of the smallest division.

For evaluation of reading error on analog readout a rule of thumb is to use half of the smallest division (in case of a meter stick with millimeter divisions it is 0.5 mm), but only the observer can ultimately decide what is his/her limitation in error evaluation. It is also to be noted that it would be wrong to assume that is always half of the smallest division of the scale. For example, the uncertainty for a person with a poor vision might be greater than one millimeter while using the same ruler, if the scale markings are relatively large say, 1 cm. In such case, one may reasonably decide that the length could be read to one-fifth or one-fourth of the smallest division.

Indirect measurements, there are other sources of uncertainty that can be much more important. For example, to measure the distance between two points, the major problem is to decide where those two points are really lying. Similarly, in an optic experiment, it is frequently necessary to measure the distance between the center of the lens and the position of the focused image. Locating the center of a thin lens, several millimeters thick is a difficult task. Moreover, the image itself may appear to be focused not at a point, but its location may span a range of several millimeters.

Another significant source of a reading error is parallax. The reading depends on the line of sight. In a laboratory, the instruments having a digital readout is used. For many digital instruments, it is assumed that the reading error is $\pm 1/2$ of the last digit displayed. If the reading of the timer in an experiment is 401.10 ms (millisecond), the error can be assumed to be ± 0.05 ms and it should be quoted as 401.10 ± 0.05 ms. However, it is the random error that determines the precision and gives an idea about the scatter that might be expected in the readings. Thus, the '$\pm$ digit' quoted by the manufacturer might be a better estimate of the random error. It is usually difficult or impossible to reduce the inherent reading error in an instrument. In some cases, it is possible to reduce the reading error by repeating measurements of exactly the same quantity and averaging them, where the reading error of the instrument approximates a 'random error distribution'.

Random Error

Random Error refers to the spread in the values of a physical quantity from one measurement of the quantity to the next. This is caused by random fluctuations in the measured value. For example, in repeating measurements of the time taken for a ball to fall through a given height, the varying initial conditions, random fluctuations in air motion, the variation of the observer's reaction time in starting and stopping a watch, etc., will cause a significant spread in the times measured. This type of error also affects the precision of the experiment.

Other sources may be the method adopted, an instrument used, and personal skill. These are briefly described below.

2.2   TYPES OF ERRORS

The errors that can affect the experimental result may be divided into two categories – determinate and indeterminate.

Determinate error

The determinate or constant error can be avoided, and their magnitude can be determined. Primarily there are five types of determinate error.

- *Operational error*: This error is mostly physical in nature and occurs when an efficient and correct analytical technique is not followed. For example, in various steps of an analysis the material may be lost due to mechanical processes – (1) improper washing (under washing or over washing) of the precipitates, (2) precipitates may not be ignited at correct temperatures, (3) before weighing the crucibles are insufficiently cooled, (4) hygroscopic materials are allowed to absorb moisture before or during weighing, and (5) reagents containing harmful impurities are used.

- *Personal error*: Such an error occurs when an analyst is not responsible or is not properly aware of the procedure or method in concern. The inability of an individual analyst is the major reason for personal error. It may be inherent such as color blindness or due to wrong practices for which the analyst fails to observe or record some findings accurately. For example, in volumetric titrations, the color changes at the endpoint due to an indicator present. Persons having color blindness cannot judge the color change sharply. As a result, the titer values noted are not correct. Similarly, observing the meniscus and noting burette or pipette reading, observing the swings of the pointer of a balance cannot be correctly made. However, at present digital balance has replaced the -called chemical balance.

  Instrumental and reagent error: This type of error occurs due to faulty construction of balance, uncalibrated or improperly calibrated weights, volumetric apparatuses, and other instruments. Sometimes some reagents can interact with glass wares, porcelain, etc. and the sample may be contaminated with foreign materials (products of above interaction). At very high-temperature platinum volatilizes and may be mixed with the sample.Besides all these, the error may arise when the reagents used contain impurities.

- *The error of method*: Incorrect samples and incomplete reaction are the major sources of this type of error. In the gravimetric analysis the error comes out of (1) precipitate obtained do have some solubility in the solvent, (2) coprecipitation and post-precipitation, (3) decomposition, (4) during ignition or weighing volatilization of material, and (5) precipitation of substance other than the intended one.

In case of titrimetric analysis, the possible sources of error may be due to (1) incompleteness of reaction, (2) occurrence of induced and side reactions, (3) determination of substances other than the intended ones, and (4) variation between observed endpoint and stoichiometric end point of a reaction.

- *Additive or proportional errors*: The absolute value of an additive error does not depend on the amount of the component present in the determination. For example, when a crucible containing a precipitate is ignited and error in weight is taken place. Such an error is known when samples of different weights are measured.

On the other hand, the absolute value of a proportional error does not depend on the amount of the component. The impurity present in a standard substance is responsible for a proportional error and is also responsible for incorrect normality or molarity of a standard solution. Some proportional errors do not vary linearly with the amount of component. However, proportional error increases with the amount of component present. For example, aluminium oxide when ignited at 1200°C produces anhydrous and non-hygroscopic aluminium oxide. But, when various amounts of it are heated at lower temperature a proportional error is observed.

Indeterminate or Accidental Error

Slight variations in successive measurements made by the same person or analyst produce this type of error in spite of taking utmost care and carrying out the analyses under almost same conditions. The reasons for such variations are not under the control of the analyst. Generally, these are so insubstantial that the analysis cannot be carried out. If a large number of observations are made and the frequencies of observations are plotted against the magnitude of errors, a plot is obtained as shown in the figure. The figure 2.1 shows that (1) small errors occur more commonly than the large ones, (2) large errors occur relatively occasionally, (3) occurrence of positive and negative errors almost equally with same numerical magnitude.

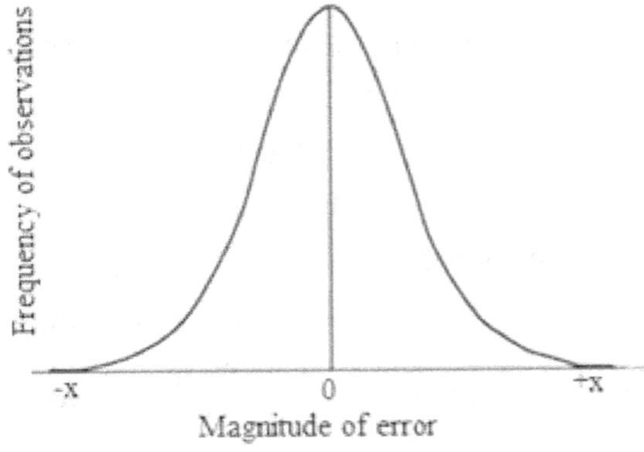

Figure 2.1 Plot of frequency distribution vs magnitude of the error.

2.3   METHODS OF MINIMIZING ERRORS

Between determinate or constant error and indeterminate or accidental error efforts are to be made to minimize the extent of determinate error which is mostly person based. Indeterminate error, on the other hand, is mostly not under the control of an analyst. There are about seven methods for minimizing errors. In some cases, the degree of determinate errors can be reduced if the following methods are used.

(i) *Calibration of apparatus and application of corrections*: All instruments and apparatuses such as balance, weights, pH meter, pipettes, burettes, flasks, etc., must be calibrated. Thereafter necessary corrections are to be applied to the original measurements. When the error cannot be eliminated, a correction for the effect it produces can be applied. For example, the impurity present in a weighed precipitate is determined and its weight can be deducted from the weight of the precipitate.

(ii) *Using a blank determination*: To determine the effect of impurities introduced through the reagents and container, a blank determination is carried out. In some cases where the unknown sample is estimated by titrimetric method, excess of standard solution is added to determine the correct endpoint. In such cases, a determination is carried out without using sample or standard (blank) but all the reagents are to be added sequentially as per the procedure and the blank titer value is deducted from the sample as well as standard titer value. Large blank correction is not desired, because it becomes uncertain to find out the correct value and precision of the analysis is reduced.

(iii) *Use of control test*: In this test, a standard or reference substance is parallelly analyzed by the same method as is used for the analysis of the sample. The standard contains the same constituent as the sample and purity of the standard is also known. The purity of the sample is then calculated as follows;

$$\frac{\text{Result obtained for standard}}{\text{Result obtained for sample}} = \frac{\text{Declared potency of the standard}}{\text{Potency of the sample}}$$

Or, Potency of sample

$$= \frac{\text{Declardt potency of the standard} \times \text{Result obtained for sample}}{\text{Result obrained for standard}}$$

Example 2: Say, the titer value for the sample is 24.90mL

The titer value for the standard is 25.05mL

The potency of the standard is 99.98%

If the weight of the sample titrated = the weight of standard titrated

Then, potency of sample $= \dfrac{24.90\text{ml}}{25.00\text{ml}} \times 99.98\% = 99.58\%$

(iv) *Use of independent methods of analysis*: In some cases, the sample is analyzed by two different methods and the results are compared. If the results of the two methods are the same, it is accepted that the values (results) are correct within small limits of error. For example, a sample of iron is analyzed gravimetrically by precipitating as ferric hydroxide. The interfering elements are removed, and the precipitate is ignited to ferric oxide and the content of iron in the sample is calculated. The sample is then reduced to ferrous state and analyzed by titrimetric (volumetric) method with a standard solution of ceric ammonium sulphate or potassium dichromate. The content of iron in the sample is then calculated.

(v) *Performing parallel determinations*: By performing these tests the result of a single determination is checked for the precision of the analysis. The results obtained for the sample containing a moderately high amount of constituent do not vary among themselves by more than 0.3%. If there is a larger variation, the analysis must be repeated until concurrent results are obtained. Forgetting concurrent results duplicate or triplicate determinations would be sufficient. However, it must be kept in mind that good agreement among the results (precision) does not justify that the result is correct. There may be a constant or determinate error. The good agreement among the determinations merely indicates that the accidental errors, or variations of the determinate errors in the parallel determinations, are the same or almost the same.

(vi) *Recovery test or addition of standard*: In this method, two samples are parallelly analyzed - one is of sample alone and other is a mixture of sample and known amount of the constituent present in the sample. The difference between the two results indicates the recovery of the constituent added. If the recovered amount is equal to the amount actually added or within the agreeable limits, the method of analysis adopted is considered accurate.

(vii) *Isotopic dilution*: In case of elemental analysis a known amount of element being determined and containing a radioactive isotope is mixed with the sample. The element is then isolated in the pure form; in practice, as a compound. The radioactivity of the isolated element is measured and compared with that of added element. Accordingly, the weight of the element in the sample can be calculated.

2.4 ACCURACY

Accuracy is a description of systematic error or a measure of the statistical bias. It can be defined in terms of a *difference between a result and a true value or trueness of a result.* According to the ISO, accuracy is defined as *the closeness of agreement between a test result and the accepted reference value.* The 'test result' refers to the observed, calculated or estimated value; while 'accepted reference value' refers to the true value. Thus, accuracy means how closely a measured value agrees with the correct value.

Trueness is the difference between the observed mean value and the reference value. True value can never be achieved repeatedly or regularly because some random variations (error) are likely to occur due to some reasons. Let us explain this through a statistical graph shown.

There are some terms relevant to accuracy and precision should be known to the reader, and hence mentioned here.

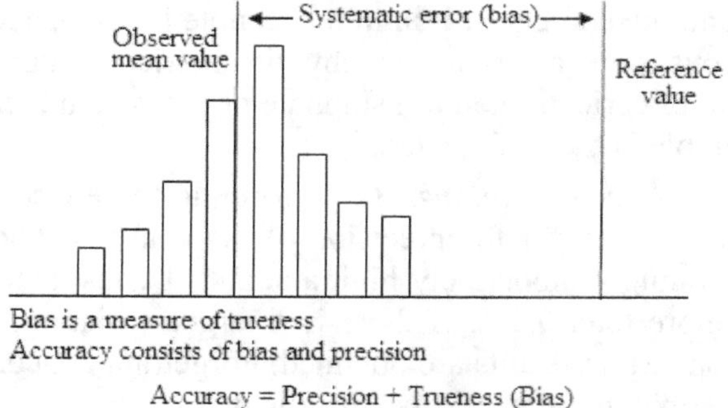

Repeatability – if the same person repeats the experiment using the same equipment; the results obtained would be close together.

Reproducibility – if the different persons carry out the experiment using different types of equipment; the results would be close together.

True value – This is an ideal value of the quantity, such as mass, volume, temperature. This can never be known exactly.

Reference value – a value very close to the true value and accepted as a point of reference. For example, a 'standard weight' measured on a balance having negligible or no error and is very close to the true value.

Errors are not the same as mistakes such as 'not reading a scale correctly' and 'incorrect graduation in the scale'.

Reliability – a judgment to be made regarding the level of mistakes or error. This is evaluated by comparing an individual result with a reference or class mean. The overall percentage error based on instrumental readings is unavoidable while mistakes (human errors) are avoidable through repeating and reproducing the results.

Anomalous point – a result which is very different from others (data point that does not match with the pattern of the graph), for example, four pH values are within the range from 4.20 – 4.30, while one is 4.75. The pH value of 4.75 is anomalous.

2.5   PRECISION AND SIGNIFICANT FIGURES

Precision

Precision may be defined as the closeness of the series of measurements of the same quantity. The mean deviation or relative mean deviation is a measure of precision. In quantitative analysis, the precision should not exceed 0.2% or 2 parts per thousand. When precision is discussed, accuracy comes. In quantitative analysis, the results may be of a high degree of precision, but it does not indicate accuracy.

This is explained through the figure 2.2. As shown in the figure there are four situations and attempts were ten. In one situation both accuracy and precision are low, in second case precision is high without accuracy, in third case accuracy is high without precision, in forth case both accuracy and precision are high.

In quantitative analysis, accuracy refers to the degree of closeness of the measurement or result or value to that of the standard or known or true value. There are two methods to determine the accuracy of an analytical method –

1. The absolute method, and
2. Comparative method.

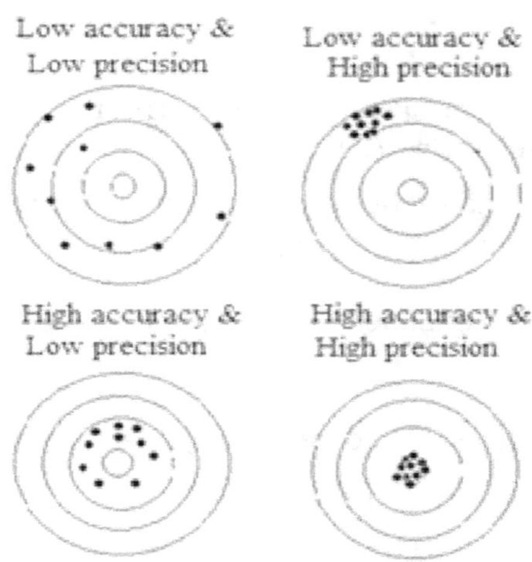

Figure 2.2 Accuracy and precision.

Example 3: A sample claims to contain 99.5 ± 0.2% of the drug. Two analysts tested the sample. The results of the two analyses are as follows;

Analyst A: 99.2%, 99.49% and 99.9%,

Analyst B: 99.63%, 99.50% and 99.78%

Solution: Analyst A: The mean value $= \dfrac{99.2 + 99.49 + 99.9}{3} = \textbf{99.55\%}$

Relative mean error $= \dfrac{(99.55 - 99.5) \times 100}{99.5} = 0.05\%$

Deviations are: 0.3, 0.06, and 0.35

Relative mean deviation $= \dfrac{(0.3 + 0.06 + 0.35)}{3} \times \dfrac{100}{99.55} = 0.237 \times 1.004 = \textbf{0.238\%}$

Analyst B: The mean value $= \dfrac{99.63 + 99.50 + 99.78}{3} = 99.64\%$

Relative mean error $= \dfrac{(99.64 - 99.5) \times 100}{99.5} = 0.14\%$

Deviations are: 0.13, 0.00, and 0.28

$$\text{Relative mean deviation} = \frac{(0.13 + 0.00 + 0.28)}{3} \times \frac{100}{99.64} = 0.137 \times \frac{100}{99.64} = \mathbf{0.137\%}$$

The results of **analyst A are more accurate and precise**; the results of analyst B are more precise. (Ans.)

Note: If a series of observations are arranged in ascending order of magnitude such as x_1, x_2, x_3, x_4, ... x_{n-1}, x_n.

$$\text{The arithmetic mean (simply mean)} = \frac{x_1 + x_2 + x_3 + ... x_n}{n} = \bar{x}$$

$$\text{The standard deviation, } \delta = \sqrt{\frac{(x_1 - \bar{x})^2 + (x_2 - \bar{x})^2 + (x_3 - \bar{x})^2 + ... + (x_n - \bar{x})^2}{n-1}}$$

and

$$\text{Coefficient of variation} = \frac{\delta \times 100}{\bar{x}}$$

Absolute method: In this method, a known amount of reference or certified substance is added to the sample. The purity of the reference substance is known. The method in question is used to analyze. The amount of reference substance used is varied, because the error may depend on the amount used. The substance is tested in the presence of other substances because it is necessary to know the effect of these substances on the method used.

Course, this requires conducting a number of experiments to standardize the method. However, the number of such tests can be reduced since a specified amount of active substance remains present and the composition is almost fixed. Usually, the active substance is separated before estimation or such a method is used which is strictly specific to the substance being tested. Whatever method is used, the accuracy depends either on the method of separation or on the efficiency of the specific method used.

Comparative method: Sometimes it is not possible to prepare and use solid synthetic samples of desired composition for analysis of a mineral. It is then necessary to opt for standard samples of the material under consideration (mineral, ore, alloy, etc.) in which the content of the constituent to be tested has been determined by one or more evidently accurate methods of analysis. This comparative method using secondary standard is very useful for analysis. Standard samples are collected from the govt. approved specific sources.

If different methods such as gravimetric, titrimetric, spectrophotometric, or spectrographic methods are available for determination of a specific compound or element, at least two of these methods which are principally different but can determine the component accurately, should be selected for the determination.

Significant Figures

Significant figure *is a digit that represents the amount of the quantity in the place in which it is present.* The digit zero is a significant figure expect when it is the first figure in a number. For example, in the quantities 2.5640g and in 2.0054g, the zero is significant and both the numbers contain five significant figures. While in the quantity 0.0056g the zeros are not significant figure, they indicate only the location of the decimal point and can be omitted by changing unit such as 5.6mg. The last quantity contains two significant figures.

In most of the analysis, weights are measured to the nearest tenth of a milligram, such as 1.2597g. This means that the weight is less than 1.2598g and more than 1.2596g. Similarly, the quantity 1.256g is nearest to one milligram, between 1.255g and 1.257g. *The digits of a number which are required to express the precision of the measurement from which the number was derived are known as significant figures.* For computation some rules are to be followed. The rules are;

- Observed quantities should be recorded with only one uncertain figure. Thus, the weight in between 10.4kg and 10.6kg should be recorded as 10.5kg, not as 10.50kg. The latter indicates that the weight is in between 10.49kg and 10.51kg. Similarly, a weight 1.5700g, nearest to 0.1mg should be written as 1.5700g, not as 1.570g or 1.57g. The quantity 1.57g is nearest to one centigram, 1.570g is nearest to one milligram.

- In rounding off quantities to the correct number of significant figures, add one to the last figure retained if the following figure (which has been rejected) is 5 or over. Thus, the average of 0.2628, 0.2623, and 0.2626 is $0.26257 \approx 0.2626$.

- In addition or subtraction, there should be in each number only as many significant figures as there are in the least accurately known number. Thus, the addition, $168.11 + 7.045 + 0.6832$ should be written as $168.11 + 7.05 + 0.68 = 175.84$.

- The sum or difference of two or more quantities cannot be more precise than the quantity having the largest uncertainty.

- In multiplication or division, retain in each factor one more significant figure than is contained in the factor having the largest uncertainty. The percentage precision of a product or quotient cannot be greater than the percentage precision of the least precise factor entering into the calculation. Thus, the multiplication, $1.26 \times 1.236 \times 0.6834 \times 24.8652$ should be obtained by using the values as $1.26 \times 1.236 \times 0.683 \times 24.87$

A. MULTIPLE CHOICE QUESTIONS

1. The difference between the true value and observed or measured value is called
   (a) Absolute error
   (b) Relative error
   (c) Accuracy
   (b) True value

2. The reliability of the experimental result depends on
   (a) The magnitude of the difference between the true value and observed/experimental value.
   (b) The difference between the true value and observed/experimental value.
   (c) The true value
   (d) None of the above

3. The closeness between a series of results is measured by
   (a) Geometric mean deviation.
   (b) Arithmetic mean deviation
   (c) Absolute error
   (d) True value

4. Reding error includes
   (a) Instrument reading error
   (b) Personal error
   (c) Both
   (d) None of the above

5. If millimeter (mm) marking on a scale is the smallest marking, then a reasonable estimate of the uncertainty would be
   (a) $\Delta l = \pm 0.05$ mm
   (b) $\Delta l = \pm 0.005$ mm
   (c) $\Delta l = \pm 0.025$ mm
   (d) $\Delta l = \pm 0.5$ mm

6. For evaluation of reading error on analogue readout a rule of thumb is to use
   (a) Half of the smallest division
   (b) One fourth of the smallest division
   (c) Two third of the smallest division
   (d) One third of the smallest division

7. In repeating measurements of the time taken for a ball to fall through a given height, the varying initial conditions are:
   (a) Random fluctuations in air motion,
   (b) The variation of the observer's reaction time in starting and stopping a watch,
   (c) Reflex of the person,
   (d) All of the above

8. If the reading of the timer in an experiment is 401.10 ms (millisecond), the error can be assumed to be
   (a) $+0.05$ ms
   (b) -0.05 ms
   (c) ± 0.05 ms
   (d) ± 0.5 ms

9. The sources of error may be
   (a) The method adopted,
   (b) Instrument used,
   (c) Personal skill
   (d) All of the above

10. Determinate or constant error
    (a) Can be avoided
    (b) Cannot be avoided
    (c) Is a source of error
    (d) All of the above

11. In spite of taking utmost care and carrying out the analyses under almost same conditions, slight variations in successive measurements made by the same person is called
    (a) Determinate error
    (b) Indeterminate error
    (c) Personal error
    (d) Instrumental error

12. Personal error, error of method, and additive or proportional errors are called as
    (a) Personal error
    (b) Indeterminate error
    (c) Determinate error
    (d) All of the above
13. Calibration of apparatus and application of corrections reduces or eliminates
    (a) Determinate error
    (b) Indeterminate error
    (c) None of the above
14. Accuracy can be defined as
    (a) The closeness of the series of measurements of same quantity
    (b) Difference between a result and a true value or trueness of a result
    (c) All of the above
    (d) None of the above
15. The same person repeats the experiment using same equipment; if the results obtained are close together, it is called
    (a) Repeatability
    (b) Reproducibility
    (c) Reliability
    (d) True value
16. In absolute method a known amount of reference or certified substance is added to the sample. The purity of the reference substance is known.
    (a) To determine accuracy
    (b) To determine precision
    (c) To determine accuracy and precision
    (d) To reduce error
17. The zero is significant in
    (a) 2.540g
    (b) 0.0254g
    (c) 0.0025g
    (d) 0.0002g

B. SHORT QUESTIONS

1. What is meant by the term error?
2. What are absolute error and relative error?
3. Name the major sources of error.
4. What is reading error?
5. What is random error?
6. What are determinate and indeterminate errors?
7. Name the errors categorized as determinate error.
8. Name the errors categorized as indeterminate error.
9. What is the basic difference between determinate and indeterminate errors?
10. How the error can be minimized? Name the methods.
11. What is the outcome of minimizing error?
12. What is accuracy?
13. What is precision?

14. What are the methods used to measure the accuracy of an analytical method?
15. What do you mean by significant figure?

C. LONG QUESTIONS

1. Explain the term accuracy and precision.
2. Explain the importance of accuracy in pharmaceutical analysis.
3. Discuss briefly the types of error.
4. Describe the sources of determinate error.
5. Explain how indeterminate error takes place.
6. Explain how the errors can be minimized.
7. Explain the term-significant figure. How it is important in pharmaceutical analysis?

CHAPTER 3

Acid-Base Titration

INTRODUCTION

The reader should recapitulate the fundamentals concepts of the theory of acid-base titration. It involves a quantitative reaction between an acid and a base. A measured volume of aqueous solution of acid or base (sample) is titrated with a solution of base or acid of definite concentration (titrant) using suitable indicator till equilibrium is attained. The volume of titrant is noted and the concentration of the solution of unknown substance is calculated by using Law of mass action. Such a titration between acid and base is called acid-base titration.

For example, 25.00mL of a solution of hydrochloric acid is titrated with a 0.1N standard solution of anhydrous sodium carbonate using methyl red. The color changes from red to yellow. Say, 25.15mL of sodium carbonate solution is consumed. Then, the strength of hydrochloric acid solution is calculated as;

$$= \frac{25.15\text{mL} \times 0.1\text{N}}{25.00} = 0.1006\text{N}$$

To understand the concept of acid-base titration one should have the knowledge about acid, base, and law of mass action.

Theories of Acids and Bases

An *acid* is defined as a substance which dissociates when dissolved in water and form hydrogen ion, as shown

$$HCl \leftrightarrow H^+ + Cl^-$$

LEARNING OBJECTIVES

After studying the chapter the students familiarize themselves with the following concepts:

- ✓ Electrochemical Cell
- ✓ Construction and working of reference electrodes (standard hydrogen, silver chloride electrode and calomel electrode)
- ✓ Construction and working of indicator electrodes (metal electrodes and glass electrode)
- ✓ Methods to Determine End Point of Potentiometric Titration Applications

$$HNO_3 \leftrightarrow H^+ + NO_3^-$$

In aqueous solution hydrogen ion, H^+ (proton) cannot exist in free state. Each hydrogen ion combines with one molecule of water and form hydroxonium ion, H_3O^+. The hydroxonium ion, H_3O^+ can be called as a hydrated proton. Hence, the above reactions can be rewritten as;

$$HCl + H_2O \leftrightarrow H_3O^+ + Cl^-$$

$$HNO_3 + H_2O \leftrightarrow H_3O^+ + NO_3^-$$

According to the above reactions, hydrochloric acid and nitric acid are monobasic acids and are almost completely dissociated in aqueous medium. These are strong acids. This can be detected by freezing point measurement and by other methods.

Polybasic acids ionize in stages. Sulphuric acid, a dibasic acid ionizes when mixed with water and releases one hydrogen ion in the first step. In this step sulphuric acid ionizes completely.

$$H_2SO_4 \leftrightarrow H^+ + HSO_4^-$$

Or, $$H_2SO_4 + H_2O \leftrightarrow H_3O^+ + HSO_4^-$$

In the second step, HSO_4^- ionizes partially, except in very dilute solution

$$HSO_4^- + H_2O \leftrightarrow H_3O^+ + SO_4^{2-}$$

Phosphoric acid is a tribasic acid; it ionizes in three stages, primary, secondary, and tertiary ionizations as shown below;

$$H_3PO_4 + H_2O \leftrightarrow H_3O^+ + H_2PO_4^- \text{ (primary ionization)}$$

$$H_2PO_4^- + H_2O \leftrightarrow H_3O^+ + HPO_4^{2-} \text{ (secondary ionization)}$$

$$HPO_4^{2-} + H_2O \leftrightarrow H_3O^+ + PO_4^{3-} \text{ (tertiary ionization)}$$

The primary ionization is greater than the secondary and secondary ionization is much greater than the tertiary ionization.

Acid such as acetic acid ionizes slightly in water. Its aqueous solution gives a normal freezing point depression. Hence, acetic acid is a weak acid.

A ***base*** is defined as a substance which dissociates and forms hydroxide ion, OH^- when dissolved in water. Sodium hydroxide, potassium hydroxide, and the hydroxides of alkaline earth metals dissociate completely in aqueous solution.

$$NaOH \rightarrow Na^+ + OH^-$$

$$Ba(OH)_2 \rightarrow Ba^{2+} + 2OH^-$$

These are strong bases. Aqueous solution of ammonia on the hand produces small amount of hydroxide ion and thus, is a weak base.

$$NH_3 + H_2O \leftrightarrow NH_4^+ + OH^-$$

Lowery-Bronsted theory of acids and bases

According to Bronsted, an acid is a substance having a tendency to lose a proton, and it is represented as;

$$Acid \leftrightarrow Proton + Conjugate\ base$$

Or, $A \leftrightarrow H^+ + B$ .....(3.1)

It may be noted that H^+ represents 'proton' not the hydrogen ion. Other ionic species may be written accordingly such as H_3O^+, NH_4^+, $CH_3CO_2H_2^+$, $C_2H_5OH_2^+$, etc. This definition does not depend on the nature of the solvent.

Thus, acid may be neutral molecule such as HCl, H_2SO_4, CH_3CO_2H, etc. and an anion such as HSO_4^-, $H_2PO_4^-$, and $HOOC-COO^-$

Similarly, a base is a substance that accepts the proton from the acid. This is expressed as

$$B_1 + H+ \leftrightarrow A_1$$ .....(3.2)

By combining the equations 1 and 2

$$A + B_1 \leftrightarrow A_1 + B$$ .....(3.3)

$A–B$ and $A_1–B_1$ are two conjugate acid-base pairs. For reaction between acids and bases the equation 3 is most important. According to this equation proton is transferred from A to B or from A_1 to B_1.

If $A–B$ is stronger acid-base pair, $A_1–B_1$ would be the weaker acid-base pair and the reaction would complete. The stronger acid loses its proton more readily than the weaker one. Similarly, stronger base accepts the proton immediately compared to weaker base.

In an aqueous solution of Bronsted acid, A ionizes as;

$$A + H_2O \leftrightarrow H_3O^+ + B$$

If A is strong acid the above equilibrium will virtually shift to the right; so that [A] is almost zero. Similarly, for a strong base, B, the equilibrium concentration of B, [B] would be zero except hydroxide ion. Thus, according to the strength acids may be arranged as HCl, HBr, HI, HNO_3, $HClO_4$, etc.

On the other hand, the typical weak acids such as acetic acid (CH_3COOH), propionic acid (C_3H_7COOH) ionize slightly in water and the reaction proceeds slightly to the right. For example;

$$CH_3COOH + H_2O \leftrightarrow H_3O^+ + CH_3COO^-$$

$$A \qquad\quad B_1 \qquad A_1 \qquad\quad B$$

The typical strong acid in aqueous system is the hydrated proton (H_3O^+) and the role of conjugate base is minor, if it is sufficiently weak base such as Cl^-, Br^-, ClO_4^-. Accordingly, the basic ionization constant of a conjugate base, $K_{B.conj} = K_W/K_{A.conj}$, where K_W is the ionic product of water.

Lewis Theory

According to G.N. Lewis an acid is a substance that accepts a pair of electrons and the base is defined as a substance that donates a pair of electrons. The electrons form a covalent bond even a proton may be involved. Solution of BF_3, BCl_3, $AlCl_3$, or SO_2 in inert solvent can change the color of an indicator similar to HCl, and the color of the indicator is reversed by addition of solution of base. Thus, these substances are called Lewis acids or electron acceptor.

The law of Mass Action

In 1867 Guldberg and Waage stated the law of mass action, alternatively called law of chemical equilibrium as; the velocity of a chemical reaction is proportional to the product of the active masses of the reacting substances. The term, 'active mass' can be expressed as 'gram-molecules' or 'mole' per litre. The law can be applied to a homogeneous system such as a solution of A and B which dissociate reversibly as follows;

$$A + B \leftrightarrow C + D$$

According to the law, the velocity of the reaction between A and B is proportional to their concentrations, i.e., $v_f = k_1 \times [A] \times [B]$

Similarly, the velocity of the backward reaction, $v_b = k_2 \times [C] \times [D]$

At equilibrium when forward reaction = backward reaction or $v_f = v_b$

$$k_1 \times [A] \times [B] = k_2 \times [C] \times [D]$$

Or,
$$\frac{k_1}{k_2} = \frac{[C] \times [D]}{[A] \times [B]} = K$$

Where, k_1 and k_2 are velocity coefficient of forward and backward reaction respectively. K is the equilibrium constant of the reaction at a particular temperature. [A], [B], [C] and [D] are molecular concentration of A, B. C, and D respectively.

Activity and Activity Coefficient

It has been mentioned earlier that the effective concentrations or active masses of the components of a reaction can be expressed by the stoichiometric concentrations. According to the thermodynamics this is not exactly correct. For a binary electrolyte system, the exact equation is written as;

$$AB \leftrightarrow A^+ + B^-$$

Or
$$K_a = \frac{a_{A+} \times a_{B-}}{a_{AB}}$$

Where, a_{A+}, a_{B-}, and a_{AB} are the activity coefficient of A^+, B^-, and AB respectively. Ka is the actual or thermodynamic dissociation constant. The term 'activity' is a thermodynamic quantity. According to Lewis activity can be related to the concentration by a factor, called activity coefficient.

$$\text{Activity} = \text{molar concentration} \times \text{activity coefficient}$$

Thus, $a_{A+} = f_A \times [A^+]$, $a_{B-} = f_B \times [B^-]$ and $a_{AB} = f_{AB} \times [AB]$, where f is the activity coefficient.

Accordingly, the above equation can be rewritten as

$$Ka = \frac{[A] \times [B]}{[AB]} \times \frac{f_{A+} \times f_{B-}}{f_{AB}}$$

This is the correct expression for the law of mass action applied to the weak electrolytes. It is evident that activity coefficient varies with concentration. For ions it varies with valency, and for all dilute solutions having same ionic strength it is also same. Ionic strength is a measure of the electrical field existing in a solution. It is represented by I and is defined as – *"equal to one half of the sum of the products of the concentration of each ion multiplied by the square of its valency."* Thus, $I = 0.5 \sum c_i z_i^2$. Where, c_i is the ionic concentration in gram-molecules/L of the solution; z_i is the valency of the ion concerned. Activity coefficient depends on the total ionic strength of the solution. The important properties of activity coefficient are;

- Mostly in concentrated solutions it is relatively difficult to determine.
- In a solution containing mixture of ions of different types of valency are present, it is relatively difficult to determine.
- In solutions containing unionized molecules the activity coefficients do not differ from unity.
- In solution of weak electrolytes, the ionic concentration and thus ionic strength is small; the activity coefficient can be replaced by molar concentration of ions. This results a difference of less than 5%.
- No correction for activity coefficient is required for dilution solution of strong electrolyte since it dissociates completely.

Determination of ionization constant

Dilute solution of a weak electrolyte such as acetic acid dissociates in water as follows;

$$CH_3COOH + H_2O \leftrightarrow H_3O^+ + CH_3COO^-$$

In simple form, $CH_3COOH \leftrightarrow H^+ + CH_3COO^-$

Where, H^+ represents the hydrated hydrogen ion. By applying the law of mass action

$$K = \frac{[CH_3COO^-][H^+]}{[CH_3COOH]}$$

Where, K is the equilibrium constant at a particular temperature and is usually called as ionization or dissociation constant. Say one gm equivalent of the electrolyte is dissolved in V litre of solution,

$$V = 1/c$$

Where, c is the concentration in gm-equivalents/L;

If α is the degree of ionization at equilibrium; then the undissociated amount of electrolyte = $(1 - \alpha)$ gm-equivalents and the amount of each of the ions would be α gm-equivalents.

Thus, concentration of unionized acetic acid in the solution would be $\dfrac{(1-\alpha)}{V}$ and the concentration of each ion = α/V.

Hence, $$K = \frac{\alpha^2}{(1-\alpha)v} = \frac{c.\alpha^2}{(1-\alpha)}$$

This is known as *Ostwald's dilution law*.

Ionization and ionic product of water

Conductivity indicates the presence of ions in a liquid. In 1894 Kohlrausch and Heydweiller observed that most of the purest waters possess a small but definite conductivity.

Thus, water, even in its purest form ionizes but might be slightly. The ionization reaction may be written as;

$$H_2O \leftrightarrow H^+ + OH^-$$

The exact equation is $H_2O + H_2O \leftrightarrow H_3O^+ + OH^-$

By applying the law of mass action to this equation at any given temperature

$$\frac{a_{H^+} \times a_{OH^-}}{a_{H_2O}} = \frac{[H^+][OH^-]}{[H_2O]} \times \frac{f_{H^+} \times f_{OH^-}}{f_{H_2O}} = constant$$

Since water ionizes slightly, the ionic concentration will be small and thus, the activity of the unionized molecules may be considered as unity. The ionization reaction becomes;

$$\frac{[H^+][OH^-]}{[H_2O]} = a\ constant$$

Thus, in pure water or in dilute aqueous solutions, the concentration of unionized water may be considered constant and the above equation can be written as

$$[H^+] \times [OH^-] = K_W \qquad .....(3.4)$$

Where, K_w is the ionic product of water. It is difficult to determine the activity coefficients under normal conditions. It can be determined only under special conditions. The ionic product changes with temperature. At about 25°C the value of ionic product of water, K_w is 1×10^{-14} g-ions per lt. As per the equation 4 concentrations of hydrogen ion and hydroxide ion in pure water are equal; hence,

$$[H^+] = [OH^-] = \sqrt{K_w} = \sqrt{1 \times 10^{-14}} = 10^{-7} \text{ g-ions/lt}$$

A solution containing equal concentrations of hydrogen ion and hydroxide ion is called neutral solution. If the hydrogen ion concentration, $[H^+]$ is more than 10^{-7} the solution is acid and if it is less than 10^{-7} the solution is alkaline or basic. The values of K_w at different temperatures are given in the Table 3.1.

Table 3.1: Ionic product of pure water at different temperatures

Temp. (°C)	$K_w \times 10^{14}$	Temp. (°C)	$K_w \times 10^{14}$
0	0.12	35	2.09
5	0.19	40	2.92
10	0.29	45	4.02
15	0.45	50	5.47
20	0.68	55	7.30
25	1.01	60	9.61
30	1.47		

pH, hydrogen-ion exponent

When gram-equivalents of hydrogen ions and hydroxide ions are small, it is very difficult to measure them. In 1909 S.P.L. Sorensen proposed a very convenient method to measure the hydrogen ion concentration in solution. He defined the hydrogen ion concentration as hydrogen ion exponent, pH as shown below;

$$pH = - \log_{10}[H^+] = \log_{10} 1/[H^+]$$

or, $[H+] = 10^{-pH}$

He proposed a pH scale from 0 to 14. pH 0 to 7 is acid range while pH 7 to 14 is alkaline range. This is explained through the following examples.

Example 1: The hydrogen ion concentration in a solution is 4.0×10^{-5}, calculate the pH of the solution.

Solution: $pH = - \log_{10}[H^+] = - \log (4.0 \times 10^{-5})$

$\qquad = - [\log 4 + \log (-5)] = - [0.602 - 5.0] = - (- 4.398)$

$\qquad = \mathbf{4.398}$

3.1   THEORIES OF ACID-BASE INDICATORS

A solution of an acid is titrated with a standard solution of a base to determine the amount of acid, vice versa. The titration is continued till the equivalence point, stoichiometrical point, or theoretical end point is reached. At this point the amount of base is chemically equivalent to the amount of acid. Such a titration is called neutralization reaction and an aqueous solution of salt is produced. When both acid and base are strong electrolytes, the resultant solution will be neutral with a pH of 7. If either the acid or base is a weak electrolyte, the salt formed hydrolyzes to a certain degree. At equivalence point the solution will be either slightly alkaline or slightly acidic. The correct end point can be characterized by the actual value of hydrogen ion concentration of the solution. The value depends on the nature of the acid and base and the concentration of the solution.

To determine the end point visually a third substance called *acid-base indicator* is used. there are large number of such substances (indicators) which change their colors with change of pH (hydrogen ion concentration). The change in color does not take place suddenly but takes place within a small interval of pH. Usually this interval of pH amounts to be about two pH units which is called *color-change interval* of the indicator. In the pH scale the color-change interval varies with indicator. In an acid base titration an indicator which changes its color nearest to the end point is used.

W. Ostwald first suggested a useful theory of indicator. In general, an indicator is either a very weak organic acid or a base. In 1891 Ostwald proposed that an undissociated indicator acid (HIn) or base (InOH) possess a different color and an indicator ion possess different color. In an aqueous solution an indicator dissociates as follows;

$$HIn \quad \leftrightarrow \quad H^+ + In^-$$

and

$$InOH \quad \leftrightarrow \quad In^+ \; + \; OH^-$$

$$\text{unionized} \qquad\qquad \text{ionized}$$

$$\text{color} \qquad\qquad\qquad \text{color}$$

Let us consider that an acid indicator (HIn) is given in an acid solution. In the acid solution hydrogen ions are present in excess amount and due to the common ion (H^+) effect ionization of the indicator will be suppressed. As a result, the concentration of In^- ions will be very small. At this situation the color of the indicator would be that of its unionized form. During titration alkali solution is gradually added to the acid solution; this decreases the concentration of H^+ ions by neutralization. Thus, the concentration of In- ions will increase gradually and at end point all the H^+ ions will be neutralized. Then addition of one drop of alkali solution will make the mixture alkaline and the indicator will dissociate. The concentration of In^- ions will increase and the indicator will show the color of its ionized form.

On application of law of mass action to the ionization reaction of the acid indicator, we get

$$HIn \quad \leftrightarrow \quad H^+ + In^-$$

$$\frac{a_{H^+} \times a_{In^-}}{a_{HIn}} = \frac{[H^+][In^-]}{[HIn]} \times \frac{f_{H^+} \times f_{In^-}}{f_{HIn}} = K_{ina}$$

and $[H^+] = \dfrac{[HIn]}{[In^-]} \times K_{ina} \times \dfrac{f_{HIn}}{f_{H^+} \times f_{In^-}}$

$$= \frac{\text{Unionized form}}{\text{Ionized form}} \times K_{ina} \times \frac{f_{HIn}}{f_{H^+} \times f_{In^-}} \qquad \qquad .....(3.5)$$

Where, K_{ind} is the *ionization constant of the indicator*. If the activity coefficient is considered to be unity, the equation 5 can be reduced to

$$[H^+] = \frac{[HIn]}{[In^-]} \times K_{ina} = \frac{\text{Unionized form}}{\text{Ionized form}} \times K_{ina} \qquad \qquad .....(3.6)$$

The equation 6 shows that the actual color of the indicator depends on the ratio of concentrations of unionized and ionized forms; hence the change of color of an indicator is directly related to the hydrogen ion concentration of the solution. The logarithmic form of the equation 6 can be written as;

$$\log [H^+] = \log \left(\frac{[HIn]}{[In^-]} \times K_{ina} \right) = \log \frac{[HIn]}{[In^-]} + \log K_{ina}$$

Or, $- \log [H^+] = - \log \dfrac{[HIn]}{[In^-]} + (-\log K_{ina})$

Or, $pH = \log \dfrac{[In^-]}{[HIn]} + pK_{ina}$ $\qquad \qquad \qquad .....(3.7)$

Similarly, for a basic indicator the ionization reaction can be written as;

$$[OH\text{-}] = \frac{[InOH]}{[In^+]} \times K_{inb} \qquad \qquad .....(3.8)$$

Where, K_{inb} is the dissociation constant of a basic indicator.

We know that $K_W = [H^+] \times [OH^-]$

Or, $[H^+] = \dfrac{K_w}{[OH^-]} = \dfrac{K_w}{\dfrac{[InOH]}{[In^+]} \times K_{Inb}}$

Or, $[H^+] = \dfrac{K_w}{K_{Inb}} = \dfrac{[In^+]}{[InOH]}$ $\qquad \qquad \qquad .....(3.9)$

The Ostwald's theory for the color change of an indicator is not practically correct. It requires modification. In fact, when an indicator changes its color, its structure also changes, quinonoid and resonance forms are produced. Structural changes of phenolphthalein are shown below;

These are characteristics of all phthalein indicators. When phenolphthalein comes in contact with dilute alkali, the lactone ring in 'A' (benzenoid form) opens to form 'B'. Triphenylcarbinol structure of 'B' loses water and produces a resonating ion 'C' (quinonoid form) which gives pink color. If phenolphthalein is added to excess of alcoholic alkali, the red color immediately produced disappears. This disappearance of color is due to formation of 'D'.

The equilibrium between the acidic form, In_A and the basic form, In_B can be expressed as;

$$In_A \leftrightarrow H^+ + In_B$$

And the equilibrium constant, K_{In} as;

$$K_{In} = \frac{a_{H^+} \times a_{InB}}{a_{InA}} \quad\quad .....(3.10)$$

The visible color of an indicator is determined by the ratio of the concentrations of acidic and basic forms. This may be expressed as;

$$\frac{[In_A]}{[In_B]} = \frac{a_{H^+} \times f_{InB}}{K_{In} \times f_{InA}} \quad\quad .....(3.11)$$

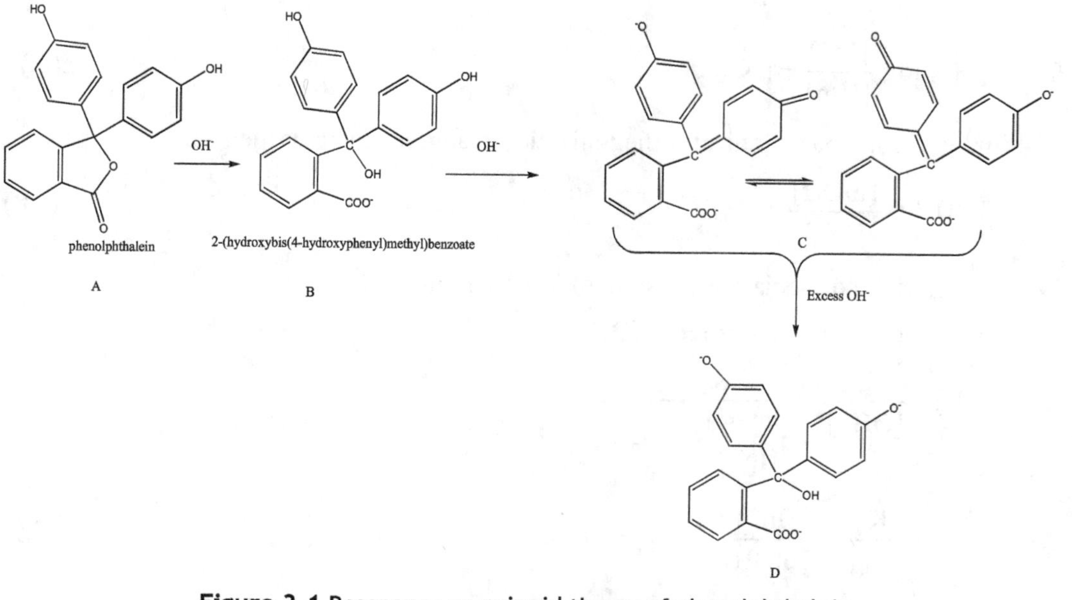

Figure 3.1 Resonance or quinoid theory of phenolphthalein

Where, f_{In_A} and f_{In_B} are the activity coefficient of acidic and basic forms of the indicator. Logarithmic form of the equation 11 is

$$\log \frac{[In_A]}{[In_B]} = \log a_{H^+} + \log \frac{f_{InB}}{f_{InA}} - \log K_{In}$$

or,

$$-\log a_{H^+} = \log \frac{[In_B]}{[In_A]} + \log \frac{f_{InB}}{f_{InA}} - \log K_{In}$$

$$pH = pK_{In} + \log \frac{[In_B]}{[In_A]} + \log \frac{f_{InB}}{f_{InA}} \qquad .....(3.12)$$

It is evident that the color of an indicator depends on the ionic strength (i.e., activity coefficient) of the solution. Thus, the pH of a solution can be determined by using a suitable indicator. When the colors of the two solutions containing same amount of indicator are same, it indicates that their pH are also same. The equation 12 can be modified to express the equilibrium at which color changes at a particular ionic strength. The modified equation is;

$$pH = pK'_{In} + \log \frac{[In_B]}{[In_A]}$$

Where, K'_{In} is the apparent dissociation constant. The value of $\frac{[In_B]}{[In_A]}$ (i.e., [Basic form]/[Acid form]) can be done visually by comparing the color. This can be done accurately by spectrophotometric method. However, at any concentration of hydrogen ion both forms remain present in the solution and both the colors are present. But one color dominates the other. Human eye has a limited ability to detect either of the two colors. It has been observed that when $\frac{[In_A]}{[In_B]}$ is more than 10, the solution will show the acid color

(color of $[In_A]$) and when $\frac{[In_B]}{[In_A]}$ is more than 10, the solution will show the basic color

(color of $[In_B]$). Thus, in the former case, $pH = pK'_{In} - 1$ (i.e., when $\frac{[In_A]}{[In_B]} > 10$).

In the latter case, $pH = pK'_{In} + 1$ (i.e., when $\frac{[In_B]}{[In_A]} > 10$).

Accordingly, the interval of color-change can be represented as $pH = pK'_{In} \pm 1$, almost two pH units. Within this pH range the color of an indicator changes from one color to other. When $\frac{[In_A]}{[In_B]} = 1$, pH of the solution becomes equal to the apparent dissociation constant of the indicator, pK'_{In}. At this point the indicator exhibits a color of mixture of acid color and basic or alkaline color. Sometimes, this is called as *middle tint* of the indicator. Table 3.2 presents a list of indicators, their color change and pH range.

Table 3.2: pH range and color change of some common indicators

pH range	Indicator	Chemical name	pK'$_{In}$	Color in Acid solution	Color in alkalin solution
0.0 – 1.0	Brilliant cresyl blue (acid)	Amino-diethyl-amino-methyl diphenazonium chloride		Red orange	Blue
0.2 – 1.8	Cresol red (acid)	α-Cresolsulphone phthalein		Red	Yellow
1.0 – 2.0	Quinaldine red	α-(p-Dimethyl-amino-phenyl-ethylene)-quinoline ethiodide		Colorless	Red
1.2 – 2.8	Thymol blue (acid)	Thymol-sulphone-phthalein	1.7	Red	Yellow
1.2 – 2.8	m-Cresol purple	m-Cresolsulphone-phthalein	1.5	Red	Yellow
1.2 – 3.2	Pentamethoxy red	2,4,2',4',2''-Pentamethoxy-triphenyl carbinol		Red-violet	Colorless
1.3 – 3.0	Tropaeolin OO	Diphenylamino-p-benzene-sodium sulphonate		Red	Yellow
2.9 – 4.0	Methyl yellow	Dimethylamino-azo-benzene	3.3	Red	Yellow
3.0 – 4.5	Ethyl orange			Red	Orange
3.0 – 4.6	Bromo-phenol blue	Tetrabromophenol-sulphone-phthalein	4.1	Yellow	Blue
3.1 – 4.4	Methyl orange	Dimethylamino-azo-benzene sodium sulphonate	3.7	Red	Orange
3.0 – 5.0	Congo red	Diphenyl-bis-azo-α-naphthylamine-4-sulphonic acid		Violet	Red
3.7 – 5.0	α-Naphthyl red	Phenylazo-1-naphthylamine		Red	Yellow
3.8 – 5.4	Bromo-cresol green	Tetrabromo-m-cresol-sulphone-phthalein	4.7	Yellow	Blue
4.2 – 6.3	Methyl red	o-Carboxybenzene-azo-dimethyl-aniline	5.0	Red	Yellow
4.5 – 6.5	Ethyl red			Red	Orange
4.6 – 6.6	Propyl red			Red	Yellow
4.8 – 6.4	Chlorophenol red	Dichloro-phenol sulphone-phthalein	6.1	Yellow	Red

Table 3.2: Contd...

pH range	Indicator	Chemical name	pK'$_{In}$	Color in Acid solution	Color in alkalin solution
5.2 – 6.8	Bromocresol blue	Dibromo-o-cresol sulphone phthalein	6.1	Yellow	Purple
5.2 – 6.8	Bromocresol red	Dibromo-phenol sulphone phthalein		Yellow	Red
5.6 – 7.6	p-Nitrophenol	p-Nitrophenol	7.1	Colorless	Yellow
6.0 – 7.6	Bromo-thymol blue	Dibromo-thymol sulphone phthalein	7.1	Yellow	Blue
6.8 – 8.0	Neutral red	Amino-dimethyl-amino-tolu-phenazonium chloride		Red	Orange
6.8 – 8.4	Phenol red	Phenol-sulphone-phthalein	7.8	Yellow	Red
7.2 – 8.8	Cresol red (base)	o-Cresolsulphone phthalein	8.2	Yellow	Red
7.3 – 8.7	α-Naphtholphthalein	α-Naphtholphthalein	8.4	Yellow	Blue
7.6 – 9.2	m-Cresol purple	m-Cresolsulphone phthalein		Yellow	Purple
8.0 – 9.6	Thymol blue (base)	Thymol sulphone phthalein	8.9	Yellow	Blue
8.2 – 9.8	o-Cresol phthalein	Di-o-cresol phthalide		Colorless	Red
8.3 – 10.0	Phenolphthalein	Phenolphthalein	9.6	Colorless	Pink
8.3 – 10.5	Thymolph-thalein	Thymolphthalein	9.3	Colorless	Blue
10.1 – 12.0	Alizaein yellow R	p-Nitrobenzene-azo-salicylic acid		Yellow	Orange red
10.8 – 12.0	Brilliant cresyl blue (base)	Amino-diethyl-amino-methyl diphenazonium chloride		Blue	Yellow
11.1 – 12.7	Tropaeolin O	p-Sulphobenzene-azo-resorcinol		Yellow	Orange
10.8 – 13.0	Nitramine	2,4.6-Trinitro-phenyl-methyl-nitroamine		Colorless	Orange brown

Note: In quantitative analysis water is commonly used solvent. The pH of water can vary from 3.7 to 7. Double distilled fresh water should have pH of 7, when it comes in contact with air its pH gradually decreases. Air contains 0.03% v/v of CO_2 and water at equilibrium with air has a pH of 5.7 and water saturated with air under normal atmospheric pressure has a pH of 3.7. Hence, one must be careful about water being used.

To improve the color change of a single indicator sometimes a suitable pH-sensitive dyestuff is added. As a result, the complement color of one of the indicator colors is produced. These are called mixed indicators. Table 3.3 provides a list of mixed indicators commonly used in volumetric titrations.

Table 3.3: pH, color change and composition of some mixed indicators

pH	Mixed indicator	Color change	Composition
4.3	Bromocresol green; Methyl orange	Orange → blue-green	0.1% of sodium salt of Bromocresol green in water and 0.2% of methyl orange in water (1:1)
6.1	Bromocresol green; Chlorophenol red	Pale green → Blue violet	0.1% of sodium salt of Bromocresol green in water and 0.1% of Chlorophenol red in water (1:1)
7.2	Bromothymol blue; Neutral red	Rose pink→ Green	0.1% solution of Bromothymol blue in alcohol and 0.1% solution of Neutral red in alcohol. (1:1)
7.5	Bromothymol blue; Phenol red	Yellow → Violet	0.1% of sodium salt of Bromothymol blue in water and 0.1% of phenol red (Na salt) in water. (1:1)
8.3	Thymol blue; Cresol red	Yellow → Violet	0.1% of sodium salt of Thymol blue in water and 0.1% of Cresol red (Na salt) in water. (3:1)
9.0	Thymol blue; Phenolphthalein	Yellow → Violet	0.1% solution of Thymol blue in 50% alcohol and 0.1% solution of Phenolphthalein in 50% alcohol. (1:3)
9.9	Thymolphthalein; Phenolphthalein	Colorless → Violet	0.1% solution of Thymolphthalein in alcohol and 0.1% solution of Phenolphthalein in water. (1:1)

Classification of volumetric titrations

In titrimetric or volumetric analysis, the reactions involved can be classified into two categories.

1. In this type or category (Type I) the valency or oxidation number of the participating element or ion does not change. The reactions involve the combination of ions. Neutralization reactions, complex formation reactions, and precipitation reactions are under this category.

2. In this type or category (Type II) of reactions the valency of the reactants or oxidation number changes due to transfer of electron.

As mentioned above type 1 titration are further classified into three types.

- *Neutralization reactions:* these titrations are alternatively called acid-base titration. These reactions involve (a) titration of free bases with standard acid (*acidimetry*), (b) titration of salts of weak acids by hydrolysis with a standard acid (*acidimetry*),

(c) titration of free acids with standard base (*alkalimetry*), (d) titration of salts of weak bases with standard base (*alkalimetry*). In these titrations hydrogen ion and hydroxyl ion combine and form water.

- *Complex formation reactions:* in this type of reactions the ions other than hydrogen and hydroxide ions combine and form complexes. The complex formed may be soluble, can be slightly dissociated ion or compound. For example, titration of a solution of a cyanide with silver nitrate or of chloride ion with mercuric nitrate solution. The reactions are shown below;

$$2CN^- + Ag^+ \leftrightarrow [Ag(CN)_2]^-$$
$$2Cl^- + Hg^{2+} \leftrightarrow HgCl_2$$

Disodium salt of ethyl ene diamine tetra acetic acid (sodium edetate) is commonly used for formation of complex in complex forming titrations or volumetric titration. Metal ion indicators are used in these titrations.

- *Precipitation reactions:* In these reactions, ions other than hydrogen and hydroxyl ions combine and form simple precipitate. For example, in the titration of chloride solution with silver nitrate a precipitate of silver chloride is formed. In this reaction there is no change of valency takes place.

- *Oxidation-reduction reactions:* this type of reactions involves change in oxidation number or transfer of electrons among the reacting substances. The standard solutions of reacting substances are either oxidizing or reducing agents. For example, potassium permanganate, potassium dichromate, ceric sulphate, manganic sulphate, iodine, potassium iodate, potassium bromate, sodium hydrochlorite, and chloramines-T. Reducing agents such as ferrous and stannous compounds, sodium thiosulphate, arsenious oxide, mercurous nitrate, titanous chloride or sulphate, etc. are commonly used in these titrations.

3.2 CLASSIFICATION OF ACID-BASE TITRATIONS

There are four types of Acid-base titrations. These are –

1. Titration of a strong acid with strong base,
2. Titration of a strong acid with weak base,
3. Titration of a weak acid with strong base, and
4. Titration of a weak acid with a weak base.

1. Titration of a strong acid with strong base,

The titration of a strong acid-strong base is conducted mainly to determine the concentration of the solution of a base by titrating it with an acid solution of known concentration, or vice-versa, until the base is completely neutralized. Since strong acid and strong base have high values of K_a and K_b respectively, both of them fully dissociate in water. That is, all the molecules of acid or base completely separate into ions. At the equivalence point, equal amounts of H^+ and OH^- ions combine to form H_2O and the anion (negative ion) produced from the dissociation of the acid combines with the cation (positive ion) produced from the dissociation of the base to form a salt. As a result, the pH of neutralized solution becomes 7.0. Therefore, the reaction between a strong acid and strong base will result in water and a salt.

Common examples of strong acids are HCl, HBr, HI, $HClO_4$, HNO_3 and H_2SO_4, etc. and of strong bases are LiOH, NaOH, KOH, RbOH, $Mg(OH)_2$, $Ca(OH)_2$, $Ba(OH)_2$, etc.

(2) Titration of a strong acid with weak base

Table 3.4: Molecular formula and pK values of some common acids

Acid	Formula	pK value
Perchloric	$HClO_4$	-7
Hydrogen Chloride	HCl	-3
Sulfuric	H_2SO_4	-3 (pK_1)
Nitric	HNO_3	-1
Hydronium	H_3O^+	0
Bisulfate	HSO_4^-	1.9 (pK_2)
Phosphoric	H_3PO_4	2.1 (pK_1)
Aquo ferric ion**	$Fe(H2O)_6^{+3}$	2.2 (pK_1)
Arsenic Acid	H_3AsO_4	2.25 (pK_1)

Results of titration of strong acid and weak base can be used to calculate the molarity and to find out acidity of a solution at various stages of the titration. To calculate the total number of moles of analyte (compound being analyzed) presents in the mixture (molar concentration) the initial and final volumes of the analyte and titrant (compound used to titrate) solutions, as well as the pH, or measure of acidity, are to be known. The data collected at various points during the titration can then be plotted to obtain the titration curve. Table3.4 shows the pK values of some strong and intermediate acids.

3. Titration of a weak acid with strong base

When a weak acid is titrated with a strong base the protons are directly transferred from the weak acid to the hydroxide or hydroxyl ion.

The reaction of the weak acid, acetic acid, with a strong base, NaOH, can be seen below. In the reaction the acid and base react in a one to one ratio.

$CH_3COOH + NaOH \rightarrow CH_3COONa + H_2O$ (4) *Titration of a weak acid with a weak base*

Weak acids and bases do not dissociate completely. Even the approach used to solve the equations related to weak acid-base is similar to those used for strong acid-base systems; the calculation of Ka becomes complicated. In most cases of this system simple assumptions are found more useful. The small pK values indicate that the concentration of the reactants is larger than that of the products; that is, the rate of forward reaction is less than that of backward reaction. For example, in some anaerobic groundwater sulfate reducing bacteria produce hydrogen sulphide. Hydrogen sulphide is a weak acid. It dissociates as;

$$H_2S \rightarrow H^+ + HS^-$$

$$Ka.1 = \frac{[H^+][HS^-]}{[H_2S]} = 10^{-7.1} \quad or, \quad pKa.1 = 7.1$$

The basic characteristic of weak acids is that the extent of their dissociation is directly related to the pH of the medium. When pH is less than pKa (pH < pK), small amount of acid dissociates. When pH increases, more acid dissociate to maintain the equilibrium. The dissociation constant of some common weak acids are shown in Table 3.5. The relationship between pH and dissociation of weak acids is expressed as:

$$pH = pKa + \log\frac{[salt]}{[acid]}$$

Table 3.5: Molecular formula and pK values of some common weak acids

Acid	Formula	pK
Hydrofluoric acid	HF	3.45
Acetic acid	CH_3COOH	4.7
Arsenic Acid	$H_2AsO_4^-$	6.77
Hydrogen Sulfide	H_2S	7.1
Dihydrogen Phosphate	$H_2PO_4^-$	7.2 (pK_2)
Hypochlorous Acid	HOCl	7.6
Hydrogen Cyanide	HCN	9.2
Boric Acid	H_3BO_3	9.3
Ammonium Ion	NH_4^+	9.3
Bicarbonate Ion	HCO_3^-	10.3
Arsenic Acid	$H_2AsO_4^-$	11.6 (pK_3)
Bisulfide	HS^-	14 (pK_2)
Water	H_2O	14

Note: When the pK = pH, the activity of the weak acid is equal to the conjugate base. Thus, at pH 7.1, $[H2S] = [HS^-]$. The pK values of some common weak acids are given in the above Table.

3.3 THEORY INVOLVED IN TITRATIONS OF STRONG, WEAK, AND VERY WEAK ACIDS AND BASES

1. Neutralization of strong acid and strong base

A strong acid or strong base is a substance which completely dissociates in water. The activity coefficients of their ions are considered 1 (unity) so that the change of pH during neutralization can be calculated easily. To understand how the pH of the acid changes during titration of a strong acid such as hydrochloric acid (HCl) with a strong base such as sodium hydroxide (NaOH) at certain points are given below. The student can know how the pH of the solution is calculated. For ease of calculation let us assume that 50mL of 1N HCl solution is being titrated with 1N NaOH solution. The pH of 1N HCl solution is zero.

- After addition of 25.00mL of 1N NaOH to 50mL of 1N HCl solution, the total volume becomes $50 + 25 = 75$mL and 25mL of 1N HCl solution remain unneutralized. So,

$$[H+] \text{ in 75 mL of solution} = 25 \times \frac{1}{75} = 3.33 \times 10^{-1} \text{ and pH} = -\log (3.33 \times 10^{-1}) = 0.48$$

- After addition of further 12.50mL of 1N NaOH to 75mL of 1N HCl solution, the total volume becomes $75 + 12.5 = 87.5$mL and 12.5mL of 1N HCl solution remain unneutralized. So, $[H+]$ in 87.5 mL of solution $= 12.5 \times \dfrac{1}{87.5} = 1.11 \times 10^{-1}$ and pH = - log $(1.43 \times 10^{-1}) = 0.94$

- After addition of 7.50mL of 1N NaOH to 87.5mL of solution, the total volume becomes $87.50 + 7.5 = 95$mL and 5mL of 1N HCl solution remain unneutralized. So,

$$[H+] \text{ in 95 mL of solution} = 5 \times \frac{1}{95} = 5.26 \times 10^{-2} \text{ and pH} = -\log (5.26 \times 10^{-2}) = 1.3$$

- Further addition of 4.90mL of 1N NaOH to 95mL of solution, the total volume becomes $95 + 4.90 = 99.9$mL and 0.1mL of 1N HCl solution remain unneutralized. So, $[H+]$ in 99.1mL of solution $= 0.1 \times \dfrac{1}{99.9} = 1.00 \times 10^{-3}$ and pH = - log $(1.00 \times 10^{-3}) = 3$

- Once 0.1mL of 1N NaOH solution is added to 99.9mL of solution, the acid is completely neutralized, and the pH of the final solution rises sharply to 7. This is the equivalence point. Provided the solution does not contain any dissolved CO_2. The solution contains only NaCl in dissolved state.

- If 0.05mL of 1N NaOH solution is added extra to this solution, then 0.05mL of 1N NaOH will remain in total volume of 100.05mL. At this stage the concentration of $[OH^-]$ will be $0.05 \times \dfrac{1}{100.05} = 4.99 \times 10^{-4}$, or pOH = 3.3 and pH = $14 - 3.3 = 10.7$

- Further addition 0.05mL of 1N NaOH solution is added extra to this solution, then 0.1mL of 1N NaOH will remain in total volume of 100.1mL, and the concentration of $[OH^-]$ will be $0.1 \times \dfrac{1}{100.1} = 9.99 \times 10^{-4}$, or pOH = 3.00 and pH = $14 - 3.0 = 11$.

The pH rises slowly. The results of the titration have been presented in Table 3.6. The Table illustrates the changes in pH after addition of 1N NaOH solution to 1N HCl solution. The Table shows that addition of even 25mL of 1 N NaOH after neutralization of 50mL of 1N HCl solution, the pH raises slowly from 7 to 13.5.

Table 3.6: Change in pH of 1N HCl after gradual addition of 1N NaOH

Vol of 1N NaOH added	pH of solution	Vol of 1N NaOH added	pH of solution	Vol of 1N NaOH added	pH of solution
0 mL	0	49.75 mL	2.6	51mL	12
25 mL	0.48	49.9 mL	3.0	52 mL	12.3
30 mL	0.60	49.95mL	4.7	53 mL	12.5
40 mL	0.96	50mL	7.0	54 mL	12.6
45 mL	1.3	50.05mL	10.7	55mL	12.7
48 mL	1.7	50.1mL	11.0	60 mL	12.96
49 mL	2.0	50.25mL	11.4	75mL	13.3
49.5 mL	2.3	50.5mL	11.4	100mL	14

Changes of pH of 1N HCl solution after addition of 1 N NaOH solution have been plotted and shown in figure 3.2. The figure comprises three neutralization plots of 0.01 N, 0.1 N and 1 N HCl solutions.

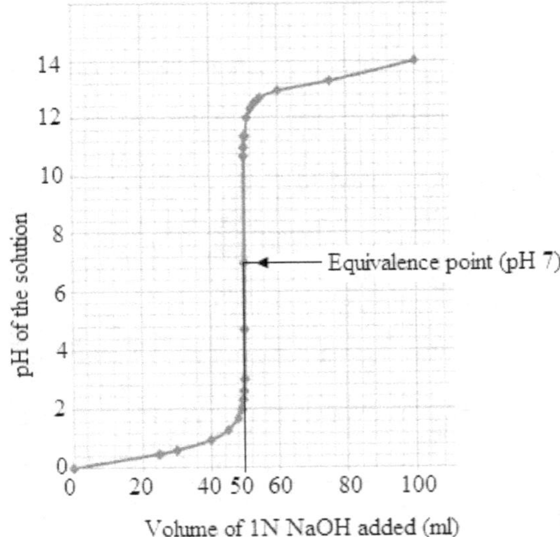

Figure 3.2 Neutralization curve

- An indicator that changes its color between pH 3 and 10.5 in titration of 1 N solution is suitable. The titration error would be negligible.
- An indicator that changes its color between pH 4.5 and 9.5 in titration of 0.1 N solution will be suitable. The titration error would be negligible. For example, methyl orange that works within the pH range of 3.1 to 4.4, if used the titration error would be 0.2%.
- An indicator that changes its color between pH 5.5 and 8.5 in titration of 0.01 N solutions will be suitable. If methyl orange is used in such titration, titration error

would be 1 – 2%. In such titration's methyl red, Bromothymol blue, phenol red can be used satisfactorily.

3.4   NEUTRALIZATION CURVES

Neutralization curve provides information about the mechanism of neutralization process. This involves the changes in hydrogen ion concentration (pH) during an acid-base titration. The change in pH in the point nearest to equivalence point is most important. It helps to select an appropriate indicator. The indicator gives the smallest titration error.

The curve produced by pH on Y-axis against the volume of alkali added (percentage of acid neutralized) on X-axis shows how the pH of the solution with gradual addition of alkali even after equivalence point is reached. Such curve produced is called *neutralization curve*. This may be evaluated by conducting experiment where the pH of the solution is determined at different stages of titration using either suitable indicator or a potentiometer (potentiometric titration). The pH of the solution can be calculated as indicated below.

Table 3.7: Change in pH of 0.1N HCl and 0.01N HCl after gradual addition of 0.1N NaOH and 0.01 NaOH

Vol of 0.1N NaOH added	pH of solution	Vol of 0.1N NaOH added	pH of solution	Vol of 0.01N NaOH added	pH of solution	Vol of 0.01N NaOH added	pH of solution
0 ml	1	50.05ml	10.7	0 ml	2	50.05ml	9.7
25 ml	1.48	50.1ml	11.0	25 ml	2.48	50.1ml	10.0
30 ml	1.60	50.25ml	11.4	30 ml	2.60	50.25ml	10.4
40 ml	1.96	50.5ml	11.4	40 ml	2.96	50.5ml	10.4
45 ml	2.3	51ml	12	45 ml	3.3	51ml	11.0
48 ml	2.7	52 ml	12.3	48 ml	3.7	52 ml	11.3
49 ml	3.0	53 ml	12.5	49 ml	4.0	53 ml	11.5
49.5 ml	3.3	54 ml	12.6	49.5 ml	4.3	54 ml	11.6
49.75 ml	3.6	55ml	12.7	49.75 ml	4.6	55ml	11.7
49.9 ml	4.0	60 ml	12.96	49.9 ml	5.0	60 ml	11.96
49.95ml	5.7	75ml	12.3	49.95ml	6.7	75ml	12.3
50ml	7.0	100ml	12.5	50ml	7.0	100ml	12.5

For example, 50 mL of 0.1N hydrochloric acid is being titrated with 0.1N sodium hydroxide solution. The pH of 0.1N hydrochloric acid is one. After addition of 25 mL of 0.1N sodium hydroxide, the pH becomes 1.48. Similarly, after addition of 50 mL of 0.1N sodium hydroxide (at the equivalence point) the pH of the 100 mL of solution sharply changes to 7. If 50.10 mL of 0.1N sodium hydroxide is added, the hydroxyl ion concentration, [OH⁻] increases and pH of the solution becomes 11.0.

These results indicate that the pH of the solution increases slowly with progression of titration till equivalence point is reached. After attainment of the equivalence point, addition of alkali shows sharp rise in pH from 7 as shown in the Table 3.7 and fig.3.3. Titrations of 0.1N and 0.01N HCl with 0.1N and 0.01N NaOH give similar curve with appropriate changes in values.

Similar trend is found in titration of 0.01N HCl with 0.01N sodium hydroxide solution. The titration curves are shown in Fig. 3.3. These curves are called as neutralization curves.

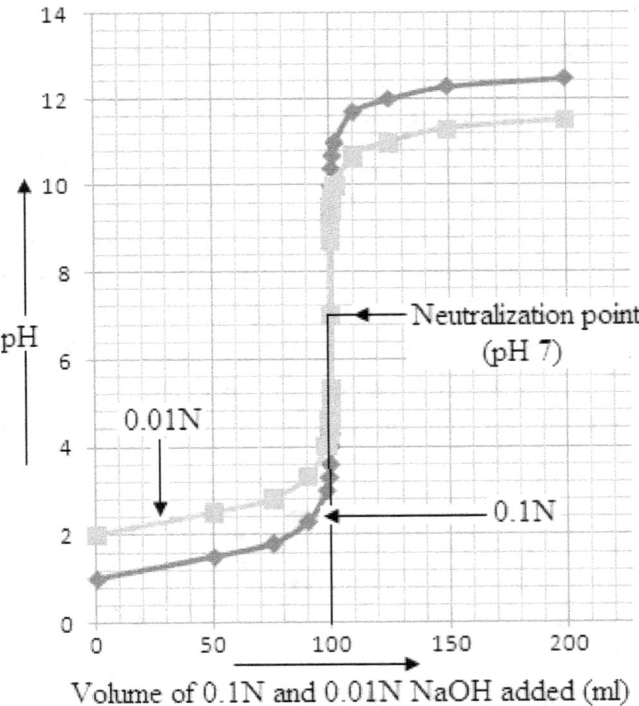

Figure 3.3 Neutralization curves

In practice there may be little deviation from the required values. Such change is due to the presence of carbon dioxide in the solution. The gas remains in equilibrium with carbonic acid. Both are weak electrolytes. The source of carbon dioxide may be two;

- Sodium hydroxide used may contain traces of carbonate, and
- Water may contain dissolved carbon dioxide.

A. MULTIPLE CHOICE QUESTIONS

1. Which one of the following statements is correct?
   (a) An acid donates H^+ ions
   (b) An acid donates proton
   (c) An acid accepts a pair of electron
   (d) All of the above

2. Which one of the following statements is correct?
   (a) A base donates OH^- ion
   (b) A base receives H^+ ions
   (c) A base donates a pair of electron
   (d) All of the above

3. Which one of the following is a tribasic acid?
   (a) Hydrochloric acid
   (b) Phosphoric acid
   (c) Sulphuric acid
   (d) Nitric acid

4. Acetic acid is a
   (a) Weak acid
   (b) Strong acid
   (c) Salt of a weak acid
   (d) Salt of a weak base

5. According to Lowery-Bronsted theory
   (a) An acid donates proton
   (b) An acid receives proton
   (c) An acid donates hydrogen ion
   (d) An acid receives hydrogen ion

6. Perchloric acid is
   (a) Stronger than hydrochloric acid
   (b) Weaker than hydrochloric acid
   (c) Stronger than nitric acid
   (d) Stronger than hydroiodic acid

7. Which one of the following statements is correct?
   (a) A strong acid ionizes completely in water
   (b) A weak acid does not ionize completely in water
   (c) A weak acid ionizes completely in alkaline solution
   (d) All of the above

8. Which one of the following statements is correct?
   (a) Polybasic acid ionizes in water completely in a single stage
   (b) Polybasic acid ionizes in water in stages
   (c) Polybasic acid does not ionize in water completely in stages
   (d) All of the above

9. Which one of the following statements is correct?
   (a) The change in color does not take place suddenly.
   (b) The change in color takes place within a small interval of pH.
   (c) The change in color takes place with change in pH
   (d) All of the above

10. The ionic product of pure water depends on
    (a) Temperature
    (b) Pressure
    (c) Temperature and pressure both
    (d) None of the above

11. Which one of the following statements is correct?
    (a) Activity and activity coefficient are same
    (b) Activity is the product of molar concentration and activity coefficient
    (c) Activity is the ratio of molar concentration to activity coefficient
    (d) None of the above

12. Which one of the following statements is correct?
    (a) $[H^+] = [OH^-] = \sqrt{K_w}$
    (b) $[H^+] = \sqrt{K_w}$
    (c) $[OH^-] = \sqrt{K_w}$
    (d) All of the above

13. Which one of the following statements is correct?
    (a) Acid-base indicators areionizable substances
    (b) Acid form of indicators has different color
    (c) Basic form of indicators has different color
    (d) All of the above

14. When an acid is titrated with a base,
    (a) The pH of the solution increases with addition of base solution
    (b) The pH of the solution decreases with addition of base solution
    (c) The hydrogen ion concentration increases gradually
    (d) The hydroxyl ion concentration increases gradually

15. Which one of the following statements is correct?
    (a) The strength of acid depends on the type of medium in which it is present
    (b) The strength of acid is independent of the medium used
    (c) The strength of acid depends on its conjugate base
    (d) None of the above

16. The pHs of 1N solution of an acid in water at 25oC are given below; which of the following is strongest?
    (a) 1.7
    (b) 3.5
    (c) 0.99
    (d) 3.1

B. SHORT QUESTIONS

1. What is an acid and what do you mean by strong acid?
2. What is a base and what do you mean by strong base?
3. What are polybasic and polyprotic acids?
4. Write down the Lowery-Bronsted theory of acid and base.
5. Define acid and base according to the Lewis theory.
6. Define the terms activity and activity coefficient.
7. Write down the law of mass action for acid-base neutralization.
8. What is ionization constant of water?

9. What is Ostwald's Dilution law?
10. What are type I and type II volumetric titrations?
11. Name different types of volumetric titrations.
12. Classify the acid-base titration.
13. How does an indicator change its color in a titration?
14. What is color-change interval?
15. What is ionization constant of an indicator?

C. LONG QUESTIONS

1. Explain Lewis theory of acid and base with suitable example.
2. Explain Lowery-Bronsted theory of acids and bases with suitable example.
3. Discuss briefly the theory of acids and bases with the help of relevant example.
4. Explain the ionization of polybasic acids.
5. Explain the law of mass action with respect to acid-base neutralization.
6. Discuss ionization of water and how the ionization product is derived.
7. Explain how you can determine the ionization constant of water.
8. Classify and define different types of volumetric titrations.
9. Discuss the mechanism of ionization of an indicator.
10. Explain neutralization of a weak acid by a weak base with the help of a graph.
11. Explain neutralization of a weak acid by a strong base with the help of a graph.
12. Explain neutralization of a strong acid by a weak base with the help of a graph.
13. Explain neutralization of a strong acid by a strong base with the help of a graph.
14. Discuss the theory of indicator.
15. What do you understand by neutralization curve?

CHAPTER 4

Non-Aqueous Titration

INTRODUCTION

The apparent strength of an acid or base depends on the extent of its reaction with a solvent. In aqueous solutions all strong acids show almost equal strength; because they react with water (solvent) and undergo complete dissociation producing hydronium ion (H_3O^+) and the corresponding anion. The strength of an acid depends on the basicity of the solvent and the strength of a base depends on the acidity of the solvent. Any acid stronger than H_3O^+ can react with water and form H_3O^+.

Hence, in a weakly protophilic solvent such as acetic acid, the order of decreasing strength for acids is perchloric, hydrobromic, sulfuric, hydrochloric and nitric. While in ammonia, acetic acid dissociates completely and behaves as strong acid. The so-called levelling effect is also observed for bases. In hydrochloric acid or in acetic acid almost all bases appear to be of the same strength. Many water-insoluble compounds gain increased acidic or basic properties when dissolved in organic solvents. Thus, for the determination of a variety of such materials by non-aqueous titration the appropriate medium and titrant should be selected. The types of compounds, in a non-aqueous medium, that may be titrated as acids, usually by lithium methoxide or tetrabutyl ammonium hydroxide, include acid halides, acid anhydrides, carboxylic acids, amino acids, enols such as barbiturates and xanthines, imides, phenols, pyrroles and sulfonamides. The types of compounds, in a non-aqueous medium that may be titrated as bases by perchloric acid, include amines, nitrogen-containing heterocyclic compounds, quaternary ammonium compounds, alkali salts of organic acids, alkali salts of inorganic acids and some salts of amines. Many halide salts of weak bases and some quaternary ammonium compounds may be directly titrated in acetic anhydride using, preferably, potentiometric end-point detection or an indicator such as malachite green or crystal violet. The characteristic properties of nonaqueous titrations are:

1. Similar property is found in case of bases also follow the same rules in non-aqueous titrations.

2. By use of non-aqueous solventsa mixture of two or more acids can be determined. Separate end point in different solvent for an individual acid can be obtained.

3. The biological ingredients of a substance, acidic or basic can be selectively titrated by using the proper solvents or indicator.

4.1   SOLVENTS

Solvents used in organic chemistry are characterized by their physical characteristics. Among these the most important characteristics are whether (1) the solvents are polar or non-polar, and (2) these are protic or aprotic. Non-polar solvents are likely to be aprotic. Generally, solvents are classified on the basis of their polarity, indicated by the dielectric constant.These are either polar or non-polar. The polarity is a continuous scale and can be known by a correct question – "how polar is it", not "whether it is polar or non-polar". In general, solvents having dielectric constants greater than 5 are considered "polar" and those with dielectric constants less than 5 are considered "non-polar."

Classification of non-aqueous solvents:

The reactions involved in titrations of acids and bases in non-aqueous solvents can be explained by using the Bronsted Lowery theory of acid and bases. Accordingly, an acid is a substance which can donate a proton, and a base is a substance which can accept the proton. Substances which are weak acids or bases in aqueous solution give poor end points. These frequently give satisfactory end point when they are titrated in non-aqueous media. There are many substances which are insoluble in water; but these substances are soluble in organic solvents and hence, their titrations can be performed using non-aqueous solvents. This is an additional advantage.

According to the Bronsted lowery theory, an acid, (HB) is considered to dissociate in solution to release a proton (H^+) and a conjugate base (B^-). Whereas, a base (B) combines with the proton released to produce a conjugate acid (HB^+).

$$HB \leftrightarrow H^+ + B^-$$
$$B + H^+ \leftrightarrow HB^+$$

The ability of a substance to act as an acid or base depends very much on the choice of solvent system.

Ionic strength of some organic acids is almost similar to that of water; such substances cannot be easily titrated using

Non-aqueous solvents are classified into four groups:

1. Aprotic,
2. Protophilic,
3. Photogenic, and
4. Amphiprotic.

1. *Aprotic solvent:* Aprotic solvents are incapable of donating proton. These are chemically neutral, and almost un-reactive under experimental conditions. For example, carbon tetrachloride and toluene are in this group; these possess low dielectric constants, do not cause ionization in solutes and do not undergo reactions with acids and bases. Aprotic solvents are frequently used to dilute reaction mixture.

2. *Protophilic Solvents:* The substances that possess a high affinity for protons are called protophilic solvents. The overall reaction can be expressed as;

$$HB + S \leftrightarrow SH^+ + B^-$$

This is reversible reaction. Its equilibrium is generally influenced by the nature of the acid and the solvent. Normally weak acids are used in the presence of strong protophilic solvents. Their acidic strengths are increased and then become similar to these of strong acids. This is known as the *leveling effect*.

3. *Photogenic Solvents:* Protogenic solvents are acidic in nature and readily donate protons. Anhydrous acids such as hydrogen fluoride and sulphuric acid are in this category. This is due to their strength and ability to donate protons. As a result, the strength of weak bases is enhanced.

4. *Amphiprotic Solvents:* Amphiprotic solvents are slightly ionized and possess both protogenic and protophilic properties. These include liquids such as water, alcohols and weak organic acids. These are capable to donate protons and accept protons. Ethanoic acid exhibits acidic properties in dissociating to produce protons:

$$CH_3COOH \leftrightarrow CH_3COO^- + H^+$$

Acetic acid accepts a proton in the presence of perchloric acid which is stronger acid.

$$CH_3COOH + HClO_4 \leftrightarrow CH_3COOH_2^+ + ClO_4^-$$

The $CH_3COOH_2^+$ ion easily releases its proton to react with a base. Thus, the basic properties of a base are increased. Titrations between weak base and perchloric acid can often be accurately carried out using ethanoic acid as solvent.

5. *Leveling Solvents:* The equilibrium of the reaction can shift towards right in presence of strong protophilic solvent, and all acids show similar strength. Similarly, all bases show similar strength in presence of a strongly protogenic solvent. Solvents having this property are called *Leveling Solvents*.

Advantages of non-aqueous solvent over aqueous solvent

1. Non-aqueous titrations are simple and accurate. The method can be used to analyze drugs such as ephedrine preparations, codeine phosphate, tetracycline, anti-histamines and various preparations of piperazine.
2. The method is suitable for the organic acids and bases which are insoluble in water but soluble in non-aqueous solvent.

Some common solvents for non-aqueous titrations

For non-aqueous titrations a large number of inorganic solvents have been used; but a few are used more commonly than others. Some of the most widely used solvents or solvent systems are mentioned below. In all instances pure, dry analytical reagent quality solvent should be used so that sharp end points can be obtained.

Glacial Ethanoic Acid: Glacial ethanoic acid is the most frequently used non-aqueous solvent. The water content of the solvent should be checked before it is used. The water content should remain within 0.1% - 1.0%.

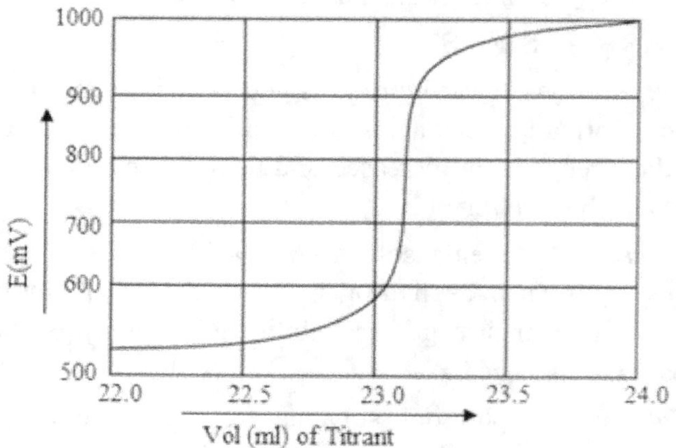

Figure 4.1 Change in potential in a potetiometric titration

Acetonitrile: Acetonitrile (methyl cyanide or cyanomethane) is commonly used with other solvents such as chloroform and phenol and especially with ethanoic acid. It produces very sharp end points in the analysis of metal ethanoates when titrated with perchloric acid.

Alcohol: Salts of organic acids, especially of soaps are determined in mixtures of glycols and alcohols or mixtures of glycols and hydrocarbons. The most common combinations are ethylene glycol (dihydroxy ethane) with propan-2-ol or butan-1-ol. These mixtures provide very good media for both the polar and non-polar ends of the molecules.

Dioxane: Dioxane is another solvent popularly used in nonaqueous titrations. This is frequently used in place of glacial ethanoic acid particularly when mixtures of substances are to be analyzed. Ethanoic acid is a leveling solvent; while dioxane is not a leveling solvent. Separate end points are obtained, depending on the individual components in the mixtures.

Dimethylformamide: Dimethylformamide (DMF) is a protophilic solvent. It is frequently used for titrations between, for example, benzoic acid and amides. However, sometimes it becomes difficult to obtain end points.

Indicators for non-aqueous titrations

Indicators used may be ionized and unionized or of different resonant forms; but depending on the nature of the titrant used in different titrations their color changes may vary at the end point. The exact colour corresponding to the correct end point may be known by conducting potentiometric titration simultaneously; so that the correct colour of the indicator at the end point is established. The appropriate colour is observed at the inflexion point of the titration curve.

A limited range of indicators are used in most of the non-aqueous titrations. Some typical examples are given here.

- **Crystal Violet:** It isused as 0.5% w/v solution in glacial acetic acid. Its colour change is from violet through blue followed by green, then to greenish yellow. In reactions in which base such as pyridine is titrated with perchloric acid.
- **Methyl Red:** It is used as a 0.2% w/v solution in dioxane. The colour changes from yellow to red.
- **Naphthol Benzein:** It is used as a 0.2% w/v solution in ethanoic acid. Its color changes from yellow to green and gives sharp end points when used for titration of weak bases against perchloric acid; particularly when ethanoic anhydride is used.
- **Quinaldine Red:** It is used as an indicator for determinations of drug content in dimethylformamide solution. A 0.1% w/v solution in ethanol gives a colour change from purple red to pale green.
- **Thymol Blue:** It is used widely as an indicator for titrations of substances that acts as acids in dimethyl formamide solution. Generally, a 0.2% w/v solution in methanol is used and at the end point a sharp colour changes from yellow to blue.

4.2 ACIDIMETRY AND ALKALIMETRY TITRATION

The apparent strength of an acid or base is measured by determining the extent to which it reacts with a solvent. In aqueous solution all strong acids react with the solvent to undergo almost complete dissociation and seem to be equally strong. While in a weakly protophilic solvent such as acetic acid, the acetonium ion ($CH_3COOH_2^+$) would be formed due to the addition of a proton. The extent of formation of the acetonium ion can provide a more sensitive method of measuring the strength of acids. The decreasing order of strength for acids is perchloric, hydrobromic, sulfuric, hydrochloric, and nitric acid.Acetic acid is weak acid because it reacts incompletely with water to form hydronium ion. But it reacts completely with a base such as ethylenediamine and behaves as a strong acid. This so-called levelling effect is observed also for bases.

The decreasing order of strength of bases used in non-aqueous titrations is potassium methoxide, sodium methoxide, lithium methoxide, and tetrabutylammonium hydroxide.

Many water-insoluble compounds when dissolved in organic solvents become more acidic or basic. Hence, these materials can be determined by non-aqueous titration by using an appropriate solvent. Pure compounds can be titrated directly. In some cases, particular part of a compound is physiologically active; by using appropriate solvent and titrant it is often possible to titrate that part. It is frequently necessary to isolate the active ingredient from its pharmaceutical preparations.

The types of compounds titrated as acids are acid halides, acid anhydrides, carboxylic acids, amino acids, enols such as barbiturates and xanthines, imides, phenols, pyrroles, and sulfonamides, etc. The types of compounds titrated as bases are amines, nitrogen-containing heterocyclic compounds, quaternary ammonium compounds, alkali salts of organic acids, alkali salts of inorganic acids, and some salts of amines. If mercuric acetate is added many salts of halogen acids may be titrated in acetic acid or acetic anhydride. Mercuric acetate removes halide ion in form of unionized mercuric halide complex. However, hydrochlorides of weak bases can be titrated in acetic anhydride without the addition of mercuric acetate, if bases do not contain acetylable groups, and malachite green or crystal violet can be used indicator. If titrations are carried out in the presence of an excess of acetic anhydride, the titrations should be carried out carefully; because acetic anhydride may react with the substance being titrated and produce low results.

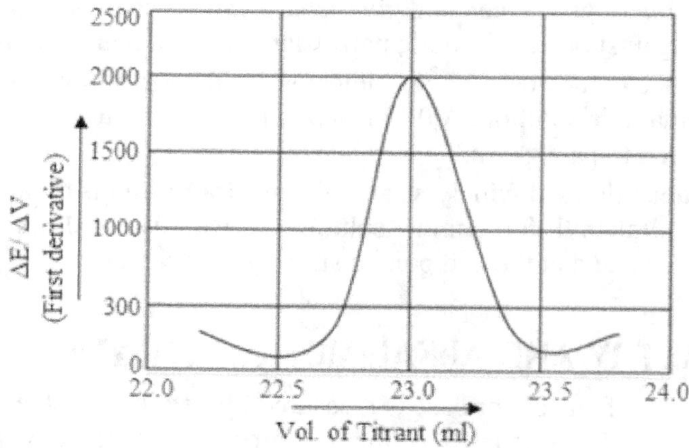

Figure 4.2 Change of dE/dV of first derivative in a potentiometric titration

Usually a basic compound is titrated with a standard solution of perchloric acid in glacial acetic; although perchloric acid in dioxane may be used in some cases. For titration of an acidic compound, a standard solution of lithium methoxide in methanol-toluene solvent is usually used. In many cases standard solution of tetrabutylammonium hydroxide in toluene is used. Earlier sodium methoxide had been widely used. However, it may cause problem if the precipitate formed in titration is gelatinous.

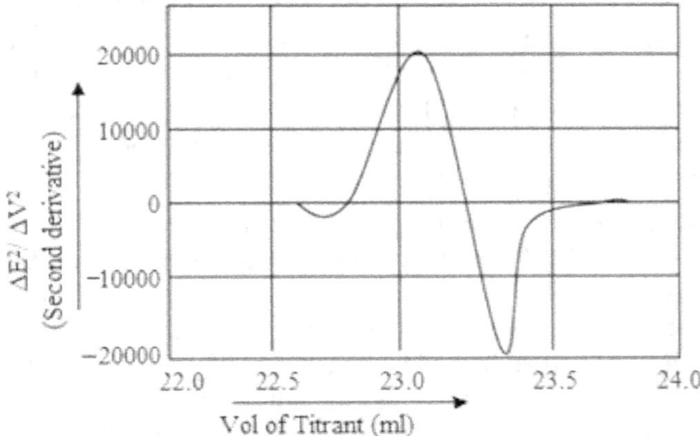

Figure 4.3 Change of dE/dV of second derivative in a potentiometric titration

Solvents for acidic compounds must be protected from excessive exposure to the atmosphere by a suitable cover or by use of an inert atmosphere during the titration, because carbon dioxide in air may interfere. A blank determination must be carried out and the titer value should not be more than 0.01 mL of a 0.1 M solution of the titrant for each mL of solvent.

The end-point can be determined either by visual observation of the color change of the indicator or by potentiometrically. It is beneficial to use the calomel reference electrode; because the aqueous potassium chloride solution in the salt bridge can be replaced by lithium perchlorate/acetic acid TS for titrations in acidic solvents, or by potassium chloride in methanol for titrations in basic solvents. It should be remembered that certain indicators, commonly used such as crystal violet, undergo a series of colour changes during a non-aqueous titration. Thus, care must be taken to ensure that the correct color change is noted at the end-point of the titration. In a potentiometric titration the end point corresponds to the maximum value of dE/dV (where E is the electromotive force and V the volume of titrant) as shown in the figures 4.1 and 4.2 with respect to first and second derivatives.

Another point should be considered that if the titrant is prepared with solvents having a relatively high coefficient of expansion, for example, glacial acetic acid, toluene, etc.; care should be taken to compensate the volume change due to differences in temperature during titration. It is safe to be standardized.

Acidimetric titration in nonaqueous solvents

Titration of Weak Bases and their salts

General method:

Prepare a solution of the substance being analyzed as specified in the monograph or dissolve in a suitable volume of glacial acetic acid. The solvent should be previously neutralized to crystal violet (in acetic acid) TS; if necessary, it should be warmed and cooled. Alternatively, the blank titration for the solvent and indicator may be done separately. If the substance is a salt of a hydrohalic acid, add 10 mL of mercuric acetate (in acetic acid) TS. Near the end-point add 2-3 drops of crystal violet/acetic acid TS to visualize the colour change and titrate slowly with perchloric acid till the specified colour change of the indicator is appeared. If in the monograph a different indicator is specified, the indicator should be used for the neutralization of the glacial acetic acid, and mercuric acetate/acetic acid TS, and the standardization of the titrant.

When the neutralization titration or standardization of the titrant is carried out potentiometrically the indicator is not required. A glass electrode and a saturated calomel cell as reference electrode are used. The calomel electrode contains potassium chloride TS (350 g/L). The junction between the titration liquid and the calomel electrode should have a sensibly low electrical resistance; transfer of liquid from one side to the other should be as minimum as possible. Unless the connections between the potentiometer and the electrode system are made in accordance with the manufacturer's instructions serious instability may result.

If the temperature at which the titration is carried out is t_2, the temperature at which the titrant is standardized is t_1, and the volume of the titrant required is v mL; then correct volume of the titrant would be: $v[1 + 0.001(t_1 - t_2)]$ mL.

Weak Bases and their salts include adrenaline acid tartrate, erythromycin stearate, metronidazole tartrate methyldopa, noradrenaline, orphenadrine citrate, prochlorperazine maleate etc.

Example 1: Assay of salt of weak base – epinephrine bitartrate

Procedure: Solution of $HClO_4$ (titrant) prepared in either glacial acetic acid or in dioxane is used for titration of weak bases. Generally, $HClO_4$ with a normality of 0.1N to 0.05N is used.

Dissolve 8.5 mL of 72% $HClO_4$ in about 900 mL glacial acetic acid with constant stirring, add about 30 mL acetic anhydride and make up the volume to 1000 mL with glacial acetic acid and keep the mixture for 24 hours.

Note:

1. Acetic anhydride absorbed all the water from $HClO_4$ and glacial acetic acid and renders the solution practically anhydrous.

2. $HClO_4$ must be sufficiently diluted with glacial acetic acid before adding acetic anhydride.

3. Reaction between $HClO_4$ and acetic anhydride is explosive.

Standardization of the prepared 0.1N $HClO_4$

Weigh accurately 500 mg of potassium hydrogen phthalate, dissolve in 25 mL of glacial acetic acid and add few drops of 5% w/v solution of crystal violet in glacial acetic acid (indicator). Titrate the solution with 0.1 $HClO_4$. The colour changes from blue to blue green.

1 mL of 0.1N $HClO_4$ = 0.020414 g of potassium acid Phthalate.

Solution of $HClO_4$ in dioxane may also be used as titrant. It is standardized in the same way as described above. The quality dioxane must be highest otherwise solution of $HClO_4$ will become dark. Dioxane can be purified by passing through resin or by shaking it with asbestos and then filtered.

Assay:

Procedure: Weigh accurately about 0.5 g of the sample into a 250 mL clean and dried conical flask; add 20mL of Glacial acetic acid, warm gently to dissolve, if necessary. Cool and titrate with 0.1 N perchloric acid using methylrosaniline chloride TS as indicator. Perform a blank determination and make necessary correction.

Each mL of 0.1N perchloric acid is equivalent to 0.03333g of $C_9H_{13}NO_3.C_4H_6O_6$

Calculation

Say, the weight of epinephrine bitartrate actually taken, w = 0.4998g,

Actual strength of $HClO_4$ solution, S = 0.10035N, and

The volume of 0.10035N $HClO_4$ solution consumed = 14.95 mL

The percentage content of epinephrine bitartrate in the sample is calculated by:

$$\frac{\text{Volume of } HClO_4 \text{ required} \times \text{Actual strength of } HClO_4 \times \text{Equivalence of the subs.} \times 100}{\text{Stated strength of } HClO4 \times \text{Actual wt of sample}}$$

Or, $\dfrac{14.95 \text{ mL} \times 0.10035N \times 0.03333g \times 100}{0.1 \times 0.4998g}$

Or, $= \dfrac{14.95 \text{ mL} \times 0.10035N \times 0.03333g \times 100}{0.4998g \times 0.1N} = \mathbf{100.04}$

Example 2:

Assay of methyldopa - The specific reaction between methyldopa and perchloric acid is expressed by the following equation:

One mol of methyldopa reacts with one mol of perchloric acid.

In other words, 211.24 g of $C_{10}H_{13}NO_4$ is equivalent to 100.45g of $HClO_4$.

Since, 1000 mL N solution of $HClO_4$ contain 100.45g of $HClO_4$,

1000 mL N solution of $HClO_4 \equiv 211.24$ g of $C_{10}H_{13}NO_4$

Or, 1 mL of 1N solution of $HClO_4 \equiv \dfrac{211.24g}{1000} = 0.2112$ g of $C_{10}H_{13}NO_4$

So, 1 mL 0.1N solution of $HClO_4 \equiv \dfrac{0.21124g}{10} = 0.02112$ g of $C_{10}H_{13}NO_4$

Procedure

Weigh accurately about 0.2 g of sample (methyldopa), transfer it into a 250 mL clean and dry conical flask, and dissolve in a mixture of 15 mL of anhydrous formic acid, 30 mL of glacial acetic acid and 30 mL of dioxane. Add 0.1 mL of crystal violet solution TS and titrate with 0.1 N perchloric acid. Perform a blank determination and make any necessary correction. Each mL of 0.1 N perchloric acid is equivalent to 0.02112 g of $C_{10}H_{13}NO_4$.

Calculation

The percentage of methyldopa present in the sample is given by:

$$\frac{\text{Volume of } HClO_4 \text{ required} \times \text{Actual strength of } HClO_4 \times \text{Equivalence of the subs.} \times 100}{\text{Stated strength of } HClO_4 \times \text{Actual wt of sample taken}}$$

Or,

$$\frac{\text{Volume of } HClO_4 \text{ required} \times \text{Actual strength of } HClO_4 \times 0.02112g \times 100}{0.1N \times \text{Actual wt of sample taken}}$$

Titration of Halogen Acid Salts of Bases

In general, the halide ions such as chloride, bromide and iodide cannot react quantitatively with acetous perchloric acid; because they are very weakly basic in character. To solve this problem, mercuric acetate is usually added to a halide salt. Mercuric acetate remains undissociated in acetic acid solution. Hence, it replaces the halide ion by an equivalent amount of acetate ion. The acetate ion works as a strong base in acetic acid as shown below:

$$2R.NH_2.HCl \leftrightarrow 2RNH_3^+ + 2Cl^-$$

$$(CH_3COO)_2Hg + 2Cl^- \rightarrow HgCl_2 + 2CH_3COO^-$$
(Undissociated)   (Undissociated)

$$2CH_3COOH_2^+ + 2CH_3COO^- \leftrightarrow 4\ CH_3COOH$$

Example 3: Assay of Amytriptyline Hydrochloride

The dissociation reaction of amytriptyline HCl and reaction between it and mercuric acetate in acetic acid are:

$$2C_{20}H_{31}ON.HCl \leftrightarrow 2C_{20}H_{31}NOH^+ + 2Cl^-$$

$$(CH_3COOH)_2Hg + 2Cl^- \rightarrow HgCl_2 + 2CH_3COO^-$$

$$2\ CH_3COOH_2^+ + 2CH_3COO^- \leftrightarrow 4CH_3COOH$$

Procedure: Weigh accurately about 1.0 g of sample (amytriptyline hydrochloride), transfer it into a 250mL clean and dry conical flask and dissolve it in 50 mL of glacial acetic acid, warm slightly; if necessary, to dissolve. Cool the solution to room temperature, add 10 mL of mercuric acetate solution, two drops of crystal violet solution TS and titrate with 0.1N perchloric acid till a green color is produced (end-point). Perform a blank determination and make any necessary correction.

The above reactions show that one mol of $C_{20}H_{31}ON.HCl$ is equivalent to one mol of $HClO_4$

That is, 337.9 g $C_{20}H_{31}ON. HCl \equiv 100.45g$ of $HClO_4$

Or, 1000 mL of 1N $HClO_4 \equiv 337.9$ g $C_{20}H_{31}ON.HCl$

Thus, each mL of 0.1N perchloric acid is equivalent to 0.03379 g of $C_{20}H_{31}ON.HCl$.

Calculation

The percentage of amytriptyline hydrochloride present in the sample is given by:

$$\frac{\text{Volume of } HClO_4 \text{ required} \times \text{Actual strength of } HClO_4 \times \text{Equivalence of the subs.} \times 100}{\text{Stated strength of } HClO_4 \times \text{Actual wt of sample taken}}$$

Or,

$$\frac{\text{Volume of } HClO_4 \text{ required} \times \text{Actual strength of } HClO_4 \times 0.02112g \times 100}{0.1N \times \text{Actual wt of sample taken}}$$

The Table 4.1 enlists acidimetric assay can be used to estimate various drug substances with perchloric acid as titrant by nonaqueous titrations, using mercuric acetate and glacial acetic acid and different indicators.

Table 4.1: List of drugs and corresponding indicators used in titrations

Sl. No	Name of drug substance	Suitable Indicator
1	Amantadine hydrochloride	Crystal violet
2	Cyproheptadiene.HCl	Do
3	Dehydroemetine.HCl	Do
4	Ephedrine hydrochloride	Do
5	Imipramine hydrochloride	Do
6	Isoprenaline hydrochloride	Do
7	Lignocaine hydrochloride	Do
8	Morphine hydrochloride	Do
9	Morphine sulphate	Do

Table 4.1: Contd...

Sl. No	Name of drug substance	Suitable Indicator
10	Phenylephrine hydrochloride	Do
11	Thiabendazole	Do
12	Phenytoin sodium	α -Naphthol benzein
13	Clonidine hydrochloride	Do
14	Chlorpromazine hydrochloride	Methyl orange
15	Promethazine hydrochloride	Do

Alkalimetric titration in nonaqueous solvents

Various weakly acidic drug substances can be titrated satisfactorily by using suitable non-aqueous solvent and with a sharp end-point. These pharmaceutical organic substances include: anhydride, acids, amino acids, acid halides, enols (viz., barbiturates), xanthenes, sulphonamides, phenols, imides and lastly the organic salts of inorganic acids. However, a weak inorganic acid e.g., boric acid, can be estimated conveniently employing ethylenediamine as the non-aqueous solvent.

Preparation of 0.1 N Sodium Methoxide: Take 150mL of methanol in a 1000 mL clean and dry volumetric flask, cool in ice bath, add 2.5g of sodium metal freshly cut into small pieces, add sufficient volume of benzene to make up 1000 mL mix thoroughly. The solution should be filled in a jar fitted with automatic burette to protect it from carbon dioxide and moisture. Otherwise the clear solution of sodium methoxide will become turbid due to reactions shown below.

The principal reactions involved in preparation and deterioration are;

$CH_3OH + Na \rightarrow CH_3ONa + H\uparrow$ (formation of sodium methoxide)

$CH_3ONa + H_2O \rightarrow CH_3OH + NaOH$ (reaction with water)

$2CH_3ONa + H_2CO_3 \rightarrow 2CH_3OH + Na_2CO_3$ (reaction with carbon dioxide)

The sodium methoxide solution, thus prepared, is standardized with anhydrous benzoic acid as follows.

Standardization of 0.1 N Sodium Methoxide solution

Procedure: Transfer 10 mL of dimethyl formamide (DMF) in a conical flask and add to it 3 to 4 drops of thymol blue and first neutralize the acidic impurities present in DMF by titrating with 0.1 N sodium methoxide in benzene-methanol. Weigh accurately 0.06g of benzoic acid, transfer immediately into a clean and dry 250mL conical flask and titrate quickly with sodium methoxide solution.

Benzoic acid interacts with dimethyl formamide and form a cation, $HCON^+H(CH_3)_2$ which subsequently reacts with CH_3O^- (methoxyl ion)

$C_6H_5COOH + H\text{-}CON(CH_3)_2 \leftrightarrow HCON^+H(CH_3)_2 + C_6H_5COO^-$

Benzoic acid   DMF

$CH_3ONa \leftrightarrow CH_3O^- + Na^+$

$HCON^+(CH_3)_2 + CH_3O^- \rightarrow HCON(CH_3)_2 + CH_3OH$

Preparation of 0.1N KOH in Methanol

Dissolve 5.6 gm of anhydrous KOH in 1000 mL of anhydrous methanol. Potassium methoxide is a titrant; but it is not as strong as sodium methoxide or lithium methoxide. The major disadvantage of it is that it reacts with acidic functional groups and produces a molecule of water, which reduces the sensitivity of titration.

Standardization: Usually standard benzoic acid AR-Grade is used to standardize these titrants. Sufficient amount of benzoic acid that would give a titer value of 20-30 mL is to be weighed accurately and transferred in a dry flask. The benzoic acid taken is to be dissolved in 25 mL dimethylformamide, 2-3 drops of 0.5% thymol blue indicator in dry methanol is to be added to the solution. A blank titration is needed to be performed in the solvent to account acidic impurity in dimethylformamide for making the correction in the titer value accordingly.

Table 4.2: Alkalimetric Assays of drug substances by Non-Aqueous Titrations using Lithium Methoxide or Sodium Methoxide either Potentiometrically or Titrimetrically

S. No.	Name of Substance	Indicator Employed
1.	Acetazolamide	Potentiometric determination
2.	Bendrofluazide	Azo violet
3.	Allopurinol	Thymol blue
4.	Mercaptopurine	-do-
5.	Amylobarbitone	Quinaldine Red
6.	Nalidixic acid	Thymolphthalein

4.3 ESTIMATION OF SODIUM BENZOATE AND EPHEDRINE HCL

Molecular formula of ephedrine HCl is $C_{10}H_{15}NO$, HCl and its molecular mass is 201.70g permol.

The method of assay of ephedrine HCl following non-aqueous titration is:

Procedure:
- Weigh accurately about 0.34g of ephedrine HCl, previously dried, and transfer it into a clean and dried 250mL conical flask,
- Add 20 mL of mercuric acetate solution, warm gently to 50°C,
- Add 100 mL of acetone, dissolve completely,
- Add 0.1 mL of saturated solution of methyl orange in acetone. Mix thoroughly,
- Titrate with standard solution of 0.1M perchloric acid until a red color is obtained, note the volume of titrant consumed (titer value).
- Repeat the titration twice more and take the average titer value for calculation.
- Perform a blank titration using all the reagents and solvent of same volume. Deduct the blank titer value from the titer value. The difference between the titer values (V mL) is used for calculating the purity of ephedrine HCl.

Each mL of 0.1M perchloric acid solution is equivalent to 0.02017g of $C_{10}H_{15}NO$, HCl.

Note: *If the temperature of the titrant at the time of assay (t_2) is different from the temperature of the titrant at the time of its standardization (t_1); then necessary correction in titer value (V mL) should be made by using the formula: V_f mL = V mL + V×0.0011 ($t_1 - t_2$)mL*

Calculation

Say, $t_1 - t_2$ is negligible; hence V mL = V_f mL

The titer value for the assay = 17.05 mL

Titer value for blank determination = 0.75 mL

Weight of ephedrine HCl taken = 0.3307g

Strength of $HClO_4$ solution = 0.1006M

$$V = V_f = 17.05 \text{ mL} - 0.75 \text{ mL} = 16.30 \text{ mL}$$

1 mL of 0.1M $HClO_4 \approx 0.02017g$ of $C_{10}H_{15}NO,HCl.$

$$1 \text{ mL of } 0.1006M\ HClO_4 \approx \frac{0.02017g \times 0.1006}{0.1} \text{ of } C_{10}H_{15}NO,HCl.$$

$$17.05 \text{mL of } 0.1006M\ HClO_4 \approx \frac{17.05 \times 0.1006 \times 0.02017g}{0.1} \text{ of } C_{10}H_{15}NO,HCl.$$

$$\text{Or, } 0.3307g \text{ of sample contains } \frac{17.05 \times 0.1006 \times 0.02017g}{0.1} \text{ of } C_{10}H_{15}NO,HCl.$$

$$\text{So, } 100 \text{ g of sample contains } \frac{17.05 \times 0.1006 \times 0.02017g \times 100}{0.1 \times 0.3307} \text{ of } C_{10}H_{15}NO,HCl$$

$$= \frac{16.30 \text{ mL} \times 0.1006M \times 0.02017g \times 100}{0.3307g \times 0.1M} = 100.01 \text{ of } C_{10}H_{15}NO,HCl$$

[Then, % purity of the sample

$$= \frac{\textbf{Final titer valte} \times \textbf{Strength of titrant} \times \textbf{Equivalence factor} \times \textbf{100}}{\textbf{Weight of sample taken} \times \textbf{Required strengh of titrant}}$$

Estimation of Sodium benzoate

The molecular formula of sodium benzoate is $C_7H_5NaO_2$ and its molecular mass is 144.1g per mol. Loss on drying should not be more than 2%. The procedure for assay of sodium benzoate by using non-aqueous titration method is given below;

Procedure

- ➢ Take about 1g of sodium benzoate in a weighing bottle, dry it at 105°C for 3 hrs/ until constant weight is obtained.
- ➢ Weigh accurately about 0.25g, transfer carefully into a clean and dry 250 mL conical flask,
- ➢ Add 20 mL of anhydrous glacial acetic acid, dissolve it by warming at about 50°C, if necessary,
- ➢ Cool the solution to room temperature,

- ➢ Add 0.1 mL of 1-naphtholbenzene indicator solution,
- ➢ Titrate the solution with standard 0.1M perchloric acid solution filled in a dry burette till end point attained,
- ➢ Note the volume of perchloric acid solution consumed (titer value),
- ➢ Repeat the process twice more and take the average titer value,
- ➢ Perform a blank titration and note the volume of 0.1M perchloric acid solution consumed,
- ➢ Deduct titer value of the blank titration from the main titer value, use the resulted value for calculation.

Calculation

Say, the final titer value = 17.15 mL

Strength of perchloric acid solution = 0.09987M,

Weight of sodium benzoate taken = 0.2506g, and

Loss on drying = 1.88%

Each mL of 0.1M perchloric acid is equivalent to 0.01441g of anhydrous $C_7H_5NaO_2$.

1 mL of 0.1M $HClO_4 \approx 0.01441g$ of $C_7H_5NaO_2$.

$$1 \text{ mL of } 0.09987M \text{ } HClO_4 \approx \frac{0.01441g \times 0.09987}{0.1} \text{ of } C_7H_5NaO_2.$$

$$17.15 \text{mL of } 0.09987M \text{ } HClO_4 \approx \frac{17.15 \times 0.09987 \times 0.01441g}{0.1} \text{ of } C_7H_5NaO_2.$$

$$\text{Or, } 0.2506g \text{ of sample contains } \frac{17.15 \times 0.09987 \times 0.01441g}{0.1} \text{ of } C_7H_5NaO_2.$$

$$100 \text{ g of sample contains } \frac{17.15 \times 0.09987 \times 0.01441g \times 100}{0.1 \times 0.2506} \text{ of } C_7H_5NaO_2.$$

$$= \frac{17.15 \times 0.09987 \times 0.01441g \times 100}{0.1 \times 0.2506} = 97.62\% \text{ of } C_7H_5NaO_2 \text{ ('as is' basis)}$$

$$\text{On anhydrous basis the \% purity of the sample} = \frac{97.62 \times 100}{100 - 1.88} = \frac{97.62 \times 100}{98.12} = \mathbf{99.49}$$

A. MULTIPLE CHOICE QUESTIONS

1. Which one of the following statements is correct?
   - (a) The strength of an acid depends on the acidity of the solvent
   - (b) The strength of an acid depends on the basicity of the solvent
   - (c) The strength of an acid does not depend on the acidity of the solvent
   - (d) The strength of an acid does not depend on the basicity of the solvent

2. Which one of the following statements is correct?
   (a) Non-polar solvents may be protophilic
   (b) Non-polar solvents may be protogenic
   (c) Non-polar solvents may be amphiprotic
   (d) Non-polar solvents may be aprotic

3. Which one of the following statements is correct?
   (a) Solvents may be polar
   (b) Solvents may be nonpolar
   (c) Solvents may be protic
   (d) All of the above

4. Nonaqueous titrations are suitable for
   (a) Insoluble organic acidic and basic substances
   (b) Soluble organic acidic and basic substances
   (c) Soluble organic acidic substances
   (d) Soluble organic basic substances

5. Which of the following solvents can be used in nonaqueous titrations?
   (a) Glacial acetic acid
   (b) Water
   (c) Formaldehyde
   (d) All of the above

6. Which of the following titrants can be used in nonaqueous titrations?
   (a) Potassium hydroxide solution
   (b) Perchloric acid solution
   (c) Sulphuric acid solution
   (d) Sodium hydroxide solution

7. Which type of substances is not analyzed by nonaqueous titration?
   (a) Enols
   (b) Carboxylic acids
   (c) Mineral acid
   (d) Amino acids

8. What is the reason for which acetic anhydride is commonly added to glacial acetic acid in nonaqueous titration?
   (a) Dilution of glacial acetic acid
   (b) Complexation with glacial acetic acid
   (c) Dissolution of solute substance
   (d) Conversion of water to acetic acid

9. The type of basic compounds titrated by perchloric acid in a non-aqueous medium includes
   (a) Amines
   (b) Alkali salts of inorganic acids
   (c) Acid salts of inorganic bases
   (d) All of the above

10. For nonaqueous titration perchloric acid is dissolved in
    (a) Water
    (b) Alcohol
    (c) Glacial acetic acid
    (d) Acetic anhydride

11. For estimation of sodium benzoate by non-aqueous titration, the moisture content of sodium benzoate should not exceed
    (a) 5%
    (b) 2%
    (c) 4%
    (d) 3%

12. Nonaqueous titrations are sometimes conducted potentiometrically, because
     (a) Change of color of the indicator is not sharp
     (b) Change of color of the indicator is very sharp
     (c) There is no end point
     (d) The end point can be detected only by a potentiometer
13. Why sodium methoxide solution becomes turbid?
     (a) Interaction with moisture
     (b) Interaction with carbon dioxide
     (c) Interaction with moisture and carbon dioxide
     (d) None of the above
14. The color change of the indicator depends on
     (a) Solvent used   (b) Titrant used
     (c) Material being titrated   (d) Room temperature
15. Correction in titer value due to variation in temperature of the titrant is calculated
     by the equation
     (a) $V_f\,ml = Vml(1 + 0.0011)(t_1 - t_2)ml$ (b) $V_f\,ml = Vml - V\times0.0011(t_1 - t_2)ml$
     (c) $V_f\,ml = V\,ml + V\times0.011(t_1 - t_2)ml$ (d) $V_f\,ml = V\,ml - V\times0.011(t_1 - t_2)ml$
16. Perchloric acid solutionmust be sufficiently diluted with glacial acetic acid before
     adding acetic anhydride; because
     (a) Perchloric acid solution will become cold
     (b) Perchloric acid solution become turbid
     (c) Strength of Perchloric acid solution will change
     (d) Perchloric acid reacts with acetic anhydride with explosion

B. SHORT QUESTIONS

1. Write down the physical characteristics of the solvents used in organic chemistry.
2. What are the advantages of non-aqueous solvent?
3. Classify the non-aqueous solvents with example of each class.
4. What is the leveling effect?
5. Name six solvents used in non-aqueous titrations.
6. Name five indicators used in non-aqueous titrations.
7. Why acetic anhydride is used in non-aqueous titrations?
8. How the end point is determined when potentiometer is used for non-aqueous titration?

C. LONG QUESTIONS

1. Discuss in short different classes of non-aqueous solvents.
2. Discuss the principle of acidimetric non-aqueous titration

3. Discuss the principle of alkalimetric non-aqueous titration
4. Explain the potentiometric non-aqueous titration curves
5. Write down the general method of non-aqueous titration of weak bases and their salts.
6. How ephedrine bitartrate is estimated?
7. Describe the method of preparation and standardization of 0.1N KOH solution.
8. Describe the preparation and standardization of 0.1 N Sodium Methoxide.
9. Describe how ephedrine hydrochloric is estimated.
10. Describe how sodium benzoate is estimated.

CHAPTER 5

Precipitation Titrations

5.1   PRINCIPLE OF PRECIPITATION

In volumetric analysis, the most common and important precipitation reaction is with silver nitrate with the anions such as chloride, bromide, iodide, and thiocyanate. Such titrations with silver salt are also known as *argentimetric titrations* because argentum is the old name of silver. Same principle can be applied to other precipitation reactions too.

The rate of reaction for silver salt precipitation is rapid. In general, the reaction takes place at a ratio 1:1 and silver salts produced are practically insoluble. The solubility products of silver salts are presented in Table 5.1.

Table 5.1: Solubility and solubility products of common silver salts

Salt	Anions	Solubility Product (Ksp)	Solubility (g/lt)
AgCl	Cl^-	1.8×10^{-10}	0.0052 (50°C)
AgBr	Br^-	5.2×10^{-13}	0.0014 (20°C)
AgI	I^-	8.3×10^{-17}	3×10^{-6} (20°C)
AgSCN	SCN^-	1.7×10^{-12}	0.00025 (21°C)
Ag_2CrO_4	CrO_4^{2+}	7.1×10^{-13}	0.0215 (20°C)

The principle can be well understood by the reaction between sodium chloride and silver nitrate. Let us consider 100mL of 0.1N sodium chloride is titrated with 0.1N silver nitrate. The solubility product of silver chloride (AgCl) at room temperature is 1.2×10^{-10}. The initial concentration of Cl^- ions is 0.1g of equivalent ions per litre or $pCl^- = 1$. Let us calculate the concentration of Cl^- ion after gradual addition of silver nitrate.

1. If 10mL of 0.1N silver nitrate solution is added to 100mL of solution of 0.1N sodium chloride, 90mL of 0.1N sodium chloride remain in a total volume of 110mL (100+10) and the strength of sodium chloride is 0.1N.

   Thus, $[Cl^-] = 90 \times \dfrac{0.1}{110} = 8.181 \times 10^{-2}$ or $pCl^- = 1.09$

2. If 90mL of 0.1N silver nitrate solution is added to 100mL of solution of 0.1N sodium chloride, the total volume becomes 190mL and remaining volume of 0.1N sodium chloride = 100mL − 90mL = 10mL, strength of the sodium chloride is 0.1N.

   Thus, $[Cl^-] = 10 \times \dfrac{0.1}{190} = 5.3 \times 10^{-3}$ or $pCl^- = 2.28$

   We know that, $[Ag^+][Cl^-] = 1.2 \times 10^{-10} = S_{AgCl}$

   so, $-\log([Ag^+][Cl^-]) = -\log(1.2 \times 10^{-10}) = -\log AgCl$

   Or, $-\log[Ag^+] + (-\log[Cl^-]) = 9.92 = p^{AgCl}$

   Or, $p^{Ag+} + p^{Cl-} = 9.92 = p^{AgCl}$

   From the last determination, $p^{Cl-} = 1.48$;

   So, $p^{Ag+} = 9.92 - 1.48 = 8.44$

In this way the concentrations of Cl^- and Ag^+ ions at different stages can be calculated or determined till the equivalence point is reached.

When equivalence point is reached, $Ag^+ = Cl^- = \sqrt{S_{AgCl}}$

Or, $p^{Ag+} = p^{Cl-} = \dfrac{1}{2} p^{AgCl} = \dfrac{9.92}{2} = 4.96$

At this point the solution would be saturated with AgCl, and there would be no excess of Ag^+ ion or Cl^- ion.

If 100.1mL of 0.1N silver nitrate ($AgNO_3$) solution is added to 100mL of 0.1N of sodium chloride (NaCl) solution, the total volume becomes 200.1mL, and the concentration of $[Ag^+] = 0.1 \times \dfrac{0.1}{200.1}$

$= 5 \times 10^{-5}$

or, $p^{Ag+} = 4.30$,

So, $pCl^- = p^{AgCl} - p^{Ag+} = 9.92 - 4.30 = 5.62$

Note: However, this value of pCl^- is not perfectly correct. Because the dissolved amount of silver chloride will produce silver and chloride ions. Hence the value of pCl- will change, may be to negligible extent.

Accordingly, the values of pCl- can be calculated after addition of 0.1N silver nitrate solution. The Table 4.2 shows the value of pCl^-, pAg^+, pI^- and of pAg^+ in the titration of sodium chloride and potassium iodide salts. Solubility product of silver chloride, S_{AgCl} $=1.2\times10^{-10}$ and solubility product of silver iodide, $S_{AgI} = 1.7\times10^{-16}$.

Table 5.2: Values of pCl^-, pAg^+, pI^- and of pAg^+ in the titration 100 mL of 0.1N sodium chloride and 0.1N potassium iodide solution

Vol (mL) of 0.1N AgNO₃ added	Titration of 0.1N NaCl solution	
	pCl⁻	pAg⁺
0	1.0	-
5	1.05	8.88
10	1.09	8.83
15	1.13	8.79
25	1.22	8.70
50	1.48	8.44
75	1.85	8.07
80	1.96	7.96
90	2.28	7.64
95	2.59	7.33
98	2.99	6.93
99	3.30	6.62
99.5	3.60	6.32
99.8	4.00	5.92
99.9	4.30	5.62
100	5.0	5.0
100.1	5.62	4.30
100.2	5.92	4.00
100.5	6.32	3.60
101	6.62	3.30
102	6.92	3.00
105	7.31	2.61
110	7.60	2.32

As per the Table 5.2 the value of pAg^+ after addition of 99.1 mL of 0.1N AgNO₃ solution is found to be 5.6 which changes to 4.3 when another 0.2mL of 0.1N AgNO3 solution is added; that is 0.1 mL of 0.1N AgNO₃ solution is added extra. This results the concentration of Ag^+ ions to change by 1.3. At the equivalence point the value of pAg^+ is 5.0 which changes to 4.3 just on addition of 0.1 mL of 0.1N AgNO₃ solution. While in case of titration of potassium iodide with 0.1N AgNO₃ solution the value of pAg^+ becomes 11.5 after addition of 99.9 mL of 0.1N AgNO₃ solution. At equivalence point this value changes to 7.9; but on addition of just 0.1 mL after the equivalence this value becomes 4.3. That is, pAg+ changes by 3.9. The larger change in silver ion concentration in the case of titration of KI solution is due to greater solubility of AgI than AgCl. This is evidenced by their solubility product values. The solubility of AgI is about 10^6 times larger than that of AgCl.

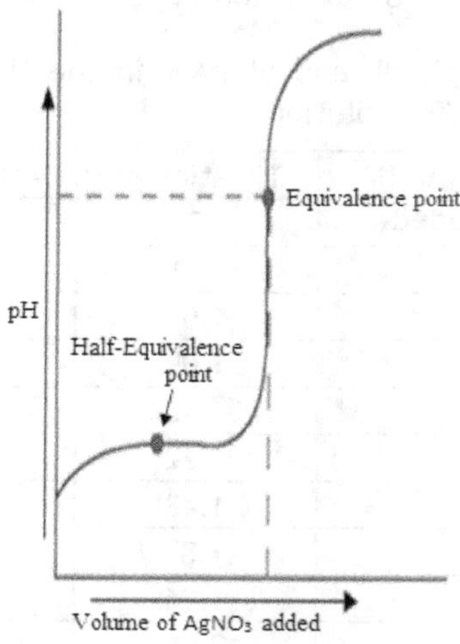

Figure 5.1 Change of pH with addition of 0.1N sodium nitrate in the titration of sodium chloride

The plot of pH versus volume (mL) of 0.1N silver nitrate solution added for titrating sodium chloride is similar to the graph shown in figure 5.1. Theoretical data of Table 5.2 when plotted on a graph paper, a graph of pCl⁻ vs. volume of 0.1N AgNO$_3$ added is obtained which is shown in fig. 5.2

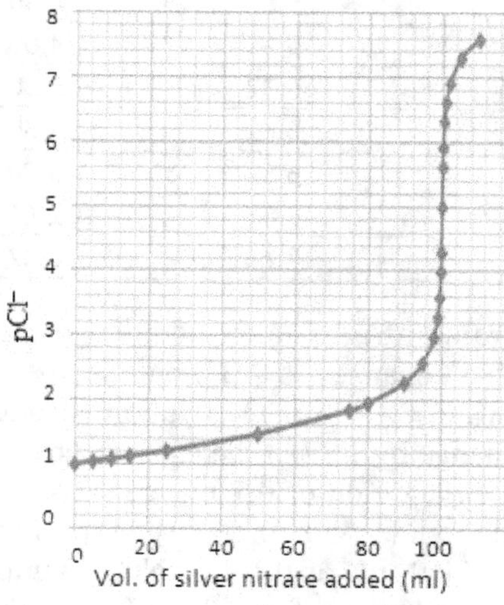

Figure 5.2 Plot of pCl- vs volume of 0.1 N AgNO$_3$ (ml)

5.2 MOHR'S METHOD

In some titrations precipitation and complex formation reactions are involved. In 1856, Mohr developed a method for determination of chloride and bromide in their salts. For example, a known amount of neutral solution of sodium chloride is titrated with standard silver nitrate (say, 0.1N) using a few mL of potassium chromate as an indicator. Silver ions of silver nitrate react with chloride ions of sodium chloride and form silver chloride (AgCl) precipitates. However, in this titration silver ions react with chromate ions of potassium chromate and form silver chromate (AgSCN) precipitate. Solubility products of AgCl and AgSCN are 1.2×10^{-10} and 1.7×10^{-12} respectively. This indicates that solubility of silver chloride is less than that of silver chromate. During beginning chloride ion concentration being more, silver chloride would be precipitated first. Appearance of red color is the end point.

When silver chromate will be formed at the first end point and just precipitate out, both silver chloride and silver chromate will remain in equilibrium in the solution.

At nearer to the end point; that is, when 99.98% of silver nitrate has been added to the solution, red color silver chromate just precipitates and at this state both silver chromate and silver chloride will remain in equilibrium. Thus,

$$[Ag^+][Cl^-] = S_{AgCl} = 1.2 \times 10^{-10}$$

$$[Ag^+]^2 [CrO_4^{2-}] = S_{Ag_2CrO_4} = 1.7 \times 10^{-12}$$

$$[Ag+] = \frac{S_{sol(AgCl)}}{[Cl^-]} = \sqrt{\frac{S_{sol(Ag_2CrO_4)}}{[CrO_4^{2-}]}}$$

Or,

$$\frac{[Cl^-]}{\sqrt{[CrO_4^{2-}]}} = \frac{S_{sol(AgCl)}}{\sqrt{S_{Ag_2CrO_4}}} = \frac{1.2 \times 10^{-10}}{\sqrt{1.7 \times 10^{-12}}} = 9.2 \times 10^{-5}$$

Thus, at equivalence point $[Cl^-] = \sqrt{S_{AgCl}} = 1.1 \times 10^{-5}$. At this point, if silver chromate is to precipitate, then chromate ion concentration should be

$$[CrO_4^{2-}] = \left(\frac{[Cl^-]}{9.2 \times 10^{-5}}\right)^2 = \left(\frac{1.1 \times 10^{-5}}{9.2 \times 10^{-5}}\right) = 1.4 \times 10^{-2}$$

Thus, 0.014M potassium chromate should be added. In fact, a slight excess of silver nitrate (at least one drop equivalent to 0.05mL) is added to get adequate visibility of the end point.

Commonly the potassium chromate solution used in titrations is more dilute, about 0.003–0.005M; because 0.01–0.02M solution of potassium chromate makes detection of endpoint difficult.

The error caused by using 0.003M potassium chromate can be calculated as follows;

With molar concentration of $[CrO_4^{2-}]$ is 0.003, silver chromate would be precipitated when

$$[Ag^+] = \sqrt{\frac{S_{Ag_2CrO_4}}{CrO_4^{2-}}} = \sqrt{\frac{1.7 \times 10^{-12}}{3 \times 10^{-3}}} = 2.4 \times 10^{-5} \qquad \dots (5.1)$$

By using the theoretical concentration of the indicator, we get

$$[Ag+] = \sqrt{\frac{1.7 \times 10^{-12}}{1.4 \times 10^{-2}}} = 1.1 \times 10^{-5} \qquad .....(5.2)$$

The difference between eqn. 1 and 2 is 1.3×10^{-5} equivalents per litre. if at equivalence point the volume of the solution is 150mL; this corresponds to $1.3 \times 10^{-5} \times 150 \times 10^{4} / 1000 = 0.02$mL of 0.1N silver nitrate. Although negligible this is the theoretical error. To detect the distinct color at end point usually 1 drop (equivalent to 0.05mL) of 0.1N silver nitrate is added extra. The calculated error (0.02mL) is less than this.

The error in titration will increase with decreasing concentration of solution being titrated. It is about 0.4% for 0.01N solutions being titrated using $0.003 - 0.005$M potassium chromate as indicator. This error can be avoided if an indicator blank titration is carried out and the blank titer value is deducted from the sample titer value for the same intensity of color at end points in both titrations.

Generally, this precipitation titration is carried out in almost neutral solutions having pH within 6.5 to 9.0.

If the acid solution is titrated following reaction would take place;

$$2CrO_4^{2-} + 2H^+ = 2HCrO_4^- = Cr_2O_7^{2-} + H_2O$$

$HCrO_4^-$ being a weak acid chromate ion concentration would be reduced and solubility product of silver chromate would not be increased.

If the solution being titrated is alkaline, silver hydroxide may be precipitated.

Hence following measures should be taken under the above situations:

1. **If the solution to be titrated is acidic:** Add excess of pure calcium carbonate or sodium bicarbonate to make the solution neutral.

2. **If the solution to be titrated is alkaline:** Acidify with acetic acid and then excess of pure calcium carbonate or sodium bicarbonate.

5.3 VOLHARD'S METHOD

Volhard in 1878 demonstrated and explained this method. This is a method of estimation of halide in its salt. In this method silver is titrated with potassium or ammonium thiocyanate in presence of free nitric acid using ferric nitrate or ferric ammonium alum as indicator. An excess amount of standard silver nitrate solution is added to the sample solution. Silver ions react with the chloride ions and form white precipitates of silver chloride.

$$Ag^+ (aq) + Cl^- (aq) \leftrightarrow AgCl(s)$$

The unreacted silver ions are then titrated with a standard solution of potassium thiocyanate in the presence of ferric ammonium sulfate solution (which acts as an indicator). During titration when thiocyanate solution is added silver ions react with thiocyanate ions and form silver-thiocyanate which precipitates in the solution. The solubility product of silver-thiocyanate is 1.7×10^{-12}.

$$Ag^+ (aq) + SCN^- (aq) \leftrightarrow AgSCN(s)$$

Once this reaction is complete, even a drop of potassium or ammonium thiocyanate if added the ferric ion of the indicator reacts with free thiocyanate ion and form a colored complex, ferri-thiocyanate ion $(FeSCN)^{2+}$.

$$Fe^{3+}(aq) + SCN^-(aq) \leftrightarrow FeSCN^{2+}(aq)$$

This colored complex produces reddish-brown color. On further addition of thiocyanate the ferri-thiocyanate complex redissolves and the reddish-brown color goes away. The titration is continued until the permanent end point is reached and reddish-brown color is produced.

This method can be used to determine the content of chloride, bromide, and iodide in their acidic solutions.

For example, in the determination of chloride following two equilibria are found when excess of standard silver nitrate is titrated with standard potassium or ammonium thiocyanate solution;

$$Ag^+ (aq) + Cl^- (aq) \leftrightarrow AgCl(s)$$
$$Ag^+ (aq) + SCN^- (aq) \leftrightarrow AgSCN(s)$$

When these two sparingly soluble salts are in equilibrium with the solution,

$$\frac{[Cl^-]}{[SCN^-]} = \frac{S_{AgCl}}{S_{AgSCN}} = \frac{1.2 \times 10^{-10}}{7.1 \times 10^{-13}} = 169$$

Thus, until the ratio of chloride ion and thiocyanate ion, $\dfrac{[Cl^-]}{[SCN^-]}$ becomes 169, thiocyanate ion will react with silver chloride and form silver thiocyanate as follows;

$$AgCl + SCN^- \leftrightarrow AgSCN + Cl^-$$

Such reaction results considerable error in titration. Silver thiocyanate, AgSCN is less soluble than silver chloride, AgCl. Thus, once the value of $\dfrac{[Cl^-]}{[SCN^-]}$ reaches 170, addition of a single drop of standard solution of potassium or ammonium thiocyanate will produce a reddish-brown color complex, $(FeSCN)^{2+}$.and the titration becomes complete.

To achieve accurate result the titration error must be reduced. Hence, it is very much necessary to prevent the reaction between AgCl and SCN^-. This can be achieved if following precautions are taken;

➢ Before back titration the solution should be filtered to remove silver chloride precipitate. Since some of Ag^+ ions remain adsorbed on to the AgCl precipitate, direct filtration may cause loss of Ag^+ ions. Hence, the solution containing AgCl precipitates should be boiled for few minutes; so that the precipitates coagulate and the adsorbed Ag^+ ions are released from the precipitates. After filtration and boiling, the cold filtrate should be titrated. However, on cooling re-adsorption of Ag^+ ions may take place.

> After addition of $AgNO_3$, potassium nitrate, KNO_3 should be added. Potassium nitrate prevents re-adsorption of Ag^+ ions and acts as coagulant.

> An immiscible liquid such as nitrobenzene can be added to coat the AgCl particles. This prevents the thiocyanate ions from interacting with AgCl. Usually 1mL of nitrobenzene is sufficient for each 50mg of chloride. The suspension containing nitrobenzene should be shaken well to coagulate the precipitated AgCl particles; then back titrated.

Similarly, bromides and iodides can be determined by the same process. When bromides are titrated with potassium or ammonium thiocyanate the equilibrium expression can be written as;

$$\frac{[Br^-]}{[SCN^-]} = \frac{S_{AgBr}}{S_{AgSCN}} = \frac{3.5 \times 10^{-13}}{7.1 \times 10^{-13}} = 0.493 \approx 0.5$$

This small value of 0.5 indicates the titration error is small. The end point can be determined without any difficulty.

Determination of HCl content of concentrated HCl

Procedure I: Usually concentrated hydrochloric acid is of 10–11N and it is diluted for determination of chloride content.

Take a 500 mL clean volumetric flask; add about 400 mL of distilled water. Accurately measure 5.00 mL of the concentrated HCl and transfer into the volumetric flask, add sufficient water to make up the volume. Mix well. Pipette out 25.00 mL of the diluted HCl into a clean 250 mL conical flask. Add 5 mL of 6N nitric acid, mix well, and then add 30 mL of 0.1 N silver nitrate standard solutions from a burette, shake well to complete precipitation and coagulation. Preferably boil the suspension for about 3 – 4 min. Filter the suspension quantitatively through sintered glass crucible (G-4) or Whatmann 42 filter paper, wash the precipitate thoroughly with 3×10 mL of 1% nitric acid. Collect the combined filtrate and washings in a clean 250 mL conical flask, add 1 mL of saturated ferric alum solution, mix well, and then titrate with 0.1 N potassium thiocyanate standard solutions from a burette until a permanent faint reddish- brown color is obtained. Repeat the titration twice more with two other 25.00 mL of diluted HCl solutions. Take the average titer value for calculation, say 7.85mL.

Calculation

Volume of 0.1 N potassium thiocyanate standard solution consumed = 7.85 mL

Strength of potassium thiocyanate standard solution = 0.10043 N, and

Strength of silver nitrate standard solution = 0.10124N

Volume of diluted HCL taken = 25.00mL

Volume of 0.10124 N silver nitrate standard solution added = 30.00 mL

Now, 1 mL of 0.1N potassium thiocyanate solution $\approx$ 1 mL 0.1N of silver nitrate solution.

So, 7.85 mL of 0.10043N potassium thiocyanate solution $\approx \dfrac{0.1N \times 7.85mL}{0.10043N} = 7.82$ mL of 0.1N silver nitrate solution.

0.1N silver nitrate solution consumed in the reaction = 30.00 mL − 7.82 mL = 22.18 mL

1 mL of silver nitrate solution ≈ 0.003546 g of Cl ≈ 0.003646 g of HCl

Or, 22.18 mL silver nitrate solution $\approx 22.18 \times 0.003646$ g of HCl = 0.08086 g of HCl

Or, 25 mL of diluted hydrochloric acid contains 0.08086 g of HCl

500 mL of diluted hydrochloric acid contains $\dfrac{0.08086 \text{ g} \times 500 \text{ mL}}{25 \text{ mL}} = 1.617$ g of HCl

That is, 5.00 mL of concentrated hydrochloric acid contains 1.617 g of HCl

So, 100 mL of concentrated hydrochloric acid contains $\dfrac{1.617 \text{ g} \times 100 \text{ mL}}{5.00 \text{ mL}} = 32.34$g of HCl

Hence, purity of concentrated hydrochloric acid is **32.34%w/v**

Procedure II:

Take a 500 mL clean volumetric flask; add about 400 mL of distilled water. Accurately measure 5.00 mL of the concentrated HCl and transfer into the volumetric flask, add sufficient water to make up the volume. Mix well. Pipette out 25.00 mL of the diluted HCl into a clean 250 mL conical flask. Add 5 mL of 6N nitric acid, mix well, and then add 30 mL of 0.1 N silver nitrate standard solutions from a burette, shake well to complete precipitation. Add 2 − 3 mL of pure nitrobenzene (A.R. grade) and 1 mL of saturated ferric alum solution (indicator), shake vigorously to coagulate the precipitate. Then, titrate the residual silver nitrate with 0.1 N potassium thiocyanate standard solutions from a burette until a permanent reddish-brown color is obtained. Repeat the titration twice more with two other 25.00 mL of diluted HCl solutions. Take the average titer value for calculation, say 6.75mL.

Calculation

Volume of 0.1 N potassium thiocyanate standard solution consumed = 6.75 mL

Strength of potassium thiocyanate standard solution = 0.1003 N, and

Strength of silver nitrate standard solution = 0.1012N

Volume of concentrated HCL taken for analysis $= \dfrac{5 \text{ mL} \times 25mL}{500mL} = 0.25$mL

Volume of 0.1012 N silver nitrate standard solution added = 30.00 mL

1 mL of 0.1N potassium thiocyanate solution $\approx$ 1 mL 0.1N of silver nitrate solution.

So, 6.75 mL of 0.1003N potassium thiocyanate solution $\approx \dfrac{0.1N \times 6.75mL}{0.1003N} = 6.73$ mL of 0.1N silver nitrate solution.

0.1N silver nitrate solution consumed in the reaction = 30.00 mL − 6.73 mL = 23.27 mL

1 mL of silver nitrate solution ≈ 0.003546 g of Cl ≈ 0.003646 g of HCl

Or, 23.27 mL silver nitrate solution ≈ 23.27 × 0.003646 g of HCl = 0.08484 g of HCl

Or, 0.25 mL of diluted hydrochloric acid contains 0.08484 g of HCl

So, 100 mL of concentrated hydrochloric acid contains $\dfrac{0.08484 \text{ g} \times 100 \text{ mL}}{0.25 \text{ mL}}$ = 33.94g of HCl

Hence, purity of concentrated hydrochloric acid is **33.94%w/v**

Procedure III:

Transfer accurately 5.00 mL of concentrated hydrochloric acid into a clean 500 mL volumetric flask containing 400 mL of water. Make up the volume with water and shake well to mix. Transfer 25.00 mL of the diluted HCl into a 250 mL clean conical flask, add 5 mL of 6N nitric acid, add 30.00 mL of 0.1N silver nitrate from a burette, and 4 – 5 drops of tartrazine solution (0.5% solution in water) as indicator. Shake vigorously for 1 – 2 min to ensure the tartrazine is adsorbed on to the precipitate as maximum as possible. Then, titrate the residual silver nitrate with 0.1 N ammonium or potassium thiocyanate from a burette until the supernatant liquid turns into a very pale-yellow color. Repeat the titration twice more with two other 25.00 mL of diluted HCl solutions. Take the average titer value for calculation.

Example 1: A sample of hydrochloric acid was tested for percent content of HCl. 25 mL of 1% v/v solution when reacted with 30.00 mL of 0.1012N silver nitrate; the residual silver nitrate consumed 6.15 mL of 0.1003N potassium thiocyanate. Calculate the percent content of HCl of the sample.

Calculation

Volume of 0.1 N potassium thiocyanate standard solution consumed = 6.15 mL

Strength of potassium thiocyanate standard solution = 0.1003 N, and

Strength of silver nitrate standard solution = 0.1012N

Volume of concentrated HCL taken for analysis = $\dfrac{1 \text{ mL} \times 25\text{mL}}{100\text{mL}}$ = 0.25mL

Volume of 0.1012 N silver nitrate standard solution added = 30.00 mL

Now, 1 mL of 0.1N potassium thiocyanate solution ≈ 1 mL 0.1N of silver nitrate solution.

So, 6.75 mL of 0.1003N potassium thiocyanate solution ≈ $\dfrac{0.1N \times 6.15\text{mL}}{0.1003\text{N}}$ = 6.13 mL of 0.1N silver nitrate solution.

0.1N silver nitrate solution consumed in the reaction = 30.00 mL – 6.13 mL = 23.87 mL

1 mL of silver nitrate solution ≈ 0.003546 g of Cl ≈ 0.003646 g of HCl

Or, 23.27 mL silver nitrate solution ≈ 23.87 × 0.003646 g of HCl = 0.08703 g of HCl

Or, 0.25 mL of diluted hydrochloric acid contains 0.08703 g of HCl

So, 100 mL of concentrated hydrochloric acid contains $\dfrac{0.08703 \text{ g} \times 100 \text{ mL}}{0.25 \text{ mL}} = 34.81$g of HCl

Hence, purity of hydrochloric acid was **34.81%w/v**

Determination of bromides

Transfer accurately 5.00 mL of hydrobromic acid into a clean 500 mL volumetric flask containing 400 mL of water. Make up the volume with water and shake well to mix. Transfer 25.00 mL of the diluted HBr into a 250 mL clean conical flask, add 5 mL of 6N nitric acid, add 30.00 mL of 0.1N silver nitrate from a burette, and 1 mL of ferric alum solution in water as indicator. Shake vigorously for 1 – 2 min. Then titrate the residual silver nitrate with 0.1 N ammonium or potassium thiocyanate from a burette until the supernatant liquid turns into a very pale-yellow color. Repeat the titration twice more with two other 25.00 mL of diluted HBr solutions. Take the average titer value for calculation.

$$1 \text{ mL of } 0.1\text{N AgNO3} \approx 0.007992 \text{ g of Br} \approx 0.008093 \text{ g of HBr}$$

The aqueous solubility of silver bromide is less than that of silver thiocyanate. Thus, silver bromide need not to be filtered during titration; while silver chloride is filtered as mentioned above. Otherwise the method of determination of bromide is similar to the method of determination of chloride.

Note: Constant boiling hydrobromic acid should be used for practice, bromine in potassium bromide can also be used for determination.

Example 2: A sample of hydrobromic acid was tested for its purity by titrating 25 mL of 1% solution of it. Volume of 0.1006N silver nitrate added was 30.00 mL and 6.42 mL of 0.0997N potassium thiocyanate was consumed by residual silver nitrate. Calculate the percentage purity of the sample tested.

Calculation

Volume of 0.0997 N potassium thiocyanate consumed = 6.42 mL

Strength of silver nitrate standard solution = 0.1006N

Volume of concentrated HBr taken for analysis $= \dfrac{1 \text{ mL} \times 25\text{mL}}{100\text{mL}} = 0.25$mL

Volume of 0.1012 N silver nitrate standard solution added = 30.00 mL

1 mL of 0.1N potassium thiocyanate solution $\approx$ 1 mL 0.1N of silver nitrate solution.

So, 6.75 mL of 0.1003N potassium thiocyanate solution $\approx \dfrac{0.1\text{N} \times 6.15\text{mL}}{0.1003\text{N}} = 6.13$ mL of 0.1N silver nitrate solution.

0.1N silver nitrate solution consumed in the reaction = 30.00 mL – 6.13 mL = 23.87 mL

1 mL of silver nitrate solution $\approx$ 0.003546 g of Cl $\approx$ 0.003646 g of HCl

Or, 23.27 mL silver nitrate solution $\approx 23.87 \times 0.003646$ g of HCl $= 0.08703$ g of HCl

Or, 0.25 mL of diluted hydrochloric acid contains 0.08703 g of HCl

So, 100 mL of concentrated hydrochloric acid contains $\dfrac{0.08703 \text{ g} \times 100 \text{ mL}}{0.25 \text{ mL}} = 34.81$ g of HCl

Hence, purity of concentrated hydrochloric acid is **34.81%w/v**

5.4 MODIFIED VOLHARD'S METHOD

Many researchers have modified the Volhard's method to improve accuracy of the result. In a review Kolthoff reported that several modifications of the Volhard's method have been done by various people, but all the methods have errors except the method proposed by Schoorl. Although this method is tedious; but it produces accurate result. Since the method requires various precautions, its application is also limited. According to this method the precipitates are to be separated from the solution before back titration.

Since some of Ag^+ ions can be adsorbed on the surface of the AgCl precipitate, direct filtration may cause loss of Ag^+ ions. Hence, the solution containing AgCl precipitates should be boiled for few minutes; so that the precipitates coagulate and the adsorbed Ag^+ ions are released from the precipitates. After filtration and boiling, the cold filtrate should be titrated. But, on cooling re-adsorption of Ag^+ ions may also take place.

Hence, after addition of $AgNO_3$, potassium nitrate, KNO_3 should be added to the chloride solution. Potassium nitrate prevents re-adsorption of Ag^+ ions and acts as coagulant. Moreover, an immiscible liquid such as nitrobenzene if added it coats the AgCl particles. Such coating prevents the thiocyanate ions from interacting with AgCl. Usually 1mL of nitrobenzene is sufficient for each 50mg of chloride. The suspension containing nitrobenzene should be shaken well to coagulate the precipitated AgCl particles; then back titrated. Official method of estimation of sodium chloride recommends the use of nitrobenzene and nitric acid.

5.5 FAJAN'S METHOD

This method is based on the use of adsorption indicator. In case of precipitation reactions K. Fajan in 1923 – 24 introduced a useful method for selection of an appropriate indicator. This type of indicators is absorbed by the precipitate at the equivalence point. During adsorption, changes occur within the indicator and the substance produced gives a color different from the color produced by the indicator itself. For this reason, these indicators are called *adsorption indicator*. Substances used as indicator are either acid dyes such as fluorescein, eosin, etc. (sodium salt) or basic dyes such as halogen salt of rhodamine.

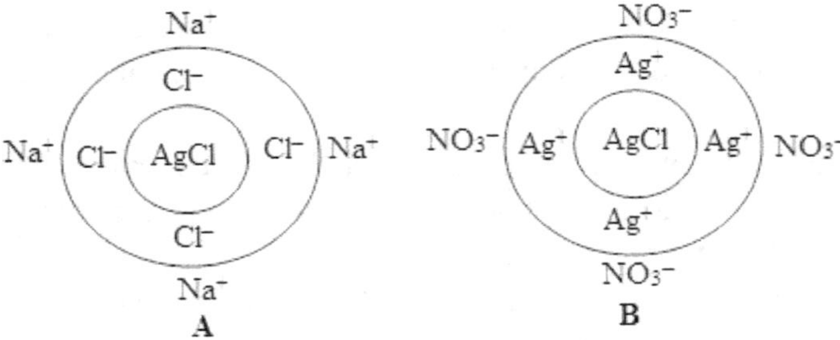

Figure 5.3 (A) when Cl⁻ ions are present in excess, and (B) when Ag+ ions are present in excess

Mechanism of action of these indicators primarily depends on properties of the colloidal precipitates. When sodium chloride is titrated with standard solution of silver nitrate, insoluble silver chloride is precipitated, and the precipitates of silver chloride adsorb Cl⁻ ions because any precipitate prefers to adsorb its own ions as shown in the figure 5.2A. This adsorption takes place in the first layer which is surrounded by a second layer of available ions in the solution.

Once the stoichiometric point is attained silver ions (Ag^+) become excess. These ions are then adsorbed in the first layer and NO_3^- ions are adsorbed in the second layer (Fig.5.2B). Under this circumstance if fluorescein is present in the solution, the negative fluorescein ions replace the NO_3^- ions and are strongly adsorbed in the second layer. Fluorescein has its own color, greenish-yellow and accordingly the solution is greenish-yellow colored. Once fluorescein ion is adsorbed by silver ion, makes fluorescein-silver complex which is pink in color. As a result, the solution becomes pink colored. This change in color takes place at the equivalence point.

This phenomenon can be explained in another way: during adsorption fluorescein ion undergoes rearrangement of its structure and form a colored substance. It is important to note that the color changes at the surface of the precipitate. At this point if Cl⁻ ions are added, the color of suspension will remain pink until the concentration of Cl⁻ ions becomes excess. Then the Ag^+ ions adsorbed will react with Cl⁻ ions and form AgCl. The freshly formed AgCl precipitate will adsorb Cl⁻ ions on their surfaces replacing fluorescein ions adsorbed already. The fluorescein ion go back to solution and color of the solution will turn to greenish-yellow.

Selection of indicator:

The factors that influence the selection of suitable indicator are;

- ➢ The precipitate particles formed should remain separated as much as possible; even the suspension may be colloidal type.
- ➢ Large amount of multivalent neutral salts should not be used; because they have coagulating effect.

➢ The solution to be titrated should not be so dilute that the amount of precipitate formed is very small. Some indicators fail to change the color sharply in very dilute solution.

➢ The indicator ions should not be adsorbed before complete precipitation of the product; but the indicator should be strongly adsorbed in secondary layer immediately after attainment of equivalence point.

➢ The precipitate particles should not adsorb the indicator ions strongly. For example, eosin (tetra bromo fluorescein) is used as indicator in the titration of chloride with silver nitrate. The eosin ions will be adsorbed in the primary or first layer of AgCl precipitates before equivalence is reached.

The major limitation of the adsorption indicators is the photosensitivity of the silver halides after adsorption of indicator ions. Hence, this type of titration should be carried out where minimum light is present. The concentration of adsorption indicator should be around 0.00025 moles per mole of silver present in the solution.

5.6   ESTIMATION OF SODIUM CHLORIDE

Chloride in neutral solution can be determined either by Mohr's method or Fajan's method. It can be done by titrating with standard 0.1N silver nitrate. If the solution of chloride is acidic, treat the solution with chloride free calcium carbonate, sodium bicarbonate, or borax. For this purpose, substance of A.R. grade should be used. If mineral acid is present in the sample, it can be removed by treating first with ammonia solution and then by excess of ammonium acetate. Chloride solution neutralized by calcium carbonate is titrated by using adsorption indicator can be easily titrated with 0.1N silver nitrate. In this case 5mL of dextrin solution, if used, can facilitate the coagulation of calcium ions.

If the chloride solution is basic it can be neutralized by treating with nitric acid using phenolphthalein as indicator.

Preparation of 0.1N silver nitrate

The purity silver nitrate A.R. grade is 99.9%. By simple heating in a hot air oven free moisture absorbed can be removed. Hence, it is used as primary standard and the strength of its solution can be calculated by weight ratio. However, for more accuracy its purity can be linked with strength as shown in calculation.

Take about 5g of silver nitrate A.R. grade in a weighing bottle. Dry it for 2 hrs at 120°C in a hot air oven. Remove the bottle and place it in a desiccator. Weigh accurately about 4.248g and transfer into a 250mL clean volumetric flask and dissolve with freshly boiled and cooled water. Shake well and transfer into a clean and dry amber-glass stoppered bottle with a proper label.

Method: *Mohrs method,*

Weigh accurately about 0.145g of sodium chloride and transfer into a clean 250mL conical flask. Add about 25mL of water and dissolve. Add 1mL of potassium chromate T.S. through a 1mL pipette. Rinse and fill a 50mL clean and dry burette with the standard solution of silver nitrate. Titrate the sodium chloride solution slowly with silver nitrate solution and swirl the flask continuously. Until reddish-brown color is formed after addition of each drop of silver nitrate and goes away after swirling. This is the indication of approaching endpoint. There after add the silver nitrate dropwise, swirl and allow the color to disappear. When the color persists even after swirling, note the burette reading as titer value.

Repeat the titration twice; make average of three titer values. Perform an indicator blank titration using 1mL potassium chromate T.S. and about 50mL of water. Add silver nitrate solution dropwise until the color of same intensity is produced. Subtract the blank titer value from the average titer value. Then calculate the content of sodium chloride in the sample.

Each mL of 0.1N silver nitrate solution is equivalent to 0.005845g of NaCl.

Calculation

Say, quantity of silver nitrate weighed = 4.2461g for 250mL solution

$$\text{Theoretically } \frac{16.988g \times 250mL}{1000mL} = 4.247g \text{ of silver nitrate should be taken}$$

$$\text{So, strength of silver nitrate solution} = \frac{\text{Practical weight}}{\text{Theoretical weight}} = \frac{4.2461g}{4.247g} = 0.9997(0.1N);$$

i.e., 0.0999N

Volume of 0.0999N silver nitrate consumed (av. Titer value) = 24.65mL

Say, quantity of sodium chloride titrated = 0.1462g

Then, % content of sodium chloride in the sample =

$$\frac{24.65mL \times 0.0999N \times 0.005845g \times 100}{0.1462g \times 0.1N} = 98.45\% \text{ ('as is basis')}$$

$$\text{The \% content of sodium chloride in the sample on dried basis} = \frac{98.45 \times 100}{98.26} =$$

100.19%

Loss on drying

Weigh accurately a clean and dry weighing bottle with its lid (xg), take about 0.5g of sodium chloride in the weighing bottle, put the lid and weigh accurately (x_1g). Place the weighing bottle in a hot-air oven; open the lid and dry the sodium chloride at 105°C for 3 hrs. Stopper the bottle and remove it from the oven and place immediately in a desiccator for cooling. Once cooled to room temperature, weigh the weighing bottle (x_2g).

Calculation

Say, Weight of empty weighing bottle (xg) = 22.0015g, and

Weight of weighing bottle + sodium chloride (x_1g) = 22.5124g

Weight of weighing bottle + dried sodium chloride (x_2g) = 22.5035g

Weight of sodium chloride taken for drying = x_1g – xg = 22.5124g - 22.5035g = 0.5109g

Loss of sodium chloride on drying = x_2g – x_1g = 22.5124g – 22.5035g = 0.0089g

$$\text{Loss on drying} = \frac{0.0089\text{g} \times 100}{0.5109\text{g}} = 1.74\%$$

Method: *Volhard's method*

Weigh accurately about 0.125g of sodium chloride previously dried at 105°C for 2 hrs; transfer it into a 250mL clean conical flask. Dissolve sodium chloride in about 25mL of water. Add 25.00mL of 0.1N silver nitrate, 1.5mL of nitric acid, 3mL of nitrobenzene, and 1mL of ferric ammonium sulphate T.S.; swirl the flask. Shake well and titrate the excess silver nitrate with 0.1N ammonium thiocyanate from a burette until reddish-brown color persists permanently. Perform a blank titration. Subtract the blank titer value from main titer value. This would the volume of ammonium thiocyanate required in back titration.

Each mL of 0.1N silver nitrate is equivalent to 5.845mg of NaCl.

Calculation

Say, amount of sodium chloride taken = 0.1248g

Volume of silver nitrate added = 25.00mL

Say. The strength of silver nitrate solution used = 0.0999N, and

Strength of ammonium thiocyanate solution = 0.0998N

Volume of ammonium thiocyanate solution required (titer value) = 3.95mL

3.95mL of 0.0998N ammonium thiocyanate $\approx \dfrac{3.95\text{mL} \times 0.0998\text{N}}{0.0999\text{N}} = 3.946\text{mL} \approx 3.95\text{mL}$ of 0.0999N silver nitrate

So, the volume of 0.0999N silver nitrate solution consumed by 0.1248g of sodium chloride

$$= 25.00\text{mL} – 3.95\text{mL} = 21.05\text{mL}$$

1mL of 0.1N silver nitrate is equivalent to 5.845mg = 0.005845g of NaCl

21.05mL of 0.1N silver nitrate is equivalent to $= \dfrac{0.0999\text{N} \times 20.95\text{mL} \times 0.005845\text{g}}{0.1\text{N}}$

$$= 0.1229\text{g of NaCl}$$

Hence, purity of sodium chloride sample $= \dfrac{0.1229\text{g} \times 100}{0.1248\text{g}} = 98.45\%$

A. MULTIPLE CHOICE QUESTIONS

1. Which one of the following statements is correct?
   (a) Argentimetric titration is the titration of silver nitrate with chloride salt
   (b) Argentimetric titration is the titration of silver nitrate with bromide salt
   (c) Argentimetric titration is the titration of silver nitrate with iodide salt
   (d) All of the above

2. Which one of the following statements is correct?
   (a) Silver iodide is less soluble than silver bromide at 20°C
   (b) Silver iodide is more soluble than silver bromide at 20°C
   (c) Solubilities of silver iodide and silver bromide are same at 20°C
   (d) None of the above

3. Concentration of potassium chromate solution used as indicator in argentimetric titration should be about
   (a) 0.003 – 0.005M
   (b) 0.01 – 0.02M
   (c) 0.1 – 0.2M
   (d) 1 – 2M

4. To titrate an acidic solution by argentimetric method, the solution should be made neutral by adding
   (a) Sodium hydroxide solution
   (b) Sodium carbonate solution
   (c) Sodium bicarbonate solution
   (d) Calcium hydroxide solution

5. Before titrating an alkaline solution by argentimetric method, the solution should be first made acidic by adding
   (a) Hydrochloric acid
   (b) Acetic acid
   (c) Sulphuric acid
   (d) None of the above

6. The molecular weights of silver nitrate and sodium chloride are 164.88 and 58.45 respectively. Each ml of 0.1M silver nitrate is equivalent to
   (a) 0.5845g of sodium chloride
   (b) 0.05845g of sodium chloride
   (c) 0.005845g of sodium chloride
   (d) 0.0005845g of sodium chloride

7. In Volhard's method the chloride solution is acidified with
   (a) Nitric acid
   (b) Sulphuric acid
   (c) Acetic acid
   (d) Citric acid

8. As per Volhard's method for determination of chloride, nitrobenzene is added to solution; because
   (a) Nitrobenzene helps nitrate to react with chloride
   (b) Nitrobenzene helps silver chloride not to dissociate
   (c) Nitrobenzene helps to coagulate silver chloride
   (d) None of the above

9. Volumetric solution of silver nitrate is standardized with
    (a) Sodium chloride
    (b) Sodium bromide
    (c) Sodium thiocyanate
    (d) None of the above

10. According to Fajan's method the argentimetric titration uses
    (a) Acid-base indicator
    (b) Adsorption indicator
    (c) Absorption indicator
    (d) None of the above

11. According to Fajan's method for the argentimetric titration
    (a) The precipitate particles formed should remain separated
    (b) Large amount of multivalent neutral salts should not be used
    (c) The solution to be titrated should not be very dilute
    (d) All of the above

12. Which of the following is adsorption indicator?
    (a) Fluorescein
    (b) Potassium chromate
    (c) Ammonium thiocyanate
    (d) None of the above

B. SHORT QUESTIONS

1. What are argentimetric titrations?
2. How can the value of pCl- be calculated?
3. Diagrammatically show the relation between pCl^- and volume of $AgNO_3$ added.
4. What measures should be taken to neutralize the chloride before estimation by Mohr's method?
5. What are the limitations of Volhard's method for estimation of chloride?
6. Why Volhard's method requires modification?
7. Write down the principle of Fajan's method.
8. What is adsorption indicator?
9. What is the limitation of an adsorption indicator?
10. What are the factors to be considered for selection of indicator?
11. Why nitric acid added in estimation of chloride?

C. LONG QUESTIONS

1. Explain the principle of argentimetric titrations.
2. Explain the principle of precipitation.
3. Discuss how the chloride can be determined by the Mohr's method.
4. Discuss the principle of Volhard's method for estimation of chloride.
5. Explain the limitations of the Volhard's method for estimation of chloride.

6. Discuss the principle of Fajan's method for estimation of chloride.
7. Explain the modified Volhard's method for estimation of chloride.
8. Describe how you can estimate the chloride content in concentrated hydrochloric acid.
9. Describe how the chloride content can be determined in a sample of sodium chloride.
10. Explain the difference between the Mohr's method and Volhard's method.

CHAPTER 6

Complexometric Titration

6.1 INTRODUCTION

The process of formation of a complex or complex ion is called *complexation* and the method used to titrate metal ions with a *complexing agent* or *chelating agent or chilons or sequestering agent* (called Ligand) is commonly called **complexometric titration**. In this method, a simple ion is transformed into a complex ion and the equivalence point is determined by using metal indicators or electrometrically. The method is alternatively called as **chilometrictitrations, chilometry, chilatometric titrations.** EDTA (Ethylene diamine tetra acetic acid) titrations have also been used for this purpose. All these terms are used to describe the same analytical method.

$$\text{Metal ion (analyte cation)} + \begin{matrix}\text{Chilon}\\\text{Chelating agent}\\\text{Complexing agent}\\\text{Ligand}\\\text{Sequestering agent}\end{matrix} \xrightarrow[\text{pM indicator}]{\text{Metal-ion indicator}} \begin{matrix}\text{Chelate}\\\text{Metal co-ordination compound}\\\text{Complex ion}\\\text{Metal complex}\\\text{Chelate compound}\end{matrix}$$

These chilons react with metal ions and form a complex known as **chelate**.

Metal ions remain solvated in solution. That is, the metal ion remains attached firmly to definite number of solvent molecules (usually 2, 4 or 6). During the formation of a metal complex or metal co-ordination compound these bound solvent molecules are replaced by other solvent molecules or ions.

The molecules or ions which displace the solvent molecules are called **Ligands**. Ligands or complexing agents or chelating agents donate electron and the ability to bind to the metal ion and produce a complex ion. This is expressed as;

$$M + C \xrightarrow[\text{pM indicator}]{\text{Metal ion-indicator}} MC$$

Where, M is metal ion (analyte, cation)

C represents chelating agent or chilons or sequestering agent or complexing agent or ligand, and

MC represents complex ion or metal complex or metal co-ordination compound or chelate or chelate compound.

For example, one Cu (II) ion binds to four molecules of ammonia in an aqueous solution and forms a complex, $[Cu(NH_3)_4]^{2+}$ as shown below:

$$[Cu(H_2O)_6]^{2+}(aq) + 4\ NH_3\ (aq) \leftrightarrow [Cu(NH_3)_4(H_2O)_2]^{2+}(aq) + 4\ H_2O(liq)\quad K_c = 1.2 \times 10^{13}$$

Bonds involved in complexes

The bonds between the metal ion and ligand are either ordinary covalent bonds or co-ordinate bonds. When the metal and the ligand contribute one electron each covalent bond is formed. On the other hand, when the pair of electrons is contributed by the ligand, it forms co-ordinate bond. Accordingly, the hexacyanoferrate ion contains three ordinary covalent bonds and three co-ordinate bonds. Cyanogens attached through co-ordinate bonds carry negative chare in the complex.

Principle of Complexometric Titration

Complexometric titrations involve various principles of acid-base titrations. In these titrations, the free metal ions are changed into complex ions. In acid-base titrations, the end point is detected by sudden change in pH. In EDTA titration, if the negative log of metal ion concentration (pM) is plotted against volume of titrant, the pM rapidly increases (decrease of log [M] as indicated in the figure) at the end point. This increase of pM takes place due to removal of traces of metal ions from solution by EDTA. The end point can be noticed either by using an indicator or instrumentally by potentiometric or conductometric (electrometric) method.

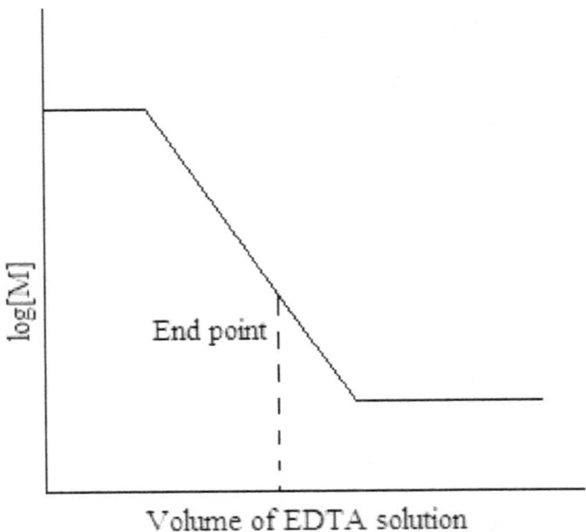

There are three important factors that influence the determination of the magnitude of break (due to increase of pM) in titration curve at end point.

- ***Stability of complex formed:***The end point becomes clear if the charge in free metal complex is large and the stability constant for complex formed is greater.
- ***Number of steps involved in complex formation:***Ifthe number of steps involved in the formation of complex is less, the break (inflexion) in titration curve at equivalent point would be greater and clear would be the end point.
- ***Effect of pH:*** During a complexometric titration, the pH must be kept constant by using a suitable buffer in the titration mixture. The concentration of H^+ ion controls the pH of the solution and plays an important role in chelation. Most of the ligands are basic in nature and bind to H+ ions throughout a wide range of pH. During chelation some of these H+ ions are sometimes displaced from the ligands (chelating agent) by the metal ions.

The general equation for complexation between metal ion and H^+ ion for ligand is expressed as:

$$M^{2+} + H_2\text{-}EDTA^{2-} \leftrightarrow M\text{-}EDTA^{2-} + 2H^+$$

Therefore, the stability of metal complex depends on the pH. When the pH of the solution is less, the stability of the complex would also be less; because more H+ ions are available to compete with the metal ions for the ligand. Metals that form very stable complexes can be titrated in acidic solution, and metals forming weak complexes can only be effectively titrated in alkaline solution.

Complexometric titration becomes easy when single complex species are formed. Schwarzenbach in 1945 observed that amino polycarboxylic acids are very good complexing agents. The most common complexing agent is ethyl ene diamine tetra-acetic acid (EDTA). The dissociation constants of EDTA in the form of zwitterions are pk_1 = 2.0, pk_2 = 2.7, pk_3 = 6.2 and pk_4 = 10.3 at 20°C. These values show that EDTA behaves as a dicarboxylic acid with strong acidic groups and one out of two ammonium protons ionizes at the pH of about 6.3 and the second at a pH of about 11.5.

There are other complexing agents (Complexones) which are sometimes used. For example, Nitrilotriacetic acid (NITA or NTA or Complex) and 1,2 diaminocyclohexane NNN'N'-tetra-acetic acid (DCYTA or DCTA or Complexone IV).

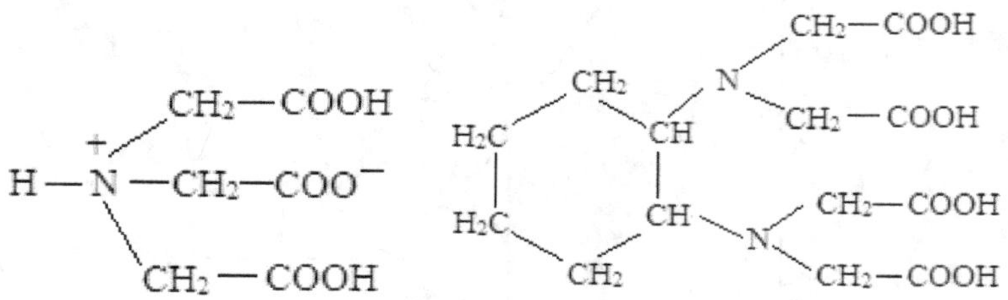

Nitrilotriacetic acid   1,2 diaminocyclohexane NNN'N'-tetra-acetic acid

As mentioned earlier thatthe complexes may be molecules such as $HgCl_2$, $Hg(SCN)_2$, or ions such as $[Ag(CN)_2]^-$, $[Cu(NH_3)^{2+}$, $[Ag(NH_3)_2]^+$, etc. which are formed step wise. For example, two ions such as Hg^{2+} and Cl^- can produce $[HgCl]^+$, $HgCl_2$, $[HgCl_3]^-$ and $[HgCl_4]^{2-}$.

The instability constants or dissociation constant characterize various equilibria among the complexes.

$$[HgCl]^+ \leftrightarrow Hg^{2+} + Cl^- \qquad k_1 = \frac{[Hg^{2+}]}{[(HgCl)^+]}$$

$$HgCl_2 \leftrightarrow Hg^{2+} + 2Cl^- \qquad k_2 = \frac{[Hg^{2+}][Cl^-]^2}{[HgCl_2]}$$

$$[HgCl_3]- \leftrightarrow HgCl_2 + Cl^- \qquad k_3 = \frac{[HgCl_2][Cl^-]}{[HgCl_3^-]}$$

$$[HgCl_4]^{2-} \leftrightarrow [HgCl_3]^- + Cl^- \qquad k_4 = \frac{[HgCl_3^-][Cl^-]}{[HgCl_4^{2-}]}$$

The overall equilibria which hold the above partial or intermediate equilibria are expressed by 'overall' dissociation constants. For example, $[HgCl_4^-] = Hg^{2+} + 4Cl^-$

$$K_4 = \frac{[Hg^{2+}][Cl^-]^4}{[HgCl_4^-]}$$

Each complex is thus characterized by the instability constant k_n or by $pk_n = -\log k_n$. The stability of the complex increases as the value of kn falls or as the value of pkn increases. The relationship between the overall and the partial constant is

$$pK_4 = pk_1 + pk_2 + pk_3 + pk_4$$

There is similarity between the dissociation of a complex (e.g., $[HgCl^+]$), and that of an acid HA. The dissociation of HA is

$$HA = H^+ + A^-; \qquad Ka = \frac{[H^+][A^-]}{[HA]}$$

Usually, a very stable complex behaves like a weak acid; while a complex of low stability behaves like a strong acid. Similar to pH, pCl can be defined as;

$$pCl = - \log [Cl^-]$$

$$= pk1 + \log \frac{[Hg^{2+}]}{[(HgCl)^+]}$$

This equation is similar to $pH = pKa + \log\frac{[Base]}{[Acid]}$

The formation of a series of complexes in titration can be applied if the titration can be stopped after the formation of a fairly stable complex MX_n. That is pkn of the complex is large enough from that of succeeding complex MX_{n+1}.

Hence, the complex would be adequately stable if its pkn is large enough such as more than 4. The stability of the complex, MX_n should be sufficiently larger than that of its succeeding complex MX_{n+1}. In fact, if $pk_n - pk_{n+1} > 4$ and $pk_n > 4$; the titration becomes accurate. Generally, titration cannot be stopped in between and should be continued till the last complex is formed; the complex should be sufficiently stable. However, there are exceptions such as complexes of mercuric ions. Titration of such ions can be stopped at intermediate stage such as at $HgCl_2$. Let the titration of mercuric perchlorate (Hg^{2+} ion) with a soluble chloride is considered. The dissociation constants for successive equilibria are $pk_1 = 6.7$, $pk_2 = 6.5$, $pk_3 = 0.8$, and $pk_4 = 1.0$. Since the difference between two dissociations constants, $pk_2 - pk_3 = 6.5 - 0.8 = 5.7$ at the point when $HgCl_2$ is formed, there shall be a point of inflexion in the titration curve and pCl at this point would be equal to $(\frac{1}{2}pk_2 + \frac{1}{2}pk_3) = 3.7$. This is similar to variation of pH during neutralization of a tetra basic acid with a base. This can be determined by potentiometric titration or by using a suitable indicator such as a mixture of diphenyl carbazone and bromophenol blue. Once the equivalence point at which $HgCl_2$ is reached diphenyl carbazone reacts with excess mercuric ion present in the solution.

Factors that influence the reaction with EDTA

- ***The nature and activity of metal ion***

  Ethylenediamine tetra-acetic acid forms complexes with complexes with most cations in a 1:1 ratio, irrespective of the valency of the ion:

$$M^{2+} + [H_2X]^{2-} \leftrightarrow [MX]^{2-} + 2H^+$$
$$M^{3+} + [H_2X]^{2-} \leftrightarrow [MX]^- + 2H^+$$
$$M^{4+} + [H_2X]^{2-} \leftrightarrow [MX] + 2H^+$$

Where, M is a metal and $[H_2X]^{2-}$ is the anion of the disodium salt (disodium EDTA) which is most commonly used. The structures of these complexes with di-, tri- and tetravalent metals contain three, four and five rings respectively:

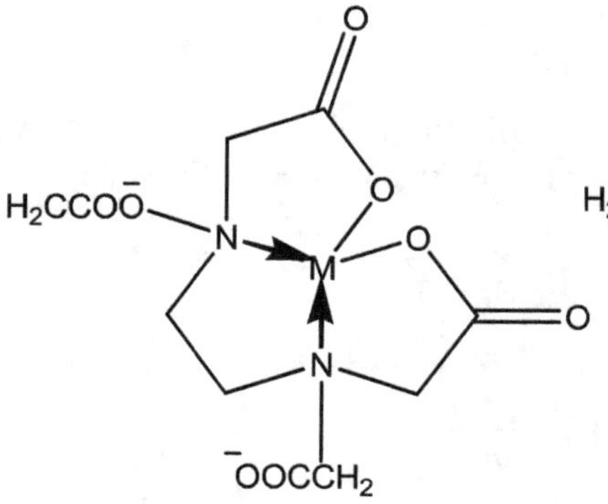

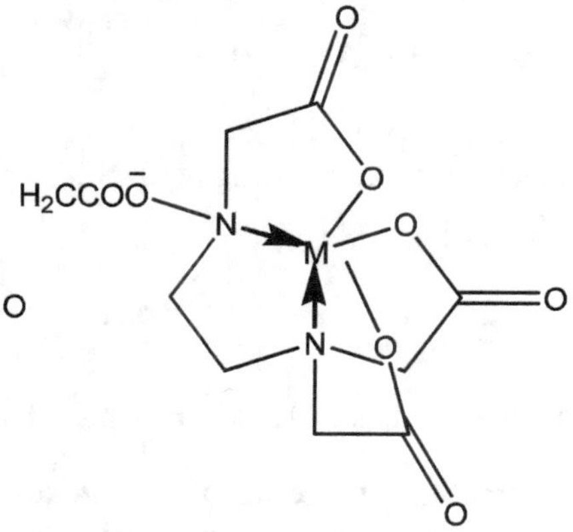

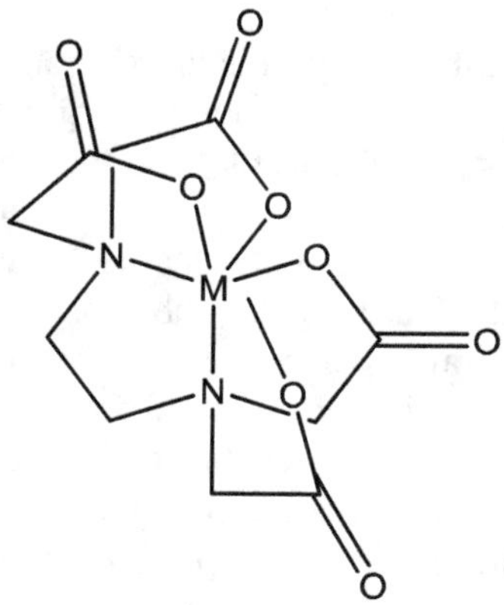

- ***The pH at which the titration is carried out***

  Ethylenediamine tetra-acetic acid ionizes in four stages (pK_1=2.0, pK_2=2.67, pK_3=6.16 and pK_4=10.26). The actual complexing species being Y^{4-}, the complexes will be formed more efficiently and would be more stable in alkaline solution. If the solubility product of the metal hydroxide is low and if the hydroxyl ion concentration is highly increased, it may be precipitated. On the other hand, at lower pH values when the concentration of Y^{4-} is lower, the stability constant of the complexes will not be greater. Complexes of most divalent metals are stable in solution of ammonia. Complexes of the alkaline earth metals, such as copper, lead and nickel, are stable at pH below 3 and hence, these can be titrated selectively in the presence of alkaline earth metals. Trivalent metal complexes are usually still more tightly bound and are stable in strong acid solutions. For example, the cobalt (III) edetate complex is stable in concentrated hydrochloric acid. Over a fair range of pH most complexes are stable, and the solutions are usually buffered at a pH at which the complex is stable and at which the colour change of the indicator is most distinct.

- The presence of interfering ions such as CN^-, Citrate, Tartrate, F^- and other complex forming agents.
- Solvent used in titration. Organic solvents also increase the stability of complex.

6.2 CLASSIFICATION OF LIGANDS

- *Unidentate Ligands:*

  When a ligand is bound to metal ion only at one place, the ligand is called unidentate ligand or one toothed ligand. For example, ammonia (NH_3) is a common unidentate ligand which forms complex with cupric ions, $[Cu(NH_3)_4]^{2+}$. This is formed in four steps as follows:

  $$\text{Step I} \qquad Cu^{2+} + NH_3 \leftrightarrow Cu(NH_3)^{2+}$$
  $$\text{Step II} \qquad Cu(NH_3)^{2+} + NH_3 \leftrightarrow Cu(NH_3)_2^{2+}$$
  $$\text{Step III} \qquad Cu(NH_3)_2^{2+} + NH_3 \leftrightarrow Cu(NH_3)_3^{2+}$$
  $$\text{Step IV} \qquad Cu(NH_3)_3^{2+} + NH_3 \leftrightarrow Cu(NH_3)_4^{2+}$$

  The overall reaction $\ Cu^{2+} + 4NH_3 \leftrightarrow Cu(NH_3)_4^{2+}$

  Other examples monodentate or unidentate are halide ion, cyanide ions.

- *Bidentate and Multidentate Ligands:*

  The ligands that contain more than one group and capable of binding with metal ions are called *multidentate ligand*. These multidentateligands or chelating agents may be bidentate ligands when contain two donor atoms, tridentate ligands when contain three donor atoms, quadridentate ligands when contain four donor atoms, etc. Thus, ethylene diamine, $H_2N\text{-}CH_2\text{-}CH_2\text{-}NH_2$ is a bidentate ligand; while ethylene diamine tetra-acetic acid, (EDTA) is a quadridentate ligand.

Ethylene diamine tetra-acetic acid, (EDTA)

Co-ordination compound or chelate compound or chelate:

When complexes are formed with the ligands (simple ligands) having only one bond are called **co-ordination compound**. The complex of a metal ion with a multidentate ligand (having 2 or more groups) is called a **chelate** or a **chelate compound**. The difference between co-ordination compound and a chelate compound is that in a chelate compound, the ring influences the stability of compound; otherwise there is no difference between these two. Therefore, a chelate possesses a heterocyclic ring structure in which a metal atom is a constituent of the ring. Generally, a chelate is usually more stable than corresponding unidentate metal complex.

- ***Chelating agent:***

Ligands having more than one electron donating groups are described as **chelating agents**. If a ligand contains ionizable amino and carboxylate groups, it becomes the most effective complexing agent. All the multidentate ligands which are important in analytical chemistry contain the structure component as follows:

$$-\!\!-N \begin{cases} CH_2COOH \\ CH_2COOH \end{cases}$$

The metal chelates containing hydrophilic groups such as COOH, SO_3H, NH_2 and OH are soluble in water. When the complex contains both acidic and basic groups, it becomes soluble over a wide range of pH. in absence of hydrophilic groups, the solubilities of both the chelating agent and the metal chelate become low; however, these are soluble in organic solvents. The chelating agents that form water-soluble complexes with bi- or poly-valent metal ions are generally called as *sequestering agent*. Although the metals remain in solution, they fail to give normal ionic reactions. Ethylenediamine tetra-acetic acid is a sequestering agent; it reacts with most polyvalent metal ions to form water-soluble complexes. The complexes formed cannot be extracted from aqueous solutions with organic solvents. Such reaction is generally used for analysis of these ions by titration with a standard EDTA solution. Such titrations are called complexometric or chilometric or EDTA titrations.

Whereas dimethylglyoxime and salicylaldoxime are chelating agents, form insoluble complexes and can be extracted with organic solvents. For example, nickel dimethylglyoxime has a sufficiently low solubility in water and is used in gravimetric assay.

The structures of EDTA, ionized and non-ionized forms are shown below:

$$HOOC.CH_2 \diagdown \atop HOOC.CH_2 \diagup N-CH_2-CH_2-N {\diagup CH_2COOH \atop \diagdown CH_2COOH}$$

Ethylenediaminetetra-acetic acid
(Non-ionized form)

$$\underset{\underset{\text{OOC.CH}_2}{\text{HOOC.CH}_2}}{\Big\rangle}\overset{+}{\text{N}}-\text{CH}_2-\text{CH}_2-\text{N}\overset{+}{\Big\langle}\underset{\text{CH}_2\text{COOH}}{\overset{\text{CH}_2\text{COO}^-}{}}$$

Ethylenediaminetetra-acetic acid
(Zwitterion - ionized form)

6.3 CLASSIFICATION OF METAL ION (ANALYTE CATION)

Schwarzenbach classified the metal ions into three categories –

1. Cations with noble gas configurations (class A),
2. Cations with completely filled *d* sub shells (class B), and
3. Transition metal ions with incomplete *d* sub shells.

Metal ions are Lewis acids (electron acceptors). He categorized the metal ions on the basis of order of electron affinity towards the electron donors in aqueous solution. The order of electron donating capacity of halogens is $F^->>Cl^->Br^->I^-$. Class A metals can form the most stable complexes with first member of each group of donor atoms in the periodic table (that is nitrogen, oxygen and fluorine).

Class B metals can form more easily the coordinate compounds with I^- than F^- in aqueous solution and form most stable complexes with the second donor (heavier) such as phosphorus, sulphur, chlorine of each group.

1. *Cations with noble gas configurations*

   The alkali metals, alkaline earths and aluminium belong to the class A metals. These metals accept electron from the donor atoms. In formation of complexes the force responsible is the electrostatic force. Hence, the small ions carrying high charge interact and form strong and stable complexes. The features of class A metal ions are;

   - Small size,

   - Oxidation state is highly positive,

   - Absence of outer electrons which are usually and easily excited to higher state.

2. *Cations with completely filled d-sub shells*

   Copper (I), silver (I) and gold (I) belong to the class B metal ions and electrons from the donor   atom. These metal ions possess greater polarizing power and form covalent bond with the atoms of a ligand. Thus, complexes are formed.

   - Large size,

   - Oxidation state is either low or zero,

   - Outer electrons of *d* sub shell can be easily excited to higher state.

3. *Transition metal ions with incomplete d- sub shells*

In periodic table the elements having class B remain in almost roughly triangular group. Where, copper remains at the apex and rhenium to bismuth remain at the base line. The elements at the left side of the group in the higher state of oxidation behave like class A elements; while the elements at the side in their higher state of oxidation behave like class B elements.

If the behaviour of class A and class B elements is characterized the principle of soft and hard acids and bases may be of use. A hard base is considered to contain the low polarizable and electronegative donor atom which is not easily oxidized. In other words, a base in which the donor atom contains tightly held electrons which cannot be easily removed or altered. Similarly, the properties of a soft base are just opposite to those of a hard base. That is, the donor atom of a hard base is highly polarizable and of low electronegativity. Thus, the donor atom of a soft base can easily oxidize. The electrons are not held tightly in its donor atom and can easily be removed or distorted.

Accordingly, class A metal ions (electron acceptor) favor to be attached to hard base such as N, O, F atoms. Similarly, class B metal ions (electron acceptor) prefer to be attached to soft bases such as P, As, S, Se, Cl, Br, I atoms. Generally, hard acids prefer to bind with hard bases and soft acids prefer to bind with soft bases. However, under certain conditions hard acids bind with soft bases and soft acids with hard bases.

6.4 DETECTION OF END POINT

Similar to other titrations success of a complexometric titration (EDTA titration) depends on the accurate determination of the end point. The end point of a complexometric titration can be detected by two methods – (1) indicator method and (2) instrumental method.

6.4.1 Instrumental Method

- *Amperometric titration:* The half-wave potential of an ion becomes more negative when metal ions are complexed. In this method the electrode potential is adjusted to a value of the half-wave potential of the free metal cation and to that of the metal complex before titration. Then the titration is carried out by slow addition of disodium EDTA solution. The diffusion current will gradually and steadily fall until it equals the residual current (that is, until the last trace of free cation has been complexed). This is taken as the end point of the titration and the amount of standard disodium EDTA solution added is considered equivalent to the amount of metal present.

- *Potentiometric titration:* Disodium edetate (EDTA) reacts preferentially with the ions of higher valency state. As a result, the redox potential is reduced according to the equation,

$$E = E_0 + \log_e [Ox]/[Red]$$

where,   E = the potential of the electrode

         E_o= the standard electrode potential

         [Ox] = activity of the ions in the oxidized state

         [Red] = activity of the ions in the reduced state

Due to the lack of suitable indicator electrodes this method has limited application. However, iron (III) and copper (II) can be titrated following this method. Excess of standard solution of disodium edetate is first added and then, the excess disodium edetate is titrated with ferric chloride in acid solution (back titration) is carried out for some ions.

- ***High frequency titrator:*** When the concentration of the solution is as low as 0.0002M, this method is suitable. The ions in buffered solution may be titrated directly or excess reagent can be added to the unbuffered solution and the liberated protons may be titrated with standard alkali. Since buffer solution and other extraneous electrolytes reduce the sensitivity of the titration, their concentration must be kept to a minimum.

- ***Spectrophotometric detection:*** When a metal ion of a complexing agent is converted to the metal complex, or when one complex is converted to another, and solution is more dilute the change can be detected more accurately in absorption spectrum more accurately. The visual method does not provide accurate result. Hence, in disodium EDTA titrations an accurate end point can be obtained using 0.001M solutions. Generally, if an indicator gives a prominent colour change, the visible region is used; but the colored ions can be titrated in absence of an indicator using spectrophotometric method. For colorless ions and complexes this method can be used to detect the end point even in the ultraviolet region.

6.4.2 Metal Ion Indicators

The metal ions complexed with dyestuffs are used in EDTA titrations. Like EDTA the dyestuff acts as chelating agent. The dyestuff molecule contains several ligand atoms which can co-ordinate compounds with metal ions. The ligand atom must have the ability to accept proton and result a change in color. Generally, the dyestuff form complex with a specific metal cation at a ratio of 1:1. However, the ratio may vary from 1:1 to 1:2 or 2:1.

The metal ion indicator can be considered not only as pM indicator but also as pH indicator. The metal ion indicators should have following characteristics:

- ➢ Near the end point when almost all the metal ions are complexed with EDTA (ligand) a strong color should be produced.
- ➢ For reaction between metal ion and indicator, the indicator should be selective and specific.
- ➢ The complex formed by metal ion with indicator must be sufficiently stable; so that a sharp change in color of the indicator (complex) is obtained. However, stability of the complex (metal-indicator) should be less than that of the metal-EDTA complex; so that at the end point the metal-indicator complexes can release the

metal ions for complexing with EDTA (principal reaction) and rapid and sharp color change at equilibrium can be detected.

➢ The color of free indicator and of metal ion-indicator must be in the range at which the titration is carried out.

As mentioned earlier that in complexometric titrations pM indicators are used, the concept of such indicators should be known and hence is briefly described below;

Say the stability constant of the metal-indicator complex is K; then

$$K = \frac{[MX]}{[M][X]}$$

Or,

$$[M] = \frac{[MX]}{K[X]}$$

Or,

$$\log [M] = \log \frac{[MX]}{K[X]} = \log \frac{[MX]}{[X]} - \log K$$

Or,

$$-\log[M] = -(\log \frac{[MX]}{[X]} - \log K) = \log \frac{[X]}{[MX]} - pK$$

Or,

$$pM = \log \frac{[X]}{[MX]} - pK$$

If a solution contains equal activities of metal complex and free chelating agent, the concentration of metal ions will remain roughly constant; that is $[X] = [MX]$, then $pM = -pK$ (or $pM = pK'$, where K' = dissociation constant). This indicates that solution should be buffered in the same way as hydrogen ions in a pH buffer. However, chelating agents are also bases and equilibrium in a metal-buffer solution is frequently affected by a change in pH. Generally, in case of chelating agents of the amino acid type such as edetic acid and ammonia triacetic acid, if $[X] = [MX]$, pM increases with pH until it reaches up to 10 and it remains almost constant. Thus, the titrations of metals with chelating agents in buffered solutions should be preferably carried out at this pH.

This has been mentioned earlier that pM indicator is a dye and such dye can act as a chelating agent to produce a dye-metal complex. Colour of the latter is different from that of the dye itself. It also has a low stability constant than the chelate-metal complex. Therefore, the colour of the solution remains that of the dye complex until the end point is reached. At this point when the slightest excess of EDTA is added, the metal-dye complex decomposes to produce free dye and the color changes.

More than 200 organic compounds form colored chelates with ions in a pM range that is unique to the cation and selected dye. The color of dye-metal chelates is visible even at concentration of 10^{-6} to 10^{-7} M.

The typical properties of acid-base indicators are similar to those of many of these indicators. The colour changes as a result of displacement of the H^+ ion by metal ion.

Metal ion indicators must have the following properties:

➢ Chelates must be chemically stable throughout the titration.

➢ The metal should form complex with the indicator at a ratio of 1:1 and the complex must be weaker than the metal chelate complex.

➤ The colors of the indicator and the metal complexed indicator must be different.
➤ Color reaction should be selective for the metal being titrated.
➤ The indicator should not compete with the EDTA

Mechanism of action of indicator:

Let M stands for the metal and I for indicator, and CH stands for the chelate. At the beginning of the titration, the reaction mixture contains the metal-indicator complex (MI) and excess of metal ion. When EDTA (titrant) is gradually added to the medium, a competitive reaction takes place between the free metal ions and EDTA. Since the metal-indicator complex (MI) is weaker than the metal-EDTA chelate (CH). When EDTA is added during the titration it forms complex with the free metal ions in solution at the expense of the MI complex. At the end point, EDTA removes the last traces of the metal from the metal-indicator complex and the color of the indicator changes from its complexed color to its metal free color. The overall reaction is expressed as:

$$MI + M + EDTA \rightarrow M\text{-}EDTA + I$$

(Color of the metal-
indicator complex)   (Color of free indicator)

Structures of some important indicators used in complexometric titrations are given below. Many compounds have been used as indicators as shown in Table below.

➤ Triphenyl methane dyes
➤ Phthalein and substituted phthalein
➤ Azo dyes
➤ Phenolic compounds

S. No	Name of the indicator	Color change	pH range	Metals detected
1	Eriochrome black T	Red – Blue	6 – 7	Ca, Mg, Ba, Zn, Cd, Mn, Pb, Hg
	Solochrome black T			
	Mordant black II			
2	Murexide or Ammonium purpurate	Violet – Blue	12	Ca, Cu, Co
3	Catechol violet	Violet – Red	8 – 10	Mn, Mg, Fe, Co, Pb
4	Methyl blue	Blue – Yellow	4 – 5	Pb, Zn, Cd, Hg
	Thymol blue	Blue – Grey	10 – 12	
5	Alizarin	Red – Yellow	4.3	Pb. Zn, Co, Mg, Cu
6	Sodium Alizaeinsulphonate	Blue – Red	4	Al, Th
7	Xylenol orange	Lemon yellow – Yellow	1 – 3	Bi, Th
			4 – 5	Pb, Zn
			5 – 6	Cd, Hg

Structure of some pM indicators

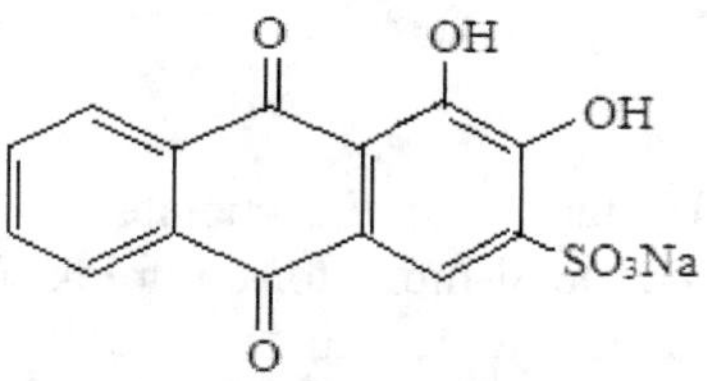

Sodium Alizarin sulphonate

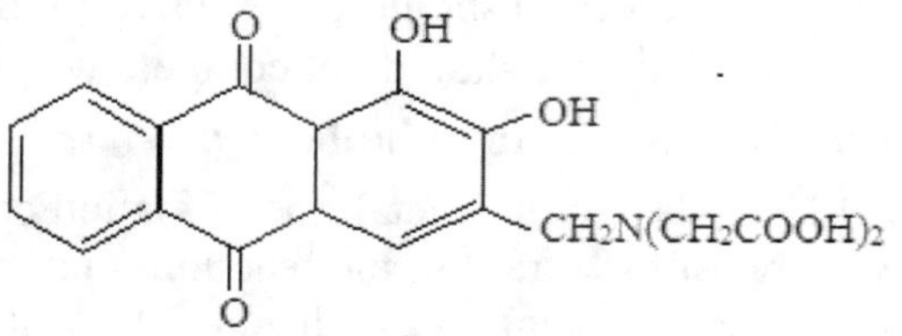

Alizarin fluorine blue (alizarin complexone)

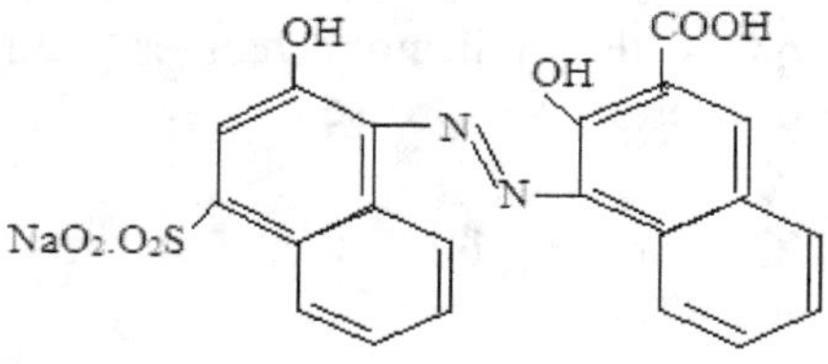

Calcone carboxylic acid

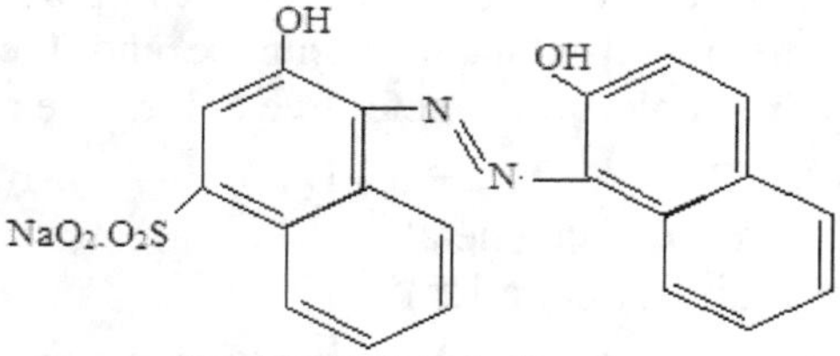

Mordant black 17 (calcone)

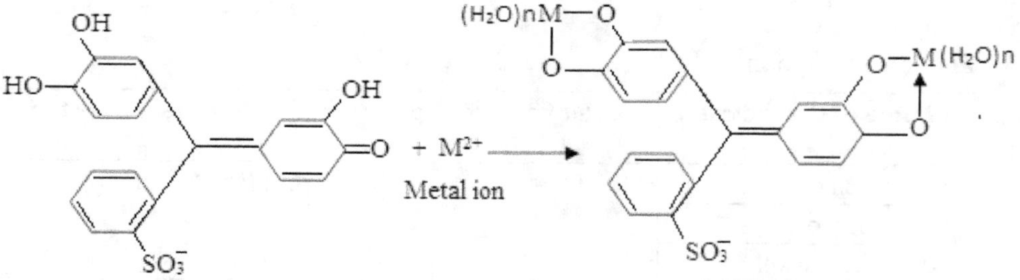

Catechol violet $+ M^{2+}$
                               Metal ion

Metal-indicator complex

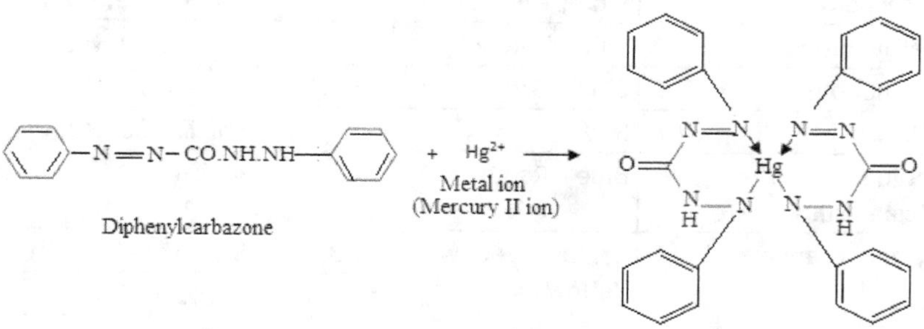

Diphenylcarbazone $+$ Hg^{2+}
                         Metal ion
                         (Mercury II ion)

Metal-indicator complex

Murexide

(HCOOH₂C)₂.NH₂C

Xylenol Orange

6.5 MASKING AND DEMASKING REAGENTS

Sometimes samples contain mixture of metal ions and each metal ion present in such sample is analyzed. Say a mixture of metal A, B and C is to be tested to determine the amount of each of A, B and C present in the mixture. To analyze the metal A others (B and C) are to be made nonresponsive or nonreactive. Similarly, to determine content of B, other metals (A and C) are to be made nonresponsive or nonreactive and the metal B is to be made active. There are substances which can make the metal ions nonresponsive or nonreactive (Masking agent) and there are substances which can make the masked-metal ion responsive or reactive (Demasking agent). *The process in which a substance or its reaction product is transformed without being separated physically or does not enter into a particular reaction is called masking.* In complexometric titrations by using the masking agentssome of themetal ions can be masked or blocked so that these cations cannot react with EDTA or with the indicator. The masking agents form insoluble complex with the metal ion and can precipitate the complex formed. These complexes would be more stable than the interfering ion-EDTA complex. General equation expressing complexation between the masking agents such as cyanide ion and a metal ion is:

$$M^{2+} + 4CN^- \rightarrow [M(CN)_4]^{2-}$$

Some of masking agents are mentioned below;

- ➤ *Masking by Precipitation:*The heavy metals such as Co, Cu and Pb can be separated either in the form of insoluble sulphides using sodium sulphide, or as insoluble complexes using thioacetamide. These can be filtered, decomposed and titrated with disodium EDTA. There are other precipitating agents commonly used. For example, sulphate for Pb and Ba; oxalate for Ca and Pb; fluoride for Ca, Mg and Pb; ferrocyanide for Zn and Cu, and 8-hydroxy quinoline for many heavy metals. To mask Cu by precipitation in the assay of lotions containing Cu and Zn thioglycerol (CH₂SH.CHOH.CH₂OH) is used.

- ➤ *Masking by Complex formation:*With the interfering metal ions masking agents form more stable complexes. The most important feature is that the masking agent does not form complexes with the metal ion which are being analyzed. The few masking agents used are:

1. Ammonium fluoridemasks aluminium, iron and titanium by complex formation.

2. Ascorbic acidis commonly used reducing agent for iron (III) which is subsequently masked by complexing as the very stable hexacyanoferrate (II) complex which is more stable and less intensely colored than the hexacyanoferrate (III) complex.

3. 2,3-Dimercaptopropanol, $CH_2SH.CHSH.CH_2OH$ (Dimercaprol)react with mercury, cadmium, zinc, arsenic, tin, lead and bismuth in weakly acidic solution to form precipitates. These precipitates are soluble in alkaline solution.

4. All these complexes are stronger than the corresponding edetate-complexes and are almost colorless. Under the above conditions' cobalt, copper and nickel form intense yellowish-green complexes. Dimercaprol can replace cobalt and copper from their edetate complexes, but not nickel.

➢ ***Potassium cyanide***: With silver, copper, mercury, iron, zinc, cadmium, cobalt and nickel ions react with potassium cyanide and form complexes in alkaline medium. In this case the complexes are more stable than the corresponding edetate-complexes. Hence, other ions such as lead, magnesium, manganese and the alkaline earth metals can be analyzed in their presence. Aldehydes such as formaldehyde or chloral hydrate prefer to form complex, cyanohydrins; thus, the metals in the first group of periodic table such as zinc and cadmium can be demasked from their cyanide complexes and can be selectively titrated.

➢ ***Potassium iodide:*** It is specific for mercury and is used to mask the mercury (II) ion as $(HgI_4)^{2-}$. Hence, can be used in the assay of mercury (II) chloride.

➢ ***Disodium catechol-3,5-disulphonate (Tiron):***Aluminium and titanium can be masked as colorless complexes by tiron. However, it forms highly colored complex with iron forms and is used to mask as hexacyanoferrate (II) complex.

➢ ***Triethanolamine*** $[N(CH_2CH_2OH)_3]$**:** Triethanolamine forms a colorless complex with aluminium and yellow complex with iron (III). The yellow colour of complex with iron is almost discharged if sodium hydroxide solution is added to it. Mordant black II is oxidized by the green manganese (III) complex. Therefore, if murexide is used in the presence of iron and manganese, these can be best masked with triethanolamine and mordant black II can be used safely in the presence of triethanolamine-aluminium complex.

Kinetic masking:

There are certain metal ions which are kinetically inert and do not effectively participate in the complexation reaction. The process of masking utilizing this property is known as kinetic masking. Thus, *it is a special case of masking where in a metal ion does not effectively participate in the complexation reaction due to its kinetic inertness.* For example, chromium does not react with EDTA in cold condition, reacts at higher temperature. Hence, if a solution contains a mixture of iron and chromium (III), iron can be determined by cooling the solution using standard solution of EDTA (titrant) and xylenol orange (indicator), chromium shall not interfere. The titrated solution if is heated to boiling state, chromium can be determined, and iron will not interfere in determination.

Demasking:

Demasking is the process which enables the masked substance to participate again in a particular reaction. As a result, more than one metal ion present in the same solution can be determined. For example, zinc ion masked by cyanide ion (zinc-cyanide complex) can be demasked by formaldehyde in acid solution as follows;

$$[Zn(CN)_4]^{2-} + 4H^+ + 4HCHO \rightarrow Zn^{2+} + 4HO.CH_2.CN$$

After demasking zinc present in the solution can be satisfactorily determined. Similarly, a solution containing three metal ions such as Ca, Cu, and Cd can be analyzed as follows;

1. The solution is titrated with EDTA directly and total quantity of three metals present is determined.

$$\begin{array}{ll} \text{Ca} & \text{Ca-EDTA} \\ \text{Cd} + \text{EDTA} \rightleftharpoons & \text{Cd-EDTA} \\ \text{Cu} & \text{Cu-EDTA} \end{array}$$

2. By adding cyanide to the solution Cu and Cd are masked, leaving Ca free for analysis. The amount of Ca is determined by EDTA.

$$\text{Cu} + \text{Cyanide ion} \xrightarrow{\text{Masking}} \text{Cu-Cyanide complex}$$

$$\text{Cd} + \text{Cyanide ion} \xrightarrow{\text{Masking}} \text{Cd-Cyanide complex}$$

$$\text{Ca} + \text{Cyanide} \longrightarrow \text{No reaction} \xrightarrow{\text{EDTA}} \text{Ca-EDTA complex}$$

3. By adding formaldehyde or chloral hydrate on Cd is demasked and the mixture of Cd and Ca is determined. By subtracting the value obtained in (2) from that of (3) the amount of Cd present can be calculated.

$$\text{Cd-Cyanide complex} + \text{HCHO} \xrightarrow{\text{Demasking}} \text{Cd ion (free)}$$

$$\text{Cu-Cyanide complex} + \text{HCHO} \xrightarrow{\text{No demasking}} \text{No reaction}$$

$$\begin{array}{ll} \text{Ca} \\ \text{Cd} + \text{EDTA} \longrightarrow & \begin{array}{l}\text{Ca-EDTA} \\ \text{Cd-EDTA}\end{array} \end{array}$$

4. By subtracting the value of (2) from that of (1) the amount of Cu present can be calculated. Thus, all the three metal ions are quantitatively analyzed individually.

6.6 ESTIMATION OF MAGNESIUM SULPHATE

Magnesium sulphate, $MgSO_4$, $7H_2O$ has molecular mass of 246.47. The purity of it can be determined as follows:

- ➢ Weigh accurately about 0.15g of the sample and transfer it into a clean 250 mL conical flask,
- ➢ Add 50 mL of freshly distilled water,
- ➢ Add 10 mL of strong ammonia-ammonium chloride solution
- ➢ Add 0.1g of mordant black II mixture (indicator)
- ➢ Titrate the solution with 0.05M disodium edetate (standard solution) until a blue color is obtained. Note the volume of 0.05M disodium edetate solution consumed (titer value, x mL).
- ➢ Perform a blank titration; note the volume of 0.05M disodium edetate solution consumed (y mL).
- ➢ Deduct the blank titer value from the main titer value (x - y) mL.
- ➢ Each mL of 0.05M disodium edetate solution is equivalent to 0.00602g of MgSO4. Calculate the percent purity of the sample.

Calculation

Say, the actual amount of sample weighed and taken = 0.1507g

The volume of 0.05M disodium edetate consumed = ($x - y$ =24.50) mL

The strength of 0.05M disodium edetate solution = 0.05015M

Then, % purity of the sample

$$= \frac{\text{Titer value} \times \text{Actual Strength of 0.05M disodium edetate} \times 0.00602g \times 100}{\text{Weight of sample taken} \times \text{Strength of 0.05M disodium edetate (Theoretical)}}$$

$$= \frac{24.50 \text{ mL} \times 0.05015M \times 0.00602g \times 100}{0.1507g \times 0.05000M}$$

$$= 98.16$$

Reagents:

1. Strongammonia-ammonium chloride solution – dissolve 6.75g of ammonium chloride in 74 mL of strong ammonia solution and dilute the solution to 100 mL with distilled water.

2. Mordant black II is also called as Eriochrome black T or Solochrome black. Mordant black II mixture is a mixture of 1 part of mordant black II and 99 parts of sodium chloride.

6.7   ESTIMATION OF CALCIUM GLUCONATE

The molecular formula of calcium gluconate is $C_{12}H_{22}CaO_{14}$, H_2O; its molecular weight is 448.40. The purity of this material can be determined by following method.

> Weigh accurately about 0.5g of the sample and transfer it into a clean 250 mL conical flask,

> Dissolve the material in 50 mL of warm distilled water, allow to cool to room temperature,

> Add 5.00 mL of 0.05M magnesium sulphate solution,

> Add 10 mL of strong ammonia solution, mix thoroughly,

> Add 0.1g of mordant black II mixture as indicator,

> Titrate the mixture with 0.05M disodium edetate solution till blue color is produced, note the volume of 0.05M magnesium sulphate solution consumed (titer value, x mL).

> Perform a blank titration and note the volume of 0.05M magnesium sulphate solution required, ymL. Subtract the blank titer value from the main titer value for calculation $(x - y)$ mL.

> Calculate the volume of 0.05M disodium edetate solution equivalent to 5.00 mL of 0.05M magnesium sulphate; say zmL. Deduct this volume from $(x - y)$ mL; that is, $(x - y - z)$ mL. Each mL of 0.05M disodium edetate solution equivalent to 0.02242g of $C_{12}H_{22}CaO_{14}, H_2O$.

Calculation

Say, the amount of sample actually taken = a g

The volume of 0.05M disodium edetate solution consumed by the sample = $(x - y - z)$ mL

The strength of 0.05M disodium edetate solution = b M

Then, the % purity of sample =

$$\frac{(x - y - z)\text{mL} \times \text{Actual Strength of 0.05M disodium edetate} \times 0.02242\text{g} \times 100}{\text{Weight of sample taken} \times \text{Strength of 0.05M disodium edetate (Theoretical)}}$$

A. MULTIPLE CHOICE QUESTIONS

1. Complexing agent is also called as
   - (a) Chilons
   - (b) Sequestering agent
   - (c) Chelating agent
   - (d) All of the above

2. Name of product of complexometric titration is
   - (a) Chelate
   - (b) Ligand
   - (c) Sequester
   - (d) None of the above

3. The bonds between the metal ion and ligand may be
   - (a) Electrovalent bond
   - (b) Covalent bond
   - (c) Hydrogen bond
   - (d) All of the above

4. In a complexometric titration ethylenediamine tetra-acetic acid (EDTA) forms
   - (a) Cation only
   - (b) Anion only
   - (c) Zwitterions
   - (d) All of the above

5. The features of class A analyte cations are
   - (a) Smaller in size
   - (b) Oxidation state is highly positive,
   - (c) Absence of outer electrons which are usually and easily excited to higher state.
   - (d) All of the above

6. Features of class B analyte cations are
   - (a) Large size,
   - (b) Oxidation state is either low or zero,
   - (c) Outer electrons of d sub shell can be easily excited to higher state
   - (d) All of the above

7. Which one of the following is a class of analyte metal ions?
   - (a) Unidentate
   - (b) Bidentate
   - (c) Cations with completely filled d sub shells
   - (d) None of the above

8. Which one of the following is a class A analyte metal ion?
   - (a) Aluminium
   - (b) Copper II
   - (c) Silver
   - (d) Gold

9. Ethylenediamine tetra-acetic acid ionizes in
   - (a) One stage
   - (b) Two stages
   - (c) Four stages
   - (d) Three stages

10. Ligand is described as chelating agent, when it has
    - (a) More than one electron donating groups
    - (b) Only one electron donating group
    - (c) No electron donating groups
    - (d) None of the above

11. Irrespective of the valency of the ion,ethylenediamine tetra-acetic acid forms complexes with most cations
    - (a) In a 1:2 ratio
    - (b) In a 1:1 ratio
    - (c) In a 2:1 ratio
    - (d) All of the above

12. The end point of a complexometric titration can be detected by
    - (a) Amperometric method
    - (b) Potentiometric method
    - (c) Indicator method
    - (d) All of the above

13. In EDTA titration the end point is due to the
    (a) Change of color of indicator as in acid-base titration
    (b) Complexation of metal ion with EDDTA
    (c) Complexation of metal ion with dyestuff
    (d) None of the above

14. In EDTA titration masking is done to
    (a) Suppress the unpleasant odor
    (b) Suppress the metal ions other than what is being estimated
    (c) Suppress the unpleasant color
    (d) None of the above

15. In EDTA titration masking is done by
    (a) Potassium cyanide
    (b) Potassium iodide
    (c) Triethanolamine
    (d) All of the above

16. Kinetic masking is the process that
    (a) Utilizes the kinetic inertness of a metal ion
    (b) Makes a particular metal ion inert using kinetic energy
    (c) Makes a particular metal ion inert using ultrasonic rays
    (d) None of the above

17. Demasking is the process of activation of the masked substance by
    (a) Using kinetic energy
    (b) Demasking agent
    (c) Withdrawing masking agent
    (d) All of the above

18. Which of the following is used as demasking agent?
    (a) Formaldehyde
    (b) Sodium cyanide
    (c) Sodium chloride
    (d) Ammonium chloride

19. The indicator used in estimation of magnesium sulphate is
    (a) Mordant black II mixture
    (b) Eriochrome black T
    (c) Solochrome black
    (d) All of the above

20. During estimation of calcium gluconate which of following solution is added?
    (a) Sodium sulphate
    (b) Magnesium sulphate
    (c) Calcium sulphate
    (d) None of the above

B. SHORT QUESTIONS

1. What is chilometric titration?
2. What is Ligand?
3. What is chelate?
4. Express the complexometric titration in form of equation
5. What is meant by stability of a complex?

6. Classify the ligands.
7. What are chelating agents?
8. How can the analyte cations be classified?
9. What is meant by 'Cations with noble gas configurations'?
10. How can the end points of complexometric titrations be detected?
11. What do you understand by 'masking' and 'demasking' phenomena?
12. Write the importance of 'masking' and 'demasking' reagents in complexometric titrations.
13. What are kinetic masking and demasking?

C. LONG QUESTIONS

1. Explain how bonds are involved in formation of complexes.
2. Discuss briefly the principle of complexometric titration.
3. Explain the factors that influence the determination of the magnitude of break in titration   curve at end point.
4. Explain the statement, "Complexometric titration becomes easy when single complex species are formed".
5. Discuss the factors that influence the reaction with EDTA.
6. Write note on 'co-ordination-compound'.
7. Explain the classification of metal ions with appropriate example.
8. Discuss in brief about the metal ion indicators.
9. Explain how an indicator works in complexometric titration.
10. Illustrate the 'masking' and 'demasking' reagent using suitable examples.
11. Write down the method used to estimate magnesium sulphate.
12. Write down the method used to estimate calcium gluconate.

CHAPTER 7

Gravimetry

INTRODUCTION

The term gravimetry means gravi (weigh) + metry (measure). Gravimetric analysis is a quantitative method of analysis by weight. It is a process of isolating/separating a particular component from a weighed quantity of sample in a pure form and weighing.

In traditional gravimetric analysis an element or radical present in a sample is determined by transforming into a pure stable compound. The compound prepared is isolated from the sample in the form of a precipitate. The precipitate is isolated in pure form, dried or ignited and weighed. The mass of an element, ion or radical present in the known amount of sample is then calculated using atomic, ionic or radical mass.

Types of gravimetric analysis

Gravimetric analysis can be divided into four basic categories based on the method of preparation of the sample:

1. Physical gravimetry,
2. Thermogravimetry,
3. Precipitative gravimetry, and
4. Electrodeposition

1. *Physical gravimetry:* It is the most common type gravimetric analysis. This method is used in engineering. In this method the mixture of substances are physically separated on basis of

LEARNING OBJECTIVES

After studying the chapter the students familiarize themselves with the following concepts:

✓ Principle and steps involved in gravimetric analysis
✓ Purity of the precipitate: co-precipitation and post precipitation
✓ Estimation of barium sulphate

volatility and particle size. Most common analytes are total solids, suspended solids, dissolved solids, surfactants, oil and grease.

2. *Thermogravimetry:* In this method the mass of a substance is determined as a function of temperature. The substance is subjected to a controlled temperature programme. This method is used in different areas such pharmacy, foods, polymer science, glasses and volatile solids.

3. *Electrodeposition:* In this method the metal ions are electrochemically reduced at a cathode. The ions subsequently deposit on the cathode. The cathode is weighed before and after electrolysis. The difference between two weights represents the mass of analyte originally present in the sample. The method is generally used in environmental engineering analysis.

4. *Precipitative gravimetry:* Precipitative gravimetry is based on the chemical precipitation of an analyte.

The **advantages** of this method are;

➢ The method is accurate and precise when modern analytical balances are used.

➢ Since filtrates can be tested for completeness of precipitation, possible sources of error are readily controlled.

➢ The precipitates may be examined for the presence of impurities.

➢ This method involves direct measurement, does not require any calibration, except the balance.

➢ Most of the apparatuses required for the analysis are cheap except muffle furnace, and sometimes platinum crucible. Thus, the method is inexpensive.

➢ The method is macroscopic and can be performed under normal laboratory conditions.

➢ The method has good repeatability and the results can vary within 0.3 – 0.5%.

Limitation of this method

➢ Accuracy depends on careful performance

➢ It is a time-consuming method

➢ Requires thoroughly clean glassware

➢ Requires very accurate weighing

➢ Co-precipitation takes place commonly and is a major problem

Application of gravimetric method

There are various applications of this method. Most important ones are;

➢ For calibration of instruments and/or of the method, standards should be used for analysis. Hence the method can be used analysis of various components.

➢ Analyses that require high accuracy and quick completion may restrict the application of this method.

➢ Gravimetric and electro-gravimetric methods provide a very broad information/experience in laboratory procedure.

➢ Thermal analysis provides more information about chemical, biochemical structures and reactions that occur under thermal conditions.

7.1 PRINCIPLE AND STEPS INVOLVED IN GRAVIMETRIC ANALYSIS

In this method the constituent to be determined is precipitated from its solution due to various reasons such as common ion effect, change in temperature, etc. The precipitate formed is so slightly soluble that no appreciable loss of the component occurs during its separation, filtration and washing. The filtered precipitate is washed sufficiently till all the possible impurities are removed, dried or ignited, and weighed. For example, in the determination of silver from its solution, an excess of sodium chloride or potassium chloride is added, and silver chloride formed precipitates out due to common ion effect. The precipitate is filtered, washed with water repeatedly till no chloride is present, and then dried at $140 \pm 10°C$ till a constant weight is obtained. The weighed silver chloride is used to calculate the amount of silver present in the sample.

The schematic diagram of the gravimetric method is shown in figure 7.1.

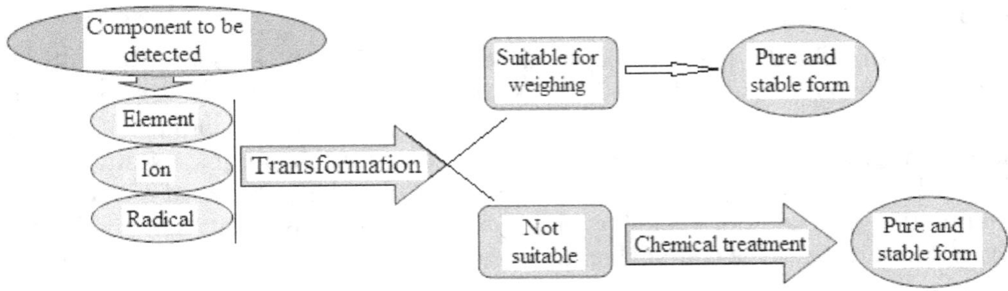

Figure 7.1 Schematic diagram of gravimetric analysis

In some cases, the compositions of precipitate and of dried precipitate are different. For example, in determining magnesium it is precipitated as magnesium ammonium phosphate [[Mg(NH$_4$)PO$_4$, 6H$_2$O]. when the precipitate is ignited the magnesium ammonium phosphate is converted to magnesium pyrophosphate [Mg$_2$P$_2$O$_7$]. According to stoichiometric reaction the amount of magnesium present in the sample is calculated.

The factors that influence successful determination of element/ion/radical by precipitation are;

> The precipitate must be insoluble in the solvent; so that no appreciable amount is lost during filtration and washing.

> The size of the particles in the precipitate must be such that these can be filtered through the filtering medium, such as Whatmann 42 or 44, and the pores of the filtering medium are not plugged with particles and the particles of the precipitate can be washed properly.

> The particles of precipitate should not be affected during washing.

> The precipitate must not be gelatinous and should not peptize in the presence of precipitant. Of course, the precipitate should not be kept longer time in presence of mother liquid to avoid peptization.

> The precipitate must be convertible into a pure substance of definite chemical composition. This may be possible either by ignition or by a simple chemical operation such as evaporation with a suitable liquid.
> The precipitate should be non-hygroscopic and non-reactive with atmosphere and preferentially should be of high molecular weight.

Problems occur when the particles of precipitates coagulate or flocculate in the form of colloidal dispersion. If the particles are very fine, these cannot be filtered through filtering medium easily. In general, the size of the particles is expressed in terms of mμ (milli-micron).

$$1\mu = 10^{-3} \text{ mm}, \ 1m\mu = 0.1 \ \mu = 10^{-6} \text{ mm, and } 1\text{Å} = 10^{-7} \text{ mm} = 0.1 \text{ m}\mu$$

The nucleation process continues to form the precipitate ultimately. The particle size increases as follows:

Ions of 10^{-8} cm size nucleate to form clusters of size range, 10^{-8} to 10^{-7} cm. These form colloidal particles of size range, 10^{-7} to 10^{-4} cm. The colloidal particles form precipitate of size more than 10^{-4} cm.

The sizes of colloidal particles lie within the range from 0.1μ to $1m\mu$. Usually, the pore size of filter paper (filtering medium) is about 10μ. Particles having size of 0.2μ are visible under microscope. If a powerful beam of light is passed through a colloidal solution and the solution is viewed at a right angle to the incident light, a scattering light is observed; this is called *Tyndall effect*. True solution contains particles of molecular size ($0.1m\mu$ or 10^{-6} mm) and does not show the Tyndall effect. Thus, a true solution is called *optically empty*. Size of the colloidal particles can be viewed by using X-ray diffraction.

Factors that influence gravimetric analysis

The factors responsible for complete analysis by precipitation are briefly mentioned here:
- Quantitative formation of precipitate.
- Formation of precipitate must be within a reasonable period of time.
- The solubility of the precipitate must be so low that it is separated quantitatively and not more than 10^{-6} mol of the substance is left in the solution.
- The precipitate obtained must be in accordance with the stoichiometric reaction and the compound is of known composition. Sometimes it is converted to a compound of stoichiometric weighable form of known composition.
- The size of the particle of the precipitate must be such that they could be filtered easily through the filtering medium and remains unaffected by the washing.
- There should not be any impurities remained in the precipitate.

Supersaturation and formation of precipitate

At a particular temperature the solubility of a substance in a given solvent is expressed as the amount of the substance remaining in equilibrium with the solvent. A supersaturated solution contains a greater concentration of solute than that of solute in its saturation at the same temperature. Therefore, super saturation is an unstable state of solution. If a crystal of the solute or of some other substance is added to a super saturated solution or a mechanical means such as shaking or stirring is applied, it brings back to a stable state of solution. In this state the solute remains in equilibrium.

von Weimarn stated that super saturation is important for determination of particle size of a precipitate. According to him the initial velocity of precipitation is proportional to $\frac{(Q-S)}{S}$

Where, Q is the total concentration of the substance which is precipitated and S is the equilibrium solubility, and (Q – S) represents the supersaturation at the time when precipitation starts. However, the equation is applicable when Q >> S. For crystalline precipitate with least adsorption and easy filtration, $\frac{(Q-S)}{S}$ would be very small. However, by increasing S the value of $\frac{(Q-S)}{S}$ can be reduced. For example, the solubility of barium sulphate (BaSO$_4$) in 2N HCl is 50 times more than in water. If 0.1N solutions of barium chloride (BaCl$_2$) and 0.1N solution of sulphuric acid (H$_2$SO$_4$) are prepared in 2N boiling HCl and the solutions are mixed, typical crystalline particles of barium sulphate will precipitate slowly from the solution. Hence, the above concepts are applied in gravimetric method of analysis as mentioned below.

- ➢ Since the solubility of a substance increases with increase in temperature, precipitation should be carried out in hot solution.
- ➢ The reagents should be added slowly with continuous stirring and precipitation should take place from dilute solution. If the reagent is added slowly the particles first added act as seed or nuclei. Subsequently these seeds grow further with addition of the particles (reagent).
- ➢ Sometimes to increase the solubility of the precipitate suitable reagent is added; so that larger primary particles are formed which there after precipitating out.

The steps involved in gravimetric analysis are shown in figure 7.2 and the steps involved in precipitation are shown in the figure 7.3.

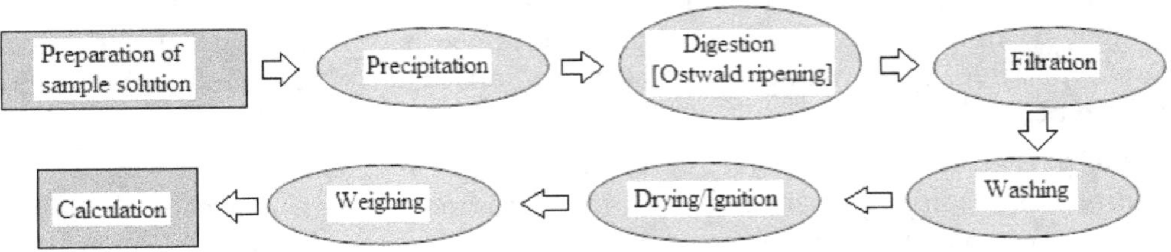

Figure 7.2 Steps involve in the formation of precipitate in gravimetric analysis

Factors affecting precipitation

Choice of precipitant: The precipitating agent (precipitant) should produce a completely insoluble precipitate i.e. solubility product should be within 10^{-6} mol. The structure of the precipitate formed should allow rapid filtration and washing. Organic precipitating agents are very useful in inorganic analysis because these have following advantages;

➢ The chelate compounds are mostly insoluble in water; this facilitates precipitation of metal ions quantitatively.

➢ Most of the organic precipitants have high molecular weights. Hence, a small amount of metal may yield a large weight of precipitate and the weighing errors minimizes.

➢ Some of the organic reagents are fairly selective and yield precipitates with only a limited number of cations. When the factors such as pH and the concentration of masking agents are properly controlled, the selectivity of the organic reagent can be greatly enhanced.

➢ The precipitates obtained with organic reagents are sometimes coarse and bulky; hence these can be easily handled.

➢ Mostly the chelates of metal are anhydrous in nature. The precipitates dry quickly. The process of drying can be made faster by washing the precipitate with alcohol.

Amount of precipitant: The amount of precipitant added is important. The effects of amount of precipitant on the precipitate are briefly mentioned here.

- If the amount of precipitant added is much large, the solubility of the precipitate increases and the precipitate formed redissolves.

- If just sufficient amount is added as per stoichiometric calculation, then precipitation reaction may not be completed; since some amount of precipitant is required to attain the required solubility product value.

- For completion of precipitation reaction, a reasonably excess amount of precipitant is to be added. The excess precipitant gives excess of common ions and the solubility of precipitate is decreased. For similar reason, the precipitate should be washed with a solution containing common ions.

Effect of temperature: At a particular temperature the solubility product of a substance is constant. Usually with the increase in temperature the solubility increases. If the precipitation reaction is carried out at higher temperature, crystal structure of the precipitate becomes better; thus, the precipitate formed is of high purity. For this reason, wherever possible, precipitation should be carried out at higher temperature; but it should be cooled before filtration.

Effect of pH: As such the solubility of a solute changes with pH of the solvent. Thus, the solubility of a precipitate changes if pH of the solution changes. However, the effect of pH depends on the type of precipitate. In general, the precipitate of metal hydroxides and those of sparingly soluble salts of weak acids are precipitated only in alkaline or neutral pH ranges. *Smaller the dissolution constant for the acid, higher is the pH required for practically complete precipitation of its salt.* By controlling the pH the effect of organic reagents can always be improved.

Effect of complex formation: Sometimes the desired component form complex ions in the presence of certain ions. These ions have higher dissociation constants and may result to incomplete precipitation. Hence, the unwanted ions should either be masked or eliminated to prevent them from getting precipitated. Masking of such common ions is done by keeping them in solution. In fact, this procedure is usually followed.

7.2 PURITY OF THE PRECIPITATE: CO-PRECIPITATION AND POST PRECIPITATION

A precipitate separating out from its solution may not be perfectly pure. The purity of the precipitate depends on (1) the nature of the precipitate itself and (2) conditions of precipitation. The precipitate is contaminated with substances (impurities) which are usually soluble in the mother liquor. Such contamination of precipitate with soluble impurities is called *co-precipitation*. Depending on how the impurities are mixed with precipitate, the co-precipitation may be of two types –

1. Adsorption of impurities present in the mother liquor over the surface of the particles of precipitate exposed to the solution; and

2. Occlusion of impurities when the primary particles undergo *crystal growth* for precipitation.

In general, surface adsorption takes place due to three reasons – (1) particle size/ surface area, (2) relative solubility, and (3) extent of dissociation.

1. The surface adsorption is more common when the precipitate is gelatinous in nature. Since gelatinous precipitate contains very fine particles, total surface area of the precipitate is much more than that of macroscopic crystalline precipitate. This increases the extent of adsorption over surface.

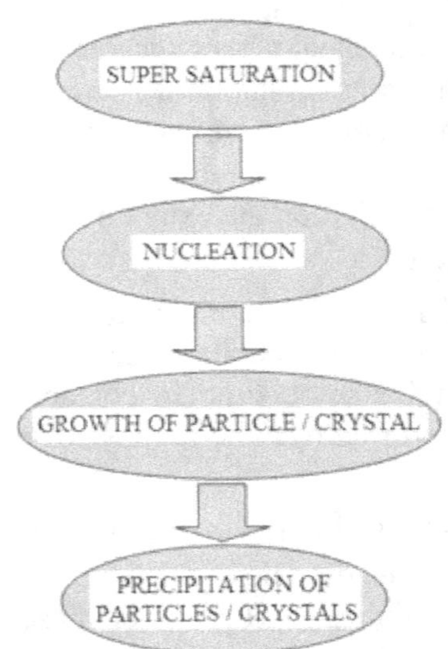

Figure 7.3 Steps involved in precipitation

2. Optimum adsorption may occur due to relative solubilities two ions. For example, calcium ion (Ca^{2+}) prefers to be adsorbed over magnesium ion (Mg^{2+}), because calcium sulphate ($CaSO_4$) is less soluble than magnesium sulphate ($MgSO_4$). Similarly, silver acetate prefers to be absorbed over silver iodide between silver iodide and silver nitrate, because silver acetate is less soluble than silver nitrate.

3. Third reason for adsorption is extent of dissociation. When a compound is less dissociable, it has more tendencies to be adsorbed. For this reason, metallic sulphides adsorb hydrogen sulphide (H_2S) strongly.

Post precipitation

Post precipitation introduces appreciable error. It occurs on the surface of the precipitate which is first precipitated after formation. Usually this happens with sparingly soluble substances which form super saturated solution. Such substance contains a ion in common with the primary precipitate. If it is allowed to stand in the mother liquid for some time, it precipitates some other substances. For example, in the presence of magnesium, magnesium oxalate, calcium oxalate, precipitate out gradually. If the precipitate is allowed to remain in contact with the solution, the extent of error will increase. Similarly, if copper sulphide or mercury sulphide from 0.3N hydrochloric acid in the presence of Zn^{2+} ion; ZnS is precipitated slowly as post precipitate. The difference between post-precipitation and co-precipitation are;

- ➢ In post-precipitation the contamination increases with time of contact with mother liquor.
- ➢ In case co-precipitation the contamination decreases with time of contact with mother liquor.
- ➢ In post-precipitation the contamination increases with the rate of agitation either by mechanical means such as shaking or stirring or by thermal means such as heating.
- ➢ In co-precipitation the contamination decreases with the rate of agitation either by mechanical means such as shaking or stirring or by thermal means such as heating.
- ➢ Extent of contamination may be much in case of post-precipitation. In co-precipitation the extent of contamination is less.

Digestion

Usually for complete precipitation digestion is carried out. The precipitate is allowed to stand at room temperature for 12 – 24 hrs or overnight. In some cases, the precipitate is warmed for some time in contact with mother liquor. Both the processes are called digestion or aging. The purpose of digestion is to complete precipitation and to facilitate filtration.

Advantages of aging or digestion of the precipitate:

- ➢ Fine particles which precipitate initially go into solution due to their greater solubility. There after these fine particles redeposit on the larger particles and precipitate out. Thus, co-precipitation of fine particles would be eliminated and total co-precipitation on the final precipitation would be reduced.
- ➢ The precipitate which is formed rapidly contains particles of irregular shape with larger surface area. On digestion these particles become more regular in shape and dense. This will result decrease in surface area and extent of adsorption would also be reduced.

Thus, digestion reduces the extent of co-precipitation, increases the particle size, and facilitates filtration.

Conditions of precipitation

In fact, there is no ideal conditions for precipitation which can be considered as universal conditions. Situation to situation these may vary. Since following conditions are applicable to many of the cases these are mentioned below.

1. Based on solubility of the precipitate, time required for filtration, and subsequent treatment on the filtrate, precipitation should be carried out in dilute solution. Thus, the error due to co-precipitation would be reduced.
2. During precipitation the reagents should be added slowly with constant stirring. This will reduce the degree of supersaturation and help growth of large particle. Generally, the reagent is added in slight excess. However, in some cases large

amount of reagent is required in some cases the order of mixing of reagents is changed.

3. Depending on the solubility and stability of the precipitate, precipitation should be carried out from the hot solution. Higher temperature increases the solubility, reduces the degree of supersaturation, favors coagulation of fine particles and reduces the formation of sol, and velocity of crystallization. Thus, crystal formation becomes better.

4. The duration of digestion of crystalline precipitate may be extended up to 12 hrs (overnight), if necessary. This is not done when post-precipitation may occur. Usually digestion is conducted over the steam bath. Digestion reduces the chances of co-precipitation and the precipitate becomes more filterable. However, on amorphous or gelatinous precipitate digestion does not exert any effect.

5. Washing of precipitate with pure water may cause peptization. The precipitate should be washed with a dilute solution of suitable electrolyte.

6. If the precipitate contains impurities due to co-precipitation or other reasons, the precipitate is dissolved in a suitable solvent and re-precipitated. By following this principle, the amount of impurities can be reduced appreciably.

Calculations

Usually in gravimetric analysis a precipitate is weighed, and from this value, the weight of the analyte in the sample is calculated using a factor called gravimetric factor (GF).

The GF is defined as the ratio of the formula weight of the substance desired to that of the substance weighed.

$$\text{Gravimetric factor (GF)} = \frac{\text{Substance desired (Formula weight)}}{\text{Substance weighed (Formula weight)}}$$

To determine the percentage of an element or ion (x) present in a sample can be calculated as:

$$x\% = \frac{\text{Weight of precipitate} \times \text{GF} \times 100}{\text{Weight of sample}}$$

7.3 ESTIMATION OF BARIUM SULPHATE

Concept

Determination of sulphate as barium sulphate: In this method the solution of sulphate is slightly acidified with hydrochloric acid. Then a dilute solution of barium chloride is slowly added to a hot solution containing sulphate.

$$Ba^{2+} + SO_4^{2-} \rightarrow BaSO_4 \downarrow$$

The precipitate formed, $BaSO_4$, is separated from the solution by filtration, washed with water carefully and thoroughly to remove completely the residual impurities such as chlorides. The precipitate is then ignited at red hot temperature till a constant weight is obtained. The ignited mass is $BaSO_4$. The percentage of SO_4 present in $BaSO_4$ (the precipitate) is then calculated.

The completeness of precipitation (determination) depends on the precipitation reaction. If the reaction conditions are not carefully controlled numerous errors may occur. The solubility of barium sulphate in water is about 3mg/L at room temperature. In the presence of mineral acid, the solubility increases due to formation of bisulphite ion ($SO_4^{2-} + H^+ \rightarrow HSO4^-$).

In fact, the solubility at room temperature increases from 3mg/L to 10mg/L in presence of 0.1N hydrochloric acid, in presence of 0.5N hydrochloric acid it increases to 47mg/L, in 1.0N hydrochloric acid it becomes 87mg/L, while in 2N hydrochloric acid the solubility increases up to 101mg/L. However, in presence of Ba2+ ions the solubility decreases. In general, precipitation is carried out in weakly acid solution to prevent the formation of barium salts of anions such as chromate, carbonate, phosphate, etc. Salts of these anions may be present in commercial samples. Barium salts of these anions are insoluble in neutral solution. The precipitate thus formed or obtained contains large crystals which can be easily filtered.

The following conditions should be maintained.

- The precipitation reaction should be carried out at boiling temperature because at higher temperature the relative supersaturation is less.
- The solubility of barium sulphate ($BaSO_4$) depends on the concentration of hydrochloric acid. Usually 0.5N HCl is suitable for required solubility. At this pH or acidity negligible amount of $BaCl_2$ remain present.
- The precipitate should be washed with cold water; so that the solubility of the precipitate in water is negligible.

During precipitation of $BaSO_4$ there may be co-precipitation. The amount of salt co-precipitated depends on the nature of the salt present. For example, $BaCl_2$ and $Ba(NO_3)_2$ can readily co-precipitate. Presence of these salts increases the weight of the $BaSO_4$ precipitate; hence, the result may be higher than the actual. Because, $BaCl_2$ does not change on ignition while $Ba(NO_3)_2$ is converted to BaO.

The error due to chloride can be greatly reduced if hot dilute solution of $BaCl_2$ is slowly added to the solution with continuous stirring. Removal of nitrate ion is not possible in this way. It can be removed by evaporating the solution with addition of large excess of HCl before precipitation. Chlorate can also be removed in similar way as nitrate.

Cations such as sodium, potassium, lithium, calcium, aluminium, chromium and iron are likely to be present in commercial variety and these can co-precipitate in form of sulphate salts. As a result, the result may show error. The error cannot be removed unless these interfering ions are removed. The obtained result would be less than the actual. Aluminium, chromium and iron can be removed by precipitation. It is not possible to remove other ions by precipitation method. Their effect can be reduced appreciably by diluting the solution considerably and subsequent digestion of the precipitate. The method of re-precipitation would not be applicable here to obtain greater purity because only sulphuric acid can be used for precipitation. No other reagent can be used.

When pure barium sulphate is heated in dry air, it is not decomposed. Barium sulphate decomposes only at $1400°C$ and above.

$$BaSO_4 \rightarrow BaO + SO_3$$

The precipitate ($BaSO_4$) can be easily reduced to sulphide when heated in presence of carbon (carbon of filter paper) at about $600°C$ or above. The reaction is as follows;

$$BaSO_4 + 4C = BaS + 4CO$$

Reduction of $BaSO_4$ can be avoided if the filter paper is charred with inflaming and then, the carbon is slowly burnt off at low temperature in presence of air. However, the reduced precipitate (BaS) can be oxidized to $BaSO_4$ by treating BaS with H_2SO_4. The excess acid is then volatilized and reheated. $BaSO_4$ thus obtained is to be ignited at temperature not more than $600 - 800°C$. In place of filter paper vitreosil or porcelain filtering crucible should be used to avoid reduction of $BaSO_4$.

Procedure

The estimation of barium sulphate in a given sample can be done as follows;

- ➤ Weigh accurately about 0.5g of the sample (solid).
- ➤ Transfer the weighed material into a 500mL beaker.
- ➤ Add 25mL of water, stir, add $0.3 - 0.6$mL of concentrated HCl and dissolve to make solution.
- ➤ Dilute the solution to 225mL.
- ➤ Heat the solution to boiling.
- ➤ From a burette or pipette add $10 - 12$mL of warm 5% $BaCl_2$ solution (5g of $BaCl_2$, $2H_2O$ in 100mL of water) drop wise with constant stirring.
- ➤ Allow the precipitate to settle for $1 - 2$ min and a clear solution remains as supernatant.
- ➤ Test the supernatant for sulphate by adding few drops of $BaCl_2$ solution; if the supernatant liquid is found to remain clear, it indicates completion of precipitation. If the supernatant liquid becomes turbid add further 3mL of $BaCl_2$ solution with constant stirring.
- ➤ Allow the precipitate to settle. Test the supernatant liquid for presence of sulphate by following the above-mentioned method.
- ➤ Put the cover over the beaker. Keep the hot solution over a boiling water bath for about 1 hr to ensure complete precipitation. The volume of the solution should not fall below 150mL.
- ➤ Remove the cover, wash the inner wall with hot water and add the washing to the beaker.
- ➤ Allow the precipitate to settle.
- ➤ Filter the precipitate either through an ash less filter paper such as Whatmann 42 or 44, or through a porcelain filter disc. Wash the filter repeatedly with small amount of water till the filtrate becomes free from chloride.
- ➤ Test the filtrate for chloride; if the filtrate is found to be free from chloride, proceed further for ignition.

➤ Take a porcelain or silica crucible which is pre-cleaned. Ignite it to red hot temperature, cool in air to moderately hot, keep it in a desiccator till it cools down to room temperature, weigh the crucible.

➤ Take out the moist filter into the tared crucible, cover loosely with the lid, and place it over a small flame to dry the paper.

➤ Increase the temperature to char the paper and to expel volatile matters, after complete charring uncover the crucible.

➤ Increase the temperature to red heat and ignite the content in the crucible for 15min, allow the crucible to cool in air to moderately hot, and then transfer the crucible into a desiccator to attain room temperature. Remove the crucible from the desiccator and weigh.

➤ Heat the crucible again to red heat temperature for 10min and allow it to cool in air, put the crucible in desiccator to cool to room temperature and weigh. Repeat the same process till two consecutive weights become same.

A. MULTIPLE CHOICE QUESTIONS

1. Which of the following steps is involved in gravimetric analysis?
    (a) Titration
    (b) Precipitation
    (c) Extraction by solvent
    (d) Chromatography

2. Which of the following is analyzed in traditional gravimetric analysis
    (a) Element
    (b) Ion
    (c) Radical
    (d) All of the above

3. In physical gravimetric analysis the mixture of substances are physically separated on basis of
    (a) Particle size
    (b) Chemical reaction
    (c) Solubility
    (d) All of above

4. Thermogravimetry is used in which areas such as
    (a) Pharmacy
    (b) Foods
    (c) Polymer science
    (d) All of the above

5. Electrodeposition is generally used in
    (a) Mechanical engineering
    (b) Chemical engineering
    (c) Environmental engineering
    (d) Thermal engineering

6. Gravimetric method requires calibration of
    (a) Balance
    (b) Burette
    (c) Pipette
    (d) All of the above

7. Accuracy of the gravimetric analysis depends on
    (a) Accuracy of weighing balance
    (b) Completeness of precipitation
    (c) Presence of impurities in the precipitate
    (d) All of the above

8. What are the factors that influence the success of gravimetric determination
    (a) Quantitative formation of precipitate
    (b) Quick formation of precipitate
    (c) Precipitate must be insoluble, filterable and stable
    (d) All of the above

9. For complete precipitation in a gravimetric analysis
    (a) The reagent must added slowly with continuous agitation
    (b) The reagent must added slowly without agitation
    (c) The reagent must added as fast as possible with continuous agitation
    (d) The reagent must added as fast as possible without agitation

10. Which one of the following statements is correct?
    (a) To reduce coprecipitation, dilute solution should be used
    (b) To reduce coprecipitation, concentrated solution should be used
    (c) Precipitation should be carried out from cold solution
    (d) Precipitation should be carried out from the solution at room temperature

11. In gravimetric analysis precipitation depends on
    (a) Amount of precipitating solution   (b) Temperature
    (c) pH of the solution   (d) All of the above

12. Which one of the following statements is correct?
    (a) Post precipitation does not have any effect on the extent of error
    (b) Post precipitation occurs on the surface of the precipitate
    (c) Post precipitation occurs and super-saturation of the precipitate are not related
    (d) Post precipitation occurs with soluble substances

13. Which one of the following statements is correct?
    (a) In post-precipitation the contamination increases with time of contact with mother liquor.
    (b) In post-precipitation the contamination decreases with time of contact with mother liquor.
    (c) In post-precipitation the contamination is not related to time of contact with mother liquor.
    (d) In co-precipitation the contamination increases with time of contact with mother liquor.

14. Which one of the following statements is correct?
    (a) In post-precipitation the contamination decreases with the rate of agitation
    (b) In post-precipitation the contamination increases with the rate of agitation
    (c) In co-precipitation the contamination increases with the rate of agitation
    (d) All of the above

15. Which one of the following statements is correct?
    (a) Digestion helps co-precipitation
    (b) Digestion helps post-precipitation
    (c) Digestion helps precipitation to complete
    (d) Digestion does not help complete precipitation.
16. Which one of the following statements is correct?
    (a) Heating increases contamination in post-precipitation
    (b) Cooling increases contamination in post-precipitation
    (c) Heating does not affect contamination in post-precipitation
    (d) Cooling does not affect contamination in post-precipitation

B. SHORT QUESTIONS
1. Define the term 'gravimetry'.
2. What are different types of gravimetric analysis?
3. Write down the advantages of gravimetric analysis.
4. What are the limitations of gravimetric method of analysis?
5. What are the applications of gravimetric method of analysis?
6. Explain the terms – saturated and supersaturated solutions.
7. What are co-precipitation and post-precipitation?
8. Explain the term 'gravimetric factor'.
9. What are reasons for adsorption of other substances present in the titration mixture on the surface of precipitate?

C. LONG QUESTIONS
1. Explain the principle of gravimetric analysis.
2. Describe in brief different types of gravimetric analyses.
3. Explain the factors that influence successful determination of element/ion/radical by precipitation method.
4. Explain the factors that influence precipitation in a gravimetric analysis.
5. Discuss the steps involved in gravimetric analysis with suitable example.
6. Explain the term ageing of precipitation and its effect on analysis.
7. Explain the conditions for precipitation.
8. Write down the principle involved in determination barium sulphate.
9. Write down the method of determination barium sulphate.

CHAPTER 8

Redox Titrations

8.1 CONCEPTS OF OXIDATION AND REDUCTION

In each oxidation-reduction reaction one reactant will undergo oxidation and one will undergo reduction simultaneously because two reactions are complementary to one another. The reactant undergoing oxidation is called reducing agent or reductant and the reactant that undergoes reduction is called oxidizing agent or oxidant.

In oxidation-reduction reactions electrons are transferred from reducing agent to the oxidizing agent. In other words, reducing agent donates electrons and oxidizing agent accepts the electrons. This is the basis of *ion-electron* method used for balancing ionic equations.

Thus, oxidation is a process in which loss of electrons by atoms or ions takes place and reduction is a process in which gain of electron takes place. Each oxidation-reduction reaction is expressed by two partial equations - one represents oxidation and other reduction. These reactions take place in aqueous solution. In addition to the ions supplied by the oxidant and reductant, the molecules of water (H_2O), hydrogen ion (H^+), and hydroxyl ion (OH^-) are involved in these reactions. The unit change in such reactions is a charge of one electron, denoted by **e**.

For example, when ferric chloride is formed from ferrous chloride the Fe^{2+} ion donates one electron and oxidized to Fe^{3+}. The electron released is accepted by Cl^- ion and get reduced to molecular iodine (Cl_2).

$$FeCl_2 \rightarrow [Fe^{2+} + 2Cl^-] \rightarrow FeCl_3$$

Thus, the oxidation reaction is $2Fe^{2+} - 2e \rightarrow 2Fe^{3+}$ and the reduction reaction is $2Cl^- + 2e \rightarrow Cl_2$. There are some substances which ionize slightly such as water, silver chloride, barium sulphate, etc. In general, the molecular formulas of these substances are written because these are present mainly in undissociated form.

The rules for application of ion-electron method are;

1.   The products of the reaction are to be determined.
2.   Partial equation for oxidation is to be arranged.
3.   Partial equation for reduction is to be arranged.
4.   Multiply each of the partial equations by a factor so that when these reactions are added the number of electrons involved can compensate each other.
5.   The partial reactions are to be added and the substances appear on the both sides of the equation are to be cancelled.

Example 1: Reduction of potassium permanganate ($KMnO_4$) in dilute sulphuric acid by ferrous sulphate ($FeSO_4$)

Partial equation for reduction: $MnO_4^- \rightarrow Mn^{2+}$

After balancing the equation electrically, it becomes

$$MnO_4^- + 8H^+ + 5e = Mn^{2+} + 4H_2O \qquad .....(8.1)$$

Partial equation for oxidation: $Fe^{2+} \rightarrow Fe^{3+}$

After balancing the equation electrically, it becomes

$$Fe^{2+} = Fe^{3+} + e \qquad .....(8.2)$$

The equation 2 is multiplied by 5 and equation 1 is multiplied by 1, then these are added

$$MnO_4^- + 8H^+ + 5e = Mn^{2+} + 4H_2O$$
$$\underline{5Fe^{2+} = 5Fe^{3+} + 5e}$$
$$MnO_4^- + 8H^+ + 5Fe^{2+} = Mn^{2+} + 4H_2O + 5Fe^{3+}$$

Example 2: Reaction between potassium dichromate ($K_2Cr_2O_7$) and potassium iodide (KI) in presence of dilute sulphuric acid.

Partial equation for reduction: $Cr_2O_7^{2-} \rightarrow Cr^{3+}$

Or, $Cr_2O_7^{2-}\ 14H^+ \rightarrow 2Cr^{3+} + 7H_2O$

After balancing the equation electrically, it becomes

$$Cr_2O_7^{2-} + 14H^+ + 6e = 2Cr^{3+} + 7H_2O \qquad .....(8.3)$$

Partial equation for oxidation: $I^- \rightarrow I_2$

$$2I^- \rightarrow I_2$$

After balancing the equation electrically, it becomes $2I^- = I_2 + 2e$ .....(8.4)

The equation B is multiplied by 3 and equation A is multiplied by 1, then these are added

$$Cr_2O_7^{2-} + 14H^+ + 6e = 2Cr^{3+} + 7H_2O$$
$$6I^- = 3I_2 + 6e$$
$$\overline{Cr_2O_7^{2-} + 14H^+ + 6I^- = 2Cr^{3+} + 7H_2O + 3I_2}$$

Equivalent weight of oxidizing and reducing agents

The equivalent weight of oxidizing and reducing agents is calculated by dividing the molecular weight by the number of electrons gained or lost by each mol of the substance.

Example 3:

1. $MnO_4^- + 8H^+ + 5e = Mn^{2+} + 4H_2O.$

   The number of electrons gained by each molecule of $KMnO_4$ is 5.

   Hence, the equivalent weight of $KMnO_4 = \dfrac{\text{Mol wt of } KMnO_4}{5} = \dfrac{158.03}{5} = 31.61$

2. $Cr_2O_7^{2-} + 14H^+ + 6e = 2Cr^{3+} + 7H_2O.$

   The number of electrons gained by each molecule of $K_2Cr_2O_7$ is 6.

   Hence, the equivalent weight of $K_2Cr_2O_7 = \dfrac{\text{Mol wt of } K_2Cr_2O_7}{6} = \dfrac{294.18}{6} = 49.03$

3. $Zn^{2+} + 2e = Zn$

   The number of electrons gained by each molecule of $ZnSO_4$ is 2.

   Hence, its equivalent weight $= \dfrac{\text{Mol wt of } ZnSO_4}{2} = \dfrac{161.47}{2} = 80.73$

4. $Fe^{2+} = Fe^{3+} + e.$

   The number of electrons lost by each mol of $FeCl_2$ is 1.

   Hence, equivalent weight of $FeCl_2 = \dfrac{\text{Mol wt of } FeCl_2}{1} = \dfrac{126.75}{1} = 126.75$

5. $SO_3^{2-} + H_2O = SO_4^{2-} + 2H^+ + 2e.$

   The number of electrons lost by each mol of Na_2SO_3 is 2.

   Hence, its equivalent weight of $Na_2SO_3 = \dfrac{\text{Mol wt of } Na_2SO_3}{2} = \dfrac{126.04}{2} = 63.02$

Equivalent weight of these substances can be calculated by using their **oxidation numbers**. The oxidation number of an element is a number is the number which is applied to that element in a particular compound. The number indicates the amount of oxidation or reduction required to convert one atom of the element from the free-state to that in the compound. In case of oxidation, the oxidation number is (+) ive (positive) and in case of reduction (–) ive (negative).

Following rules are followed to determine the oxidation number;

➢ Oxidation number of a free or uncombined element is zero.

➢ Oxidation number of hydrogen (except in hydride) is +1.

➢ Oxidation number of oxygen (except in peroxide) is –2.

➤ Oxidation number of a metal in a compound (except in hydride) is usually (+) ive.

➤ Oxidation number of a radical or ion is same as its electrovalence with the appropriate sign attached. The value is equal to its electrical charge.

➤ Oxidation number of a compound is always zero. It is determined by adding the Oxidation number of individual atom multiplied by the number of it present in the molecule of the compound.

Equivalent weight of an oxidizing agent

Equivalent weight of an oxidizing agent can be determined by dividing the molecular weight of the compound by its oxidation number.

Example 4: Oxidation number of manganese in potassium permanganate in presence of dilute sulphuric acid (reduction) is calculated as;

$$KMnO_4 \rightarrow MnO_2 + SO_2$$

Oxidation number of element	+1	+7	-8 [4×(-2)]
Constituting element	K	Mn	O_4

+2	+6	-8 4×(-2)]
Mn	S	O_4

The change in oxidation number of Mn is from +7 to +2. That is 5 units; hence, the equivalent weight of $KMnO_4$ would be $1/5^{th}$ of its molecular weight.

Similarly, the equivalent weight of $K_2Cr_2O_7$ in presence of dilute sulphuric acid (reduction) is calculated as follows;

Oxidation number of element	+2 [2×(+1)]	+12 [2×(+6)]	-14 [7×(-1)]
Constituting element	K_2	Cr_2	O_7

+6 [2×(+3)]	-6 [3×(-2)]
Cr_2	$(SO_4)_3$

The change in oxidation number of 2 atoms of Cr is from +12 to +6. That is, by 6 units. Hence, equivalent weight of $K_2Cr_2O_7$ is $1/6^{th}$ of its molecular weight $(\frac{294.18}{6} = 49.03)$.

Equivalent weight of reducing agent

Equivalent weight of reducing agent can be determined by dividing the molecular weight of the compound by its oxidation number.

In conversion of ferrous chloride ($FeCl_2$) to ferric chloride ($FeCl_3$) or ferrous sulphate ($FeSO_4$) to ferric sulphate [$Fe_2(SO_4)_3$] (oxidation reaction) the equivalent weight of $FeCl_2$ or $FeSO_4$ can be calculated as follows:

Example 5: The oxidation number of Fe atom in $FeCl_2$ changes from +2 to +3. That is by 1 unit. Hence the equivalent weight of $FeCl_2$ would be $\dfrac{\text{Mol wt of } FeCl_2}{1}$.

Oxidation number of element	+4	-4
	[2×(+2)]	[2×(-2)]
Constituting element	2Fe	2SO₄

→

+6	-6
[2×(+3)]	[3×(-2)]
Fe₂	(SO₄)₃

Similarly, the oxidation number of Fe atom in $FeSO_4$ changes from +2 to +3 per atom. That is by 1 unit. Hence the equivalent weight of $FeSO_4$ would be $\dfrac{\text{Mol wt of } FeSO_4}{1}$.

Example 6: Oxidation of oxalic acid is another important example, it produces carbon dioxide. The equivalent weight of oxalic acid is calculated as;

Oxidation number of element	+2	+6	-8
	[2×(+1)]	[2×(+3)]	[4×(-2)]
Constituting element	H₂	C₂	O₄

→

+8	-8
[2×(+4)]	[4×(-2)]
2C	2O₂

The change in oxidation number of two atoms of carbon is from +6 to +8 or by 2 units. Hence, the equivalent weight of oxalic acid is ½ of its molecular weight. Thus,

1. The equivalent weight of an element taking part in an oxidation-reduction reaction is the atomic weight divided by the change in oxidation number.
2. If in any compound or complex molecule an atom of a constitute element undergoes oxidation or reduction, the equivalent weight of the substance is calculated by dividing its molecular weight by the change in oxidation number of that oxidized or reduced (reactive) element.
3. When the number of atoms of the reactive element present in one molecule is more than one, the equivalent weight is calculated by dividing its molecular weight by the total change in oxidation number.

The Table below shows the radicals or elements involved in common oxidation or reduction reactions and change in oxidation number.

Oxidizing agents	Radical or Element involved	Oxidation Number of reactive element	Reduction product	New Oxidation number	Change in oxidation number
$KMnO_4$ (in acidic medium)	MnO_4^-	+ 7	Mn^{2+}	+2	5
$KMnO_4$ (in neutral medium)	MnO_4^-	+ 7	MnO_2 or Mn^{4+}	+4	3
$KMnO_4$ (in strong alkaline medium)	MnO_4^-	+ 7	MnO_4^{2-}	+6	1
$K_2Cr_2O_7$	$Cr_2O_7^{2-}$	+ 6	Cr^{2+}	+ 3	3
HNO_3 (Dilute solution)	NO_3^-	+ 1	NO	+ 2	1

Contd...

Oxidizing agents	Radical or Element involved	Oxidation Number of reactive element	Reduction product	New Oxidation number	Change in oxidation number
HNO_3 (Conc. solution)	NO_3^-	$+5$	NO_2	$+4$	1
Cl_2	Cl	0	Cl^-	-1	1
Br_2	Br	0	Br^-	-1	1
I_2	I	0	I^-	-1	1
$3HCl:1HNO_3$	Cl	0	Cl^-	-1	1
H_2O_2	O_2	0	O^{2-}	-2	2
Na_2O_2	O_2	0	O^{2-}	-2	2
$KClO_3$	ClO_3^-	$+5$	Cl^-	-1	6
$KBrO_3$	BrO_3^-	$+5$	Br^-	-1	6
KIO_3	IO_3^-	$+5$	I^-	-1	6
$NaOCl$	OCl^-	$+1$	Cl^-	-1	2
$FeCl_3$	Fe^{3+}	$+3$	Fe^{2+}	$+2$	1
$Ce(SO_4)_2$	Ce^{4+}	$+4$	Ce^{3+}	$+3$	1
Reducing agents					
H_2SO_3 or Na_2SO_3	SO_3^{2-}	$+4$	SO_4^{2-}	$+6$	2
H_2S	S^{2-}	-2	S	0	2
HI	I^-	-1	I	0	1
$SnCl_2$	Sn^{2+}	$+2$	Sn^{4+}	$+4$	2
Metals, e.g., Zn	Zn	0	Zn^{2+}	$+2$	2
Hydrogen	H	0	H^+	$+1$	1
Ferrous salt, e.g., $FeSO_4$	Fe^{2+}	$+2$	Fe^{3+}	$+3$	1
Na_2AsO_3	AsO^{3-}	$+3$	AsO_4^{3-}	$+5$	2
$H_2C_2O_4$	$C_2O_4^{2-}$	$+3$	CO_2	$+4$	1
$Ti_2(SO_4)_3$	Ti^{3+}	$+3$	Ti^{4+}	$+4$	1

8.2   TYPES OF REDOX TITRATIONS (PRINCIPLES AND APPLICATIONS)

Redox titration is a titration that involves the oxidation-reduction reaction. Since there are different oxidizing and reducing agents; based on the type of reaction taking place or involved the titrations can be classified into seven categories.

1. Cerimetry

   This type of titration includes the titrations involving ceric ion.

2. Permanganometry

   It includes the titrations involving potassium permanganate.

3. Iodimetry

   This is a type of titration reaction in which standard solution of iodine is used for titration. Sometimes it is called direct (iodometric) titration.

4. Iodometry

   It includes the titrations of iodine liberated in chemical reaction. Sometimes it is called indirect (iodometric) titration.

5. Bromatometry

   It includes the titrations that use bromine directly or indirectly as in titrations involving iodine.

6. Dichrometry

   This type titration involves potassium dichromate.

   Titrations involving potassium iodate

8.2.1 Cerimetry

Ceric ion is a powerful oxidizing agent and titration procedure employing this oxidant is called cerimetry. The use of cerium (IV) salts as reagents for volumetric analysis was first proposed in the middle of 19th century. The systematic studies started since about 70 years. Cerimetry or cerimetric titration is also known as cerate oximetry. It is one of the volumetric chemical methods of analysis. It is a redox titration in which the change of color of ferroin (Fe^{2+}-1,10-phenanthroline complex) indicates the end point. If the solution is titrated with a solution of cerium sulphate (Ce^{4+} salt), ferroin gets oxidized and discolored.

Standard solutions can be prepared from different Ce^{4+} salts. Most often cerium sulphate is used. Non-stoichiometry of oxides containing several elements in oxidation states is suitable for cerimetric analysis. Cerimetric analysis is related to the Fe^{3+}/Fe^{2+} redox pair. It can be used for analyses of nonstoichiometric levels that either oxidize Fe^{2+} or reduce Fe^{3+}. In the case of oxidation, a slight excess of high-purity crystalline Mohr's salt is added for digestion of the oxide in aqueous hydrogen chloride; while in the case of reduction, an excess of 1M iron trichloride ($FeCl_3$) is added. In the both cases, this is Fe^{2+} ions are titrated subsequently. The Ce^{4+} solution is prone to hydrolysis. The titration is done in a strongly HCl-acidic solution into which some phosphoric acid is added to obtain a less colored phosphato complex of Fe^{3+}.

Cerium (IV) species are easily reduced to the +3 state.

$$Ce^{4+} + e \leftrightarrow Ce^{3+}$$

Cerimetric titrations are used for the determination of some drugs. Iron (II) solution can be accurately determined by coulometric titration with electro-generated cerium (IV), and also by gravimetric titration with a standard potassium dichromate.

The redox potentials are measured using the combined redox electrode (Pt–Ag/AgCl) in equimolar Ce^{4+}/Ce^{3+} solutions in sulfuric acid electrolyte. The Ce^{4+}/Ce^{3+} redox potential decreases significantly (shift to more negative values); if the concentration of sulfuric acid in the medium is increased. Cyclic voltammetric experiments confirm slow electrochemical kinetics of the Ce^{4+}/Ce^{3+} redox reaction on carbon glassy electrodes (CGEs) in sulfuric acid solutions.

Sequential injection analysis (SIA) technique can be used for determination of vitamin C with Ce (IV) in sulfuric acid solution using a spectrophotometer as a detector at the wavelength of 410 nm. Some titrants used for the determination of a number of reducing substances are; in the presence of iodine chloride or potassium bromide as a catalyst cerium (IV) is used to titrate sodium oxalate, iron (II), arsenic (III) and antimony (III) at room temperature. The reaction between ceric sulphate and oxalic acid is rapid in hydrochloric acid medium and in the presence of iodine monochloride as catalyst. Oxalic acid can be titrated with ceric sulphate at room temperature in IN hydrochloric acid medium using ferroin as indicator, and if barium ion is present as scavenger for sulphate ion, the reaction rates between oxalic acid and oxidized ferroin, also between oxalic acid and Ce (IV) decrease noticeably. The recent method has various advantages over that of Willard and Young. In the recently developed method the reaction can be conducted at temperature lower than 50°C, where the ferroin indicator is found to undergo some dissociation, no catalyst such as iodine monochloride is required. By this method ketotifen fumarate, Ganciclovir, propranolol hydrochloride, and ciprofloxacin can be determined using Ce (IV) as titrant. In the method, the drug is treated with a measured and excess volume of Ce (IV) in H_2SO_4 solution, the mixture is allowed to stand for 10 min. The excess amount of oxidant is determined by back titration with iron (II). Bulk drug and formulations of Methdilazine hydrochloride (MDH) are determined by titration with Ce (IV) using ferroin as indicator. The MDH is oxidized by Ce (IV) in acidic medium. At room temperature vanadium (IV) has been titrated with Ce (IV) sulphate in sulphuric acid and syrupy phosphoric acid medium, using Rhodamine 6G as an internal fluorescent indicator. A greenish-yellow fluorescence of the indicator is suddenly quenched with a slight excess of the oxidant at the equivalence point.

Potentiometric titration can also be used to titrate with Ce (IV) solution. Accurate results can be obtained by potentiometric determination of vanadium (IV) with cerium (IV) in the presence of sulfuric, hydrochloric or perchloric acid at 70 -75°C. A method has been developed for the simultaneous differential potentiometric titration of iron (II) and vanadium (IV) with Ce (IV) sulphate in a sulphuric acid medium using orthophosphoric acid as a catalyst. The method is satisfactory. Chromium (III) and iron (III) do not interfere in these titrations. The determination of norfloxacin (NRF) in bulk drug and in its dosage, forms can be done satisfactorily by potentiometric titration. This method is based on the oxidation reaction of norfloxacin with cerium (IV) in 0.3 M HCl. The reaction has been found to be quantitative.

Example 7: Determination of ascorbic acid in a sample

Preparation of 0.001M [Ce (IV)] ceric sulphate solution

Weigh accurately about 0.4044g of ceric sulphate, transfer carefully into a 100 mL volumetric flask. Add 0.26 mL of concentrated H_2SO_4 and dissolve. Dilute the solution to 100 mL with distilled water. Mix thoroughly. Pipette out exactly 10 mL of the above solution in to another 100 mL volumetric flask and made up to the mark with distilled water. The Ce (IV) stock solution is standardized with arsenic (III) oxide by using N-phenyl anthranilic acid indicator.

Amaranth dye Solution

0.003g of amaranth dye is weighed and dissolved in distilled water to make 10 mL of the solution.

Procedure

Weigh accurately the sample containing 1.0 mg of ascorbic acid, transfer carefully into a 250 mL beaker, and dissolve in 10 mL of freshly distilled water. Add 0.2 mL of amaranth dye solution. Mix well. Titrate the sample with ceric sulphate solution until the pink color disappears. Repeat the titration twice more following same method. Note the titer values. Say, the average titer value is Vs mL.

Carry out the titration (Blank) using 10 mL of distilled water; say titer value is Vb mL.

Calculation

Amount of ascorbic acid present in sample = (Vs – Vb) × M × EW

Where, M is the actual strength of ceric sulphate solution, and EW is the gram of ascorbic acid equivalent to 1 mL ceric sulphate solution.

8.2.2 Permanganometry

It is one of the most common techniques used to analyze a compound quantitatively in chemistry using potassium permanganate. It is a redox titration used to measure an analyte present in the compound.

Potassium permanganate, $KMnO_4$, is a strong oxidizing agent. Permanganate, MnO^{4-}, is a dark purple color ion. During titration the purple color permanganate ions are reduced to the colorless Mn^{2+} ions and at the equivalence point the solution turns from dark purple to a faint pink color. No additional indicator is required in this titration. Reduction of permanganate takes place in strong acidic medium. Hence, a volumetric solution of potassium permanganate with known strength is required.

Depending on the reaction conditions permanganate ion may be reduced to manganese in the 2+, 3+, 4+ or 6+ states.

1. In solutions that are 0.1 M or greater in mineral acid the common reduction product is manganese (II) ion

   $$MnO_4^- + 8H^+ + 5e^- \leftrightarrow Mn^{2+} + 4H_2O \qquad E_o = 1.51 \text{ V}$$

   This is the most widely used of the permanganate reactions.

   In solutions that are weakly acidic (above pH 4) neutral, or weakly alkaline manganese dioxide is the most common reduction product

   $$MnO_4^- + 4H^+ + 3e^- \leftrightarrow MnO_2(s) + 2H_2O \qquad E_o = 1.70 \text{ V}$$

   Titration in which manganese dioxide is the product suffer from the disadvantage that the slightly soluble **brown oxide** obscures the end point; time must be allowed for the solid to settle before an excess of the permanganate can be detected.

Some important volumetric analyses based on permanganate involve reduction to manganese ion according to the half reaction given below;

$$MnO_4^- + e^- \leftrightarrow MnO_4^{2-} \qquad E_o = 0.56\ V$$

This stoichiometry tends to predominate in solutions that are greater than 1M in sodium hydroxide. Alkaline oxidations with permanganate have proved to be most useful in the determination of organic compounds.

Standardization of 0.1N Potassium Permanganate solution

In this process the potassium permanganate solution is standardized with standard solution of sodium or potassium oxalate or of oxalic acid. Permanganate ion is reduced by oxalate ion, $C_2O_4^{2-}$ in acidic medium. At room temperature oxalate reacts very slowly; but fast in higher temperature. So, the hot solutions are to be titrated to complete the titration in adequate time. The reaction is given below;

$$MnO_4^- + C_2O_4^{2-} \rightarrow Mn^{2+} + CO_2 \text{ (acidic solution)}$$

Preparation

Dissolve 3.3g of potassium permanganate in 1000 mL of water in a clean stopper flask, stopper the flask, shake well to mix. Keep it for 2 days, filter the solution through Whatmann No.1 filter paper and standardize the solution as follows.

Procedure

Dry about 1g of sodium oxalate in a hot air oven at $110^\circ C$ for about 3 hrs to constant weight. Cool the material to room temperature in a desiccator. Weigh accurately 0.6701g of dried sodium oxalate, transfer into a 100 mL volumetric flask, and make up the volume with water; shake well. Pipette accurately 25 mL of this solution into a 250 mL of water; add 50 mL of water and 7 mL of sulphuric acid, heat the solution to about $80^\circ C$.

Rinse and fill a 50 mL burette with potassium permanganate solution. Titrate the warm solution of sodium oxalate slowly with potassium permanganate solution from the burette with constant stirring until a pale pink color is produced. The color should persist at least for 15 seconds. It is to be noted that the temperature of the solution should remain around $60 - 70^\circ C$ till completion of the titration. Note the volume of potassium permanganate solution consumed (titer value). Repeat the titration twice more and take the average titer value for calculation.

Calculation

Say, weight of sodium oxalate taken = 0.6724g (practical weight)

Weight of sodium oxalate to be taken = 0.6701g (theoretical weight)

$$\text{Strength of sodium oxalate solution } (S_1) = \frac{\text{practical weight}}{\text{theoretical weight}}$$

$$= \frac{0.6724}{0.6701} = 1.0034(N/10) = 0.1003N$$

Volume of 0.1003N sodium oxalate solution taken (V_1) = 25.00 mL

Say, the av. Titer value (V_2) = 25.03 mL

So, the strength of potassium permanganate $(S_2) = \dfrac{V_1 \times S_1}{V_2} = \dfrac{25\ mL \times 0.1003N}{25.03\ mL} = 0.10017N = \mathbf{0.1002N}$

8.2.3 Iodimetry and Iodometry

Iodine is a moderately weak oxidizing agent. When reduced it forms iodide, an anion as shown below;

$$I_2(aq) + 2e^- \leftrightarrow 2I^-(aq)$$
$$2I^-(aq) - 2e^- \leftrightarrow I_2$$

The above redox reaction is reversible and iodide ion, also a weak reducing agent, can react with an oxidizing agent to form iodine. Thus, iodine can be used to titrate a number of oxidizing and reducing agents. According to how the iodine is involved, such redox titrations can be classified into two categories –

1. Iodimetry, and

2. Iodometry.

1. **Iodimetry:** In iodimetric titrations are the reactions using standard solution of iodine. In this titration the reducing form of an analyte (A_{ox}) reacts with iodine and forms an oxidizing form of the analyte (A_{red}). The general reactions involved in iodimetry can be expressed as;

   $$A_{ox} + I_2 \rightarrow A_{red} + 2I^-$$

   Where, A_{ox} and A_{red} are the oxidized form and reduced form of analyte present in the sample. This can be expressed in other way:

   $$Reducing\ agent + I_2 \rightarrow Oxidizing\ agent + 2I^-$$

   Where the reducing agent and oxidizing agent are the two form of the analyte present in the sample.

2. **Iodometry:** The general reaction takes place in iodometry is

   $$A_{red} + (excess)2I^- \rightarrow A_{ox} + I_2$$

   According to the above equation, iodine produced in the reaction is stoichiometrically related to the amount of analyte originally present in the sample. If iodine is titrated the concentration analyte in the sample can be determined. Usually the titrant used for determining iodine is sodium thiosulfate. They react quantitatively as follows:

   $$2Na_2S_2O_3 \rightarrow 4Na^+ + 2S_2O_3^{2-}$$

   $$I_2 + 2S_2O_3^{2-} \rightarrow S_4O_6^{2-} + 2I^-$$

   Therefore, the reactions involving iodine can be used for the analysis of moderately strong reducing agents (by reacting with I_2 in iodimetry) or moderately strong oxidizing agents (through reaction with excess iodide in iodometry).

Solid iodine is not very soluble in water and is volatile. As a result, iodine solutions are usually prepared by dissolving the solid iodine in the concentrated potassium iodide solution. Iodine reacts with iodide and forms the soluble tri-iodide ion:

$$I_2(aq) + KI \leftrightarrow KI_3$$

Or, $$I_2(aq) + I^- \leftrightarrow I_3^-$$

The tri-iodide ion present in solution dissociates to form iodide ion as follows;

$$I_3^- + 2e^- \leftrightarrow 3I^- \qquad [E° = 0.545 \text{ V}]$$

Although the standard reduction potential of the above reaction, $[E° = 0.545 \text{ V}]$ indicates the accurate the oxidizing strength of iodine as titrant, thermodynamically it makes no difference. Iodine/tri-iodide solutions are unstable. Aqueous iodine exerts a significant vapor pressure. Generally, the iodine solutions are stable at neutral pH values. Under acidic conditions iodide is slowly air-oxidized to produce iodine and under alkaline conditions, iodine will disproportionately produce iodide and iodate, as follows:

$$3I_2 + 6OH^- \leftrightarrow IO_3^- + 5I^- + 3H_2O$$

Iodine titrant solutions should be standardized against a standard sodium oxalate solution.

The disproportionation reaction of iodine is fully reversible and can be used to produce standard solutions of iodine. If a solution is prepared by dissolving primary standard potassium iodate and mixed with a slight excess of iodide and acidified with sulfuric acid, a standard iodine solution is prepared by this *reverse disproportionation* reaction.

$$IO_3^- + 5I^- + 6H^+ \leftrightarrow 3I_2 + 3H_2O$$

However, the solution thus obtained can be used to standardize sodium thiosulfate titrant, or to generate a known quantity of iodine reagent *in situ*. Unfortunately, it is not stable enough for general use as a titrant as mentioned previously.

Difference between Iodometry and Iodimetry

The names, Iodimetry and Iodometry, indicate that in these methods' iodine is involved. Both the methods/titrations are based on oxidation-reduction and are used to determine the redox substances quantitatively.

➢ In Iodimetry a species is directly titrated with an iodine solution. But in Iodometry a species is titrated with an iodide solution and then the released iodine is titrated with sodium thiosulphate solution.

➢ Iodimetry is a direct method; while Iodometry is an indirect method.

➢ Iodimetry is a method used to determine the quantity of a reducing agent; while iodometry is used to determine the quantity of an oxidizing substance.

➢ Iodimetry only one redox reaction takes place; while in iodometry two redox reactions take place.

Determination of Ascorbic acid (vitamin C) by iodimetry

Ascorbic acid is a reducing agent and is considered as an anti-oxidant by pharmacists and food nutritionists.

Iodine rapidly oxidizes ascorbic acid, $C_6H_8O_6$, and produces dehydroascorbic acid, $C_6H_6O_6$.

$$C_6H_8O_6 + I_2 \rightarrow C_6H_6O_6 + 2I^- + 2H^+$$

Ascorbic acid
$[C_6H_8O_6]$

Dehydroascorbic acid
$[C_6H_6O_6]$

Ascorbic acid is readily soluble in water. Direct iodimetric titration is a standard method for the analysis of vitamin C in a variety of citrus fruits and in vitamin tablets. Actually, an iodimetric back-titration can be performed. An excess of iodine in the sample solution is generated and measured by titrating the unreacted iodine with sodium thiosulfate. Although this back titration is considered as an iodimetric titration, since it is based on the reaction of analyte with aqueous iodine. However, such a back titration allows using the same titrant (sodium thiosulfate) in the iodometric analysis of hydrogen peroxide.

Determination of Hydrogen Peroxide by Iodometry

Hydrogen peroxide is an oxidizing agent. Solutions of hydrogen peroxide are widely sold as disinfectants. Hydrogen peroxide reacts with iodide in a redox reaction:

$$H_2O_2 + 2H^+ + 2I^- \rightarrow I_2 + 2H_2O$$

The velocity of the reaction is relatively slow. If the concentration of acid is increased, the velocity increases. Addition of 3 drops of a neutral 20% ammonium molybdate solution makes the reaction almost immediate; but at the same time hydroiodic acid gets oxidized in contact with atmosphere. Thus, the titration should be conducted in presence of carbon dioxide not in air.

Commercial hydrogen peroxide contains some stabilizers such as boric acid, salicylic acid, glycerol, etc. which may affect the estimation of hydrogen peroxide. The iodometric method is better than the permanganate method because the iodometric method is not affected by these materials and can produce accurate results.

Procedure

 ➢ Pipette out accurately 10.0 mL of the sample and transfer into a 250mL volumetric flask, make up the volume with distilled water. Mix well

- ➢ Weigh accurately about 1g of pure potassium iodide and transfer into a 250mL iodine flask, add 100mL of 2N sulphuric acid and dissolve.
- ➢ Pipette out exactly 25 mL of diluted hydrogen peroxide and add gradually to potassium iodide solution with constant stirring; stopper the flask immediately and keep it for fifteen minutes.
- ➢ Rinse and fill a 50-mL burette with 0.1N standard sodium thiosulphate solution.
- ➢ Titrate the liberated iodine with the sodium thiosulfate solution until the brown color (tri-iodide color) is changed to pale straw color.
- ➢ Add about 2 mL of the starch solution (a blue color is formed) and titrate until the solution changes sharply from blue to colorless.
- ➢ Note the volume of sodium thiosulphate required.
- ➢ Repeat the titration twice more and take average of three values for calculation.
- ➢ Calculate the H_2O_2 content of the sample.

Note: Sodium thiosulphate solution requires re-standardization at every few days, or as and when it is to be used.

$$1mL \text{ of } 0.1N \text{ sodium thiosulphate} \approx 0.001701g \ H_2O_2$$

Calculation

Say, av. titer value (volume of 0.1N $Na_2S_2O_3$ consumed) $= x$ mL

Strength of $Na_2S_2O_3$ solution $= 0.0998N$

Volume of diluted sample titrated $= 25.00mL$

$$\%w/v \text{ content of } H_2O_2 \text{ of the sample} = \frac{x \times 0.0998N \times 0.001701g \times 250 \times 100}{25 \times 10}$$

8.2.4 Bromatometry

Potassium bromate is a stable compound and available with high purity even up to 99.9%. Hence, it is used as primary standard and strength of its volumetric solution is calculated by dividing the actual weight taken by the theoretical weight for making definite volume of solution.

In acid medium potassium bromate ($KBrO_3$) behaves as a strong oxidizing agent. When it reacts with a reducing agent, it is easily converted into bromide, Br^-.

$$BrO_3^- + 6H^+ + 6e^- \leftrightarrow Br^- + 3H_2O$$

Thus, equivalent weight of $KBrO_3$ is $1/6^{th}$ of its molecular weight (167.016); that is, $167.016/6 = 27.836$; hence 1N solution contains 27.836g of $KBrO_3$ per L of solution or 0.1N solution contains 2.7836g of $KBrO_3$ per L of solution.

When potassium bromate reacts with a bromide salt, bromine is formed.

$$BrO_3^- + 5Br^- + 6H^+ = 3Br_2 + 3H_2O$$

The endpoint of the titration can be detected by the appearance of yellow color of bromine. But it is better to use a suitable indicator such as methyl orange, methyl red, naphthol blue black, brilliant ponceau 5R, fuchsine, etc. These indicators exhibit their colors in acid solution and the color is lost by bromine. Since bromine produced depends quantitatively on the bromate used. Hence, for loss of bromine bromate is also lost. Although the amount of bromate consumed by the indicator is negligible; performing a blank titration this loss can be taken care of.

Sometimes, an irreversible dyestuff is used in direct titration with bromate. For this titration presence of HCl is required and the concentration of HCl should be around 1.5N. In such titrations some amount of chlorine is produced along with bromine.

$$2BrO_3^- + 10Cl^- + 12H^+ = 5Cl_2 + Br_2 + 6H_2O$$

The chlorine produced is sufficient to bleach the indicator. Titration with bromate should be done slowly to detect the color change of the indicator; because the indicator changes its color slowly. During titration if the indicator fades, 1-2 drops of indicator solution should be added till the endpoint is detected (change of indicator color is clear).

For this reason, reversible indicator such as quinoline yellow, α-naphtholflavone, þ-ethoxychrysoidine, etc. have been used. These indicators are commonly used in determination of trivalent arsenic and trivalent antimony. If a small amount of tartaric acid or potassium sodium tartrate is added along with a suitable reversible indicator to the titration mixture antimony (III) can be determined accurately with precision by titrating with bromate. This prevents hydrolysis at lower concentration.

Indicators commonly used in bromatometric titrations are given below.

Name of indicator	Type	Conc. & type of solution	Color change
Methyl orange	Irreversible	0.1% aqueous	Red to colorless or pale yellow
Brilliant Ponceau 5R	Do	0.1% aqueous	Dark red to colorless
Fuchsine	Do	0.2% aqueous	Reddish yellow to colorless
Bordeaux	Do	0.1% aqueous	Red to colorless
Naphthol Blue Black	Do	0.2% aqueous	Blue to colorless or faint pink
α-Naphthoflavone	Reversible	0.5% alcoholic	Greenish opalescence to orange brown
Quinoline Yellow	Do	0.5% aqueous	Yellow to colorless
þ-Ethoxychrysoidine	Do	0.1% alcoholic	Red to orange yellow

Some substances can react quantitatively with bromate while some react quantitatively with bromine when excess of bromine is present. Thus, Bromatometry includes the titration with potassium bromate as well as with bromine.

Reactions of some substances with potassium bromate are shown below in the form of equations:

$$BrO_3^- + 3H_3AsO_3 \xrightarrow{HCL} Br^- + 3H_3AsO_4$$

$$2BrO_3^- + 3N_2H_4 \xrightarrow{HCL} 2Br^- + 3N_2 + 6H_2O$$

$$BrO_3^- + NH_2OH \xrightarrow{HCL} Br^- + NO_3^- + H^+ + H_2O$$

$$BrO_3^- + 6[Fe(CN)6]^{4-} + 6H^+ \xrightarrow{HCL} Br^- + 6[Fe(CN)6]^{3-} + 3H_2O$$

Bromine can be prepared quantitatively by the reaction of potassium bromate with potassium bromide in presence of acid and as per the equation given

$$BrO_3^- + 5Br^- + 6H^+ = 3Br_2 + 3H_2O$$

Thus, 1 mole of potassium bromate produces 3 moles of bromine. Bromine is very volatile; hence, this titration should be done at lower temperature and using stoppered (ground-glass stoppered) conical flask. Excess of bromine can be determined iodometrically by addition of excess of potassium iodide and liberated iodine is titrated with standard solution of sodium thiosulphate.

$$2I^- + Br_2 = I_2 + 2Br^-$$

Preparation of 0.1N Potassium Bromate

Dry about 10g of powdered potassium bromate A.R. at 120°C for 2hrs. Allow to cool in desiccator. Weigh accurately about 2.784g of dried potassium bromate and transfer into a 1 L volumetric flask. Dissolve in water, make up the volume and shake well to mix. Since potassium bromate is a primary standard the strength of the solution can be calculated with respect to weight; i.e. $\dfrac{\text{Practical weight}}{\text{Theoretical weight}}$

Use of Bromatometry

Example 8: Determination of metals, e.g. aluminium (Al)

Various metals such as aluminium, iron, cadmium, copper, manganese, cobalt and magnesium form crystalline precipitate with 8-hydroxyquinoline at specific pH. The general formula of these precipitate can be written as $M(C_9H_6ON)_n$; where n is the charge on the metal ion, M.

Oxinates react with dilute HCl and produce oxine. One molecule of oxine reacts with two molecules of bromine and produces 5,7 dibromo-8-hydroxyquinoline.

$$C_9H_6ON + 2Br_2 = C_9H_5ONBr_2 + 2H^+ + 2Br^-$$

Thus, 1 mol of the oxinate of a divalent metal requires 8 equivalents of bromine and 1 mol of the oxinate of a trivalent metal requires 12 equivalents of bromine. Bromine is generated when 0.02M potassium bromate is added to excess of potassium bromide in acid solution.

$$BrO_3^- + 5Br^- + 6H^+ = 3Br_2 + 3H_2O$$

Procedure:

Prepare a 2% solution of 8-hydroxyquinoline in 2M acetic acid (ethanoic acid). Add ammonia solution until a slight precipitate is formed and remains as such. Dissolve the precipitate by warming the solution. Dilute the sample (aluminium salt) in such a way that about 0.08g of Al is present in 100mL. Pipette out 25 mL of the sample accurately and transfer into a 500mL conical flask. Add 125 mL of water, heat to 50° – 60°C, add oxine solution in excess by 20%. The concentration/volume of oxine solution should be such that 1 mL of oxine solution can precipitate 1 mg of Al. complete precipitation of Al(C₉H₆ON) by adding a solution containing 4g of ammonium ethanoate in minimum quantity of water. Stir the mixture well and then allow to cool to room temperature. Filter the precipitate through Whatmann No. 44 filter paper or sintered glass crucible (G4). Wash the precipitate with warm water to remove oxine completely.

Dissolve the precipitate in warm concentrated HCl in a ground glass stoppered 250 mL conical flask. Add 5 drops of 0.1% solution of sodium methyl red or of methyl orange. Add 1g of potassium bromide. Titrate the solution slowly with 0.2M potassium bromate until a pure yellow color is appeared. Since it becomes difficult to detect the endpoint (color change) an excess amount of 0.2M potassium bromate should be added after tentative color change. Add sufficient amount of 2M HCl to dilute the solution so that 5,7 dibromo-8-hydroxyquinoline does not precipitate during titration. Keep it for 5 – 10 min, add 10 mL of 10% solution of potassium iodide and titrate the liberated iodine with 0.1M sodium thiosulphate using starch solution as indicator. Discharge of blue color to colorless is the endpoint.

Determination of phenol

Bromine results number of substitutions in phenol. This substitution reaction is quantitative and rapid. Bromine is generated *in situ* when bromate and bromide are present in acid solution. After completion of substitution reaction with phenol, the unreacted bromine can be determined by adding excess of potassium iodide and the liberated iodine is back titrated with standard sodium thiosulphate solution.

OH + 3Br2 ⟶ OH (with Br, Br, Br substituents) + 3HBr

Other substituted phenols are 4-chlorophenol, 3-methyl phenol (m-cresol), and 2-naphthol.

Procedure

Prepare 0.02M potassium bromate by weighing accurately about 1.67g and dissolving in water in a 500 mL volumetric flask and make up the volume. Shake well to mix thoroughly.

Weigh accurately about 0.3g of phenol and transfer into a clean 250 mL volumetric flask, dissolve in sufficient water to make 250 mL. Pipette accurately 25.00 mL of this solution into each of three clean 250 mL ground-glass stoppered flasks. To each flask pipette 25.00 mL of standard solution of potassium bromate, add 0.5g of potassium bromide and 5 mL of 3M sulphuric acid; mix the contents in each flask well and allow to stand the flasks for 15 min. add rapidly 2.5g of potassium iodide to each flask and stopper each flask immediately. Swirl the flask and titrate the liberated iodine with standard 0.1N sodium thiosulphate until the color of the solution changes to pale yellow. Add 5 mL of starch solution as indicator, a blue color is produced. Continue the titration dropwise until the blue color becomes colorless. Note the titer value of each titration. Carry out a blank titration by taking all the reagents sequentially except phenol solution. Subtract the blank titer value from the average titer value for calculation.

Calculation

Say, the weight of potassium bromate taken = 1.6713g

The weight of potassium bromate to be taken = 1.67g

So, the strength of 0.02M potassium bromate solution $= \dfrac{\text{Practical weight}}{\text{Theoretical weight}}$

$= \dfrac{1.6713\text{g}}{1.67\text{g}}$

$= 1.0008$

Or, the strength of potassium bromate solution = 0.02002M

The volume of phenol solution taken = 25.00 mL

Say, the blank titer value = V_1mL

Sample titer value = V_2 mL

Difference in titer values = V_1mL – V_2 mL = V_3 mL

Each mL of 0.1N sodium thiosulphate $\approx$ 0.001569g of phenol

Or, 25.00 mL of diluted sample solution contains c of phenol

0.3g of sample contains $\dfrac{V_3 \times 0.001569\text{g} \times 250}{25} = V_3 \times 0.01569\text{g}$ of phenol

% content of phenol in the sample $= \dfrac{V_3 \times 0.01569\text{g} \times 100}{0.3} = 5.23 \times V_3$

8.2.5 Dichrometry

Titrations involving potassium dichromate are termed as Dichrometry. Compared to potassium permanganate, potassium dichromate is weaker oxidizing agent. However, it has certain advantages such as;

> ➤ It is available in pure form,
> ➤ It is stable up to its fusion point,
> ➤ It can be used as primary standard.
> ➤ The concentration of its aqueous solution does not change during storage for very long period, if protected from evaporation.
> ➤ It is not photosensitive also.

Potassium dichromate is used in acid solution and is reduced to green chromic salt rapidly even at room temperature. Cold hydrochloric acid can reduce the potassium dichromate, but the concentration of acid should be more than 2N. Organic matters which can reduce potassium permanganate cannot reduce it. Potassium dichromate is mainly used for determination of iron in iron ore. Iron ore is first dissolved in hydrochloric acid and ferric ions are reduced to ferrous ions by treating with stannous chloride solution.

$$Cr_2O_7^{2-} + 6Fe^{2+} + 14H^+ = 2Cr^{3+} + 6Fe^{3+} + 7H_2O$$

Reduction of potassium dichromate in acid solution can be expressed as;

$$Cr_2O_7^{2-} + 14H^+ + 6e = 2Cr^{3+} + 7H_2O$$

The above equation indicates that the equivalent weight of potassium dichromate is its $1/6^{th}$ of its molecular weight (294.22); that is 49.037. Thus, 0.1N solution contains 4.9037g of potassium dichromate per litre.

For determination of the endpoint in titration with potassium dichromate solution, there are three methods:

> ➤ With an external indicator,
> ➤ With an internal indicator, and
> ➤ Potentiometric titration.

Use of *external indicator* has been traditionally and widely used. This method has been practiced since when the titration of ferrous iron was started. Potassium ferricyanide on storage converts to ferrocyanide particularly in surface layer of a crystal. Hence to get a pure ferricyanide crystal, the crystal is washed several times with water to remove ferrocyanide. Then the ferricyanide crystal is dissolved in sufficient water to make a solution of less than 0.1%. a drop of this solution when placed and spread over a white tile appears colorless or pale yellow.

The acidified solution of ferrous ions is titrated with standard potassium dichromate solution. The equivalent weight potassium dichromate is $1/6^{th}$ of its molecular weight. To understand how its equivalent weight is calculated, the reader may consider the following hypothetical equations.

$$K_2Cr_2O_7 + 4H_2SO_4 = K_2SO_4 + Cr_2(SO_4)_3 + 4H_2O + 3O$$

$$K_2Cr_2O_7 + 8HCl = 2KCl + 2CrCl_3 + 4H_2O + 3O$$

After first titration potassium dichromate solution is added dropwise with swirling the solution, so that the change in color from pale yellow to deep blue, from deep blue to bluish green and then from bluish green to green can be clearly observed.

As *internal indicator* 1% diphenylamine solution was first used in this titration. Later on, 1% solution of diphenyl benzidine dissolved in concentrated sulphuric acid was used. Thereafter 0.2% aqueous solution of sodium diphenyl sulphonate has also been used. However phosphoric acid is mixed with any of the three indicators; because phosphoric acid forms a complex, $[Fe(HPO_4)]^+$ with ferric ion and reduces the oxidation potentials of ferric-ferrous systems. These indicators produce a green color in ferrous solution; then the color deepens to a blue-green when endpoint is about to reach. At the endpoint the blue-green color changes to deep purple or blue-violet color which does not change further. If N-phenylanthranilic acid or 5,6-dimethyl-1,10-phenanthroline ferrous sulphate (5,6-dimethylferroin) are used, phosphoric acid is not required.

Out of these two, N-phenylanthranilic acid is relatively cheaper and 0.1% solution is prepared by dissolving 0.1g in 5 mL of 0.1N sodium hydroxide and diluting to 100 mL with water. the color changes from green to violet-red.

For *potentiometric titration* appropriate redox indicator should be selected on the basis of theoretical concept. Two types of potentials are considered in potentiometry – standard potential and formal potential. The standard potential of the half-cell reaction is 1.33 volts.

$$Cr_2O_7^{2-} + 14H^+ + 6e = 2Cr^{3+} + 7H_2O$$

For practical purpose formal potential is to be considered. In a redox system the formal potential is necessary with unit concentrations of oxidant and reductant at a specified acid concentration. For the potentiometric titration of ferrous ion with dichromate ion, the formal potentials of the two systems – $Cr_2O_7^{2-}$, Cr^{3+} and Fe^{3+}, Fe^{2+} should be taken into consideration for selection of an appropriate indicator. It depends on the concentration of acid present in the system. Formal potentials of dichromate and iron systems in different concentrations of acids are shown below:

Acid present	$E^{o'}$, volts		Acid present	$E^{o'}$, volts	
	$Cr_2O_7^{2-}$, Cr^{3+}	Fe^{3+}, Fe^{2+}		$Cr_2O_7^{2-}$, Cr^{3+}	Fe^{3+}, Fe^{2+}
0.1M HCl	0.03	0.73	0.5M H_2SO_4	1.08	0.68
0.5M HCl	0.07	0.72	1M H_2SO_4	1.03	0.69
1M HCl	1.00	0.70	2M H_2SO_4	1.11	0.69
2M HCl	1.05	0.69	4M H_2SO_4	1.15	0.69
3M HCl	1.08	0.68	8M H_2SO_4	1.35	0.66
4M HCl	1.10	0.66	0.1M $HClO_4$	0.84	0.74
0.1M H_2SO_4	0.92	0.68	1M $HClO_4$	1.03	0.74

A redox reaction can be expressed as;

$$aOx_1 + bRed_2 \leftrightarrow bOx_2 + aRed_1$$

It is desired that near the endpoint (within 0.1%) the indicator should change its color. This helps detection of endpoint. For this color change formal potential of the indicator, E_{In} should be as follows;

$$E_1^{o'} - \frac{3 \times 0.059}{a} > E_{In} > E_2^{o'} + \frac{3 \times 0.059}{b}$$

Where E_1^{o} is the formal potential of the half-cell reaction, $Ox_1 + ae \leftrightarrow Red_1$ and $E_2^{o'}$ is the formal potential of the half-cell reaction, $Ox_2 + be \leftrightarrow Red_2$.

This has been observed that for ferric-ferrous titration 4,7-dimethyl ferroin and 5,6-dimethyl ferroin are most suitable. These provide sharp change in color at the endpoint and addition of phosphoric acid is not required. Although theoretically ferroin indicators should not be used in ferric-ferrous titration; but in practice 4,7-dimethyl ferroin gives a satisfactory result.

Preparation of 0.1N potassium dichromate

Equivalent weight of potassium dichromate is 49.035g. Potassium dichromate, A.R. with purity of 99.9% is used. Powder finely about 3g of potassium dichromate in a glass mortar pestle. Transfer the powder into a clean, dry, and tared weighing bottle. Dry the powders at about 150°C for 1 hr.; cool the dried powders in a desiccator. Weigh accurately about 1.225g of dried potassium dichromate; take it in a 250 mL volumetric flask and dissolve in sufficient water, make up the volume with water and shake well.

Determination of iron in ferric ammonium sulphate

Molecular formula of ferric ammonium sulphate $FeNH_4(SO_4)_2, 12H_2O$; molecular weight is 482.21.

Weigh accurately about 4.822g of ferric ammonium sulphate; dissolve in sufficient water to make 100 mL in a volumetric flask. Shake well to mix thoroughly. Pipette out exactly 25.00 mL of the solution in a 500 mL conical flask. Reduce the ferric solution with stannous chloride solution. Add 200 mL of 2.5% of sulphuric acid, 5 mL of phosphoric acid and 0.4 mL of sodium diphenylamine sulphonate indicator. Titrate rapidly with standard 0.1N potassium dichromate with constant swirling until a permanent violet-blue color is produced. Note the volume of 0.1N potassium dichromate consumed (titer value). Repeat the titration twice and take average titer value for calculation.

Calculation

$$\text{Strength of 0.1N potassium dichromate} = \frac{\text{Practical weight}}{\text{Theoretical weight}}$$

Each mL of 0.1N potassium dichromate is equivalent to 0.005585g of Fe.

8.2.6   Titration with Potassium Iodate

Like potassium bromate potassium is a strong oxidizing agent. Potassium iodate when reacts with a reducing agent such as potassium iodide or arsenious oxide in moderately acid solution (0.1 – 2M HCl) is reduced to iodine. The chemical equation involved is expressed as follows:

$$IO_3^- + 5I^- + 6H^+ = 3I_2 + 3H_2O$$

$$2IO_3^- + 5H_3AsO_3 + 2H^+ = I_2 + 5H_3AsO_4 + H_2O$$

In 1903 L.W. Andrews showed that in high concentration (3 – 9M) of hydrochloric acid potassium iodate is reduced to iodine monochloride as indicated below;

$$IO_3^- + Cl^- + 6H^+ + 4e = ICl + 3H_2O$$

In hydrochloric acid solution iodine monochloride forms stable complex ion with chloride ion

$$ICl + Cl^- = ICl_2^-$$

The overall half-cell reaction can be written as;

$$IO_3^- + 2Cl^- + 6H^+ + 4e = ICl_2^- + 3H_2O$$

The reduction potential is 1.23. Under these conditions potassium iodate acts as a strong oxidizing agent and its equivalent weight is $1/4^{th}$ of its molecular weight; that is 214.01/4 = 53.503g. Hence its 0.1N solution will contain 5.3503g per lt. In presence of hydrochloric acid (3 – 9M) iodate ion oxidizes in several steps

$$IO_3^- + 6H^+ + 6e \leftrightarrow I^- + 3H_2O$$

$$IO_3^- + 5I^- + 6H^+ \leftrightarrow 3I_2 + 3H_2O$$

$$IO_3^- + 2I_2 + 6H^+ = 5I^+ + 3H_2O$$

Initially free iodine is liberated by iodate ion, with further addition of iodate ion oxidation proceeds, iodine monochloride is formed and the dark color of iodine gradually fades. The overall reaction can be expressed as;

$$IO_3^- + 6H^+ + 4e = I^+ + 3H_2O$$

This reaction can be used for determination of various reducing agents. Appropriate hydrochloric acid concentration (3 – 6M) is required; but not in every case.

Detection of endpoint

At high concentration of acid starch-iodine complex is not formed; hence starch cannot be used as indicator in this titration. In place of starch few mL of chloroform or carbon tetrachloride is added to the titration mixture. The color of the insoluble organic solvent becomes blue due to solubilization of iodine produced in the reaction. For the titration ground-glass stoppered conical flask is used. As the reaction proceeds the blue color disappears gradually and finally at the endpoint the organic solvent becomes colorless.

Some dyes such as amaranth, brilliant ponceau 5R and naphthol blue black can be used at concentration of 0.2 to 0.5% in place of organic solvent. The excess of iodate destroys the dyes; hence the dye should be added near to the endpoint when the concentration of iodate is reduced in the solution. In case of amaranth the color changes from red to colorless; in case of brilliant ponceau 5R color changes from orange to colorless, and when naphthol blue black is used the color changes from green to light pink. Thus, these indicators are irreversible.

þ-ethoxychrysoidine is a reversible indicator; its 0.1% solution is used. At the endpoint the color changes from red to orange, near endpoint the color of the indicator is red-purple. A blank titration must be determined.

Preparation of 0.1N Potassium iodate

Take about 1g of potassium iodate in a weighing bottle, dry in at 120°C for about 1 hr; cool it in a desiccator. Weigh accurately about 0.5350g of dried potassium iodate and transfer into a 100 mL volumetric flask, dissolve in water to make 100 mL. Shake well. The strength of the solution would be 0.125M also and 0.1N with respect to the following reaction;

$$IO_3^- + Cl^- + 6H^+ + 4e = ICl + 3H_2O$$

Determination of iodide in KI

The reaction involved in this determination is;

$$IO_3^- + 3Cl^- + 6H^+ + 2I^- = 3ICl + 3H_2O$$

The reaction shows that one iodate ion is equivalent to two iodide ions. thus, 1mL of 0.1N $KIO_3 \approx 0.006347$g of I^-, in other words 1mL of 0.1N $KIO_3 \approx 0.0031735$g of I_2

Procedure

Weigh accurately 2g of potassium iodide, transfer in a 250 mL of volumetric flask, and dissolve in sufficient water to make 250 mL. Shake well. Pipette out 25.00 mL of potassium iodide solution accurately into a 250 mL clean glass-ground conical flask, add 25 mL of water and 60 mL of concentrated hydrochloric acid, mix and 5 mL of carbon tetrachloride. Titrate the mixture with 0.1N standard potassium iodate solution from a burette with constant shaking until carbon tetrachloride shows a faint brown color. Stopper the flask and shake vigorously and examine the color of the carbon tetrachloride. Add two drops of KIO_3 solution; stopper the flask and shake vigorously. Repeat the same until carbon tetrachloride layer acquires a pale-yellow color due to formation of iodine chloride. As such the change of color from faint-violet to pale-yellow, at the endpoint is sharp.

To know whether the titration is overshot or not, add one drop of KI solution prepared, stopper the flask and shake vigorously. The carbon tetrachloride layer will acquire a very faint violet color.

A. MULTIPLE CHOICE QUESTIONS

1. In oxidation-reduction reaction
    (a) The reactants undergo only oxidation reaction
    (b) The reactants undergo only reduction reaction
    (c) The reactants undergo oxidation and reduction simultaneously
    (d) None of the above

2. In oxidation-reduction reaction
    (a) The reducing agents undergo oxidation
    (b) The reducing agents undergo reduction
    (c) The oxidizing agents undergo oxidation
    (d) All of the above

3. In oxidation-reduction reaction
    (a) The oxidizing agents undergo oxidation
    (b) The oxidizing agents undergo reduction
    (c) The reducing agents undergo reduction
    (d) All of the above

4. In oxidation-reduction reaction
    (a) Electron is accepted by reducing agent
    (b) Electron is accepted by oxidizing agent
    (c) Electron is donated by oxidizing agent
    (d) None of the above

5. In oxidation-reduction reaction
    (a) Electron is donated by reducing agent
    (b) Electron is donated by oxidizing agent
    (c) Electron is accepted by reducing agent
    (d) None of the above

6. The rules for application of ion-electron method are:
    (a) The products of the reaction are to be determined.
    (b) Partial equations for oxidation and reduction are to be arranged.
    (c) Multiply each of the partial equations by a factor to balance, add the partial equations and cancel the substances appear on the both sides of the equation.
    (d) All of the above

7. Which one of the following statements is correct?
    (a) Oxidation number indicates the amount of oxidation or reduction required to convert one atom of the element from the free-state to that in the compound.
    (b) Equivalent weight of an oxidizing agent can be determined by dividing the molecular weight of the compound by its oxidation number.
    (c) Equivalent weight of reducing agent can be determined by dividing the molecular weight of the compound by its oxidation number.
    (d) All of the above

8. Which one of the following statements is correct?
   (a) Oxidation number of a free or uncombined element is zero.
   (b) Oxidation number of hydrogen is ± 1
   (c) Oxidation number of oxygen is ± 2
   (d) Oxidation number of oxygen is $+2$

9. Which one of the following statements is correct?
   (a) Oxidation number of oxygen in peroxide is -2
   (b) Oxidation number of hydrogen in hydride is $+1$
   (c) Oxidation number of a compound is always zero.
   (d) Oxidation number of a compound is not always zero.

10. Equivalent weight of $KMnO_4$ is (mol wt is 158.03)
    (a) 22.57   (b) 31.61
    (c) 52.68   (d) 39.51

11. Which one of the following statements is correct?
    (a) Iodometry is the titrations of iodine liberated in chemical reaction.
    (b) Iodimetry is the titrations of iodine liberated in chemical reaction.
    (c) Iodometry is the titrations with standard solution of iodine
    (d) None of the above

12. Which one of the following statements is correct?
    (a) Iodimetric titrations are used to determine the redox substances quantitatively.
    (b) Iodometric titrations are used to determine the redox substances quantitatively.
    (c) Iodimetry and iodometrytitrations are used to determine the redox substances quantitatively.
    (d) None of the above

13. Which one of the following statements is correct?
    (a) Iodimetry is a direct titration method
    (b) Iodimetry is anindirect titration method
    (c) Iodometry is a direct method
    (d) None of the above

14. The endpoint in titration with potassium dichromate solution can be determined using
    (a) An external indicator   (b) An internal indicator
    (c) A potentiometer   (d) All of the above

15. Which one of the following is an oxidizing agent?
    (a) Potassium iodide   (b) Potassium iodate
    (c) Iodide ion   (d) None of the above

16. Which one of the following requires potassium iodide for its solubilization in water?
    (a) Iodine
    (b) Potassium iodate
    (c) Potassium chromate
    (d) Potassium bromate

17. Which one of the following is not a primary standard?
    (a) Potassium iodate
    (b) Potassium bromate
    (c) Potassium permanganate
    (d) Sodium oxalate

B. SHORT QUESTIONS

1. What do you understand by oxidation and reduction?
2. What are the rules for application of ion-electron method?
3. Define oxidation number and give example.
4. What are the rules followed to determine the oxidation number?
5. Classify the titrations based on the type of oxidation-reduction reaction involved.
6. What is cerimetry?
7. What is Permanganometry?
8. Distinguish between iodimetry and iodometry.
9. What is Bromatometry?
10. What do you understand by the term dichrometry?

C. LONG QUESTIONS

1. Oxidation and reduction reactions take place simultaneously – justify the statement with relevant example.
2. Explain with example how the equivalent weight of oxidizing and reducing agents is calculated.
3. Discuss in brief the principle involved in cerimetric analysis.
4. Describe in brief the principle involved in permanganometric analysis.
5. Describe the method of preparation and standardization of $0.1N$ $KMnO_4$.
6. Explain with example iodimetry and iodometry.
7. Describe the application of iodimetry in determination of a substance.
8. Describe the application of iodometry in determination of a substance.
9. Explain the principle involved in bromatometric analysis.
10. Describe the application of bromatometry in determination of a substance.
11. Describe titration with potassium iodate.

CHAPTER 9

Conductometry

9.1 INTRODUCTION

The methods of quantitative analysis based on the measurement of electrical properties are briefly called **electrochemical methods of analysis**. The main techniques employed in these electrical methods are:

1. Conductometry
2. Potentiometry
3. Polarography
4. Coulometry
5. Electrogravimetry

Conductometry, potentiometry and polarography is discussed in this book while coulometry and electrogravimetry is out of scope of pharmaceutical analysis-I syllabus.

Conductometry is a method of analysis is based on measuring electrolytic conductance. According to the Ohm's law the current, I (amperes) flowing in a conductor is directly proportional to the applied electromotive force, E (volts) and inversely proportional to the resistance, R (Ohm) of the conductor:

$$I = \frac{E}{R}$$

The reciprocal of resistance, R is called conductance, κ. The resistance of a homogeneous material having uniform cross section can be expressed as;

$$\kappa = \frac{1}{R} = \rho . \frac{l}{a}$$

Where, ρ is the characteristic property of the material, called specific resistance; l is the length (cm), and a is the area (sq. cm). Specific conductance, κ (kappa) is the reciprocal of specific conductance.

Thus, conductivity is the ability of a solution, a metal or a gas - in short, all materials - to pass an electric current. In solutions the current is carried by cations and anions. In metals it is carried by electrons. The flow of electricity in a solution depends on the following factors:

- Concentration
- Mobility of ions
- Valence of ions
- Temperature

All substances possess some degree of conductivity. In aqueous solutions, the degree of ionic strength varies from the low conductivity such as in ultra-pure water to the high conductivity such as in solution of strong electrolyte.

The factors influencing the conductance of the solution:

- **Concentration:** The total contribution from all ions present is considered as electrical conductance of a solution. It depends on the number of ions in unit volume of solution and their nature such as the ion whether presents itself independently or not. If the number of ions increases, the conductance of the solution increases. The conductance of a concentrated solution of a strong electrolyte is less due to inter-ionic forces.

- **Mobility of ions:** The velocity or mobility of ions carrying the electric current towards the electrodes varies with their nature, such as size, molecular weight, number of charges the ion possesses and other factors.

- **Nature of the electrolyte:** The conductance of an electrolyte depends upon the number of ions present in the solution. Therefore, if the number of ions in the solution is more, the conductance of the solution will be more. Depending on its nature an electrolyte produces specific number of ions in a solution. For example, a strong electrolyte dissociates completely into ions in its solutions. Therefore, its solutions will have high conductance. On the other hand, weak electrolyte dissociates to only small extents and produces lesser number of ions. Therefore, the solutions of weak electrolytes have low conductance.

- **Temperature:** The conductance increases with increase of temperature. If the temperature is increased by $1°C$ the conductance increases by 2%. For this reason, the measurements must be carried out at a constant temperature using thermostatically controlled water bath or by using a conductometer having a device which can calibrate the temperature increase continuously during measurements

- **Resistance of the conductor:** The material carrying or conducting the current should be homogeneous material and uniform cross section. Then the resistance, R which has been defined and expressed earlier is rewritten here;

$$R = \rho . \frac{l}{a}$$

Conductive solution

Conductivity is typically measured in aqueous solutions of electrolytes. That is, the solutions of ionic salts or of compounds that can ionize in solution. The ions formed in solution carry the electric current. Electrolytes include acids, bases and salts. These can be either strong or weak. Most conductive solutions measured are aqueous solutions, because water has the capability of stabilizing the ions formed by a process called solvation.

Strong electrolytes

Strong electrolytes are substances that remain fully ionized in solution. Thus, the concentration of ions in solution is directly proportional to the concentration of the electrolyte. For example, hydrochloric acid, sodium hydroxide, sodium chloride, etc.

Solutions of strong electrolytes conduct electricity because the positive and negative ions can migrate independently under the influence of an electric field.

Weak electrolytes

Weak electrolytes are not fully ionized in solution. For example, acetic acid partially dissociates into acetate ions and hydrogen ions, so that an acetic acid solution contains both molecules and ions. A solution of a weak electrolyte can conduct electricity, but usually not equal to that of a strong electrolyte because fewer ions are there in the solution to carry the charge from one electrode to the other.

Terms used in conductivity

Resistance of a solution (R) can be calculated using Ohm's law: $V = R \times I$.

So,
$$R = \frac{V}{I}$$

Where, V = voltage (volts), I = current (amperes) and R = resistance of the solution (ohms)

Conductance

Conductance (G) is defined as the reciprocal of the electrical resistance (R) of a solution between two electrodes.

$$G = \frac{1}{R}$$

A conductivity meter measures the conductance, and displays the reading converted into conductivity.

Cell constant

The cell constant (K) is the ratio of the distance (d) between the electrodes to the area (a) of the electrodes.

$$K = \frac{d}{a}$$

K = cell constant (cm^{-1})

a = effective area of the electrodes (cm^2)

d = distance between the electrodes (cm)

Conductivity

Electricity is the flow of electrons and it has been mentioned earlier that the ions present in solution conduct electricity. Hence, conductivity (κ) is the ability of a solution to pass current. The conductivity reading of a sample changes with temperature.

$$\kappa = G \times K$$

κ = conductivity (S/cm)

G = conductance (S), where $G = \dfrac{1}{R}$ and K = cell constant (cm^{-1})

Resistivity

This is the reciprocal of the conductivity value and is measured in ohm $\times$ cm. It is generally limited to the measurement of ultrapure water, the conductivity of which is very low.

- **Equivalent conductance (Λ)**

Equivalent conductance (Λ) is defined as the conductance of one-gram equivalent of a solute when placed between two electrodes spaced one centimeter apart.

Hence, $\qquad \Lambda = \dfrac{1000\,\kappa}{C}$

Where, C is the concentration of the solute in gram equivalent per liter.

Equivalent ionic conductance (Λo)

This has been mentioned earlier that on dilution of an electrolyte solution the conductance decreases due to reduced inter-ionic interaction. Hence, at infinite dilution, interactions become nil; the overall conductance of the solution becomes equal to the sum of the individual equivalent ionic conductance

So, $\qquad \Lambda o = \lambda^{o}_{+} + \lambda^{o}_{-}$

Where, λ^{o}_{+} and λ^{o}_{-} are equivalent ionic conductance of the cation and anion of the salt at infinite dilution. Individual ionic conductance can be determined from other electrolytic measurements.

Table 9.1: Ionic conductance of some cations and anions

Cation	λ^{o}_{+}	Anion	λ^{o}_{-}
H^+	349.8	OH^-	198.3
Na^+	50.1	F^-	55.4
K^+	73.5	Cl^-	76.3
NH_4^+	73.5	Br^-	78.1
Ag^+	61.9	I^-	76.8
$\frac{1}{2}Ca^{2+}$	59.5	NO_3^-	71.5
$\frac{1}{2}Ba^{2+}$	63.6	ClO_3^-	64.6
$\frac{1}{2}Mg^{2+}$	53.1	ClO_4^-	67.4

Table 9.1: *Contd...*

Cation	λ°_{+}	Anion	λ°_{-}
$\frac{1}{2}Zn^{2+}$	52.8	BrO_3^-	55.7
$\frac{1}{2}Pb^{2+}$	69.5	IO_3^-	40.5
$\frac{1}{2}Cu^{2+}$	53.6	HCO_3^-	44.5
$\frac{1}{2}Fe^{2+}$	54	SO_3^{2-}	80
$\frac{1}{2}Co^{2+}$	55	$HCOO^-$	54.6
$\frac{1}{3}Fe^{3+}$	68.4	$\frac{1}{3}PO_4^{3-}$	80

Instruments used in conductometric determination

To carry out conductometric measurement it is necessary to measure the resistance of the solution and the conductance.

The instrument consists of two parts:

1. Conductivity Bridge, which measures the resistance; then converts it to conductivity unit.
2. Conductance cell, which contains the solution to be measured.

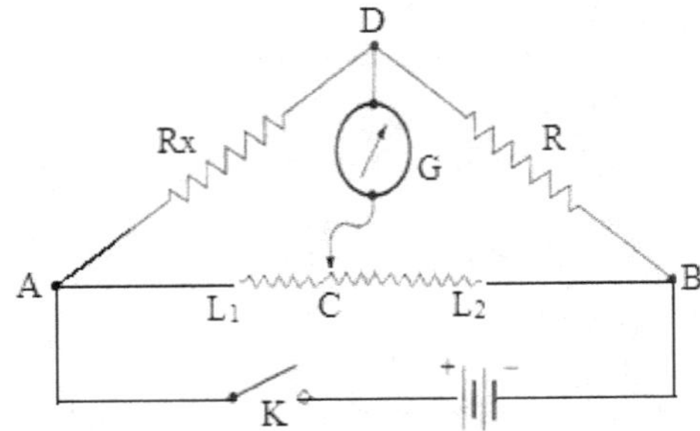

Figure 9.1 Wheatstone Bridge

Conductivity Bridge (Kohlrausch Bridge)

It consists of:

(a) Wheatstone Bridge.

(b) An oscillator.

The schematic diagram of Wheatstone bridge shown in the figure 9.1 is used to measure the resistance. The power source K provides an ac current at a potential of 6 to 10 V.

The unknown resistance Rx is placed in the upper-left arm of the bridge.

A null detector G (ac galvanometer) is employed to indicate an absence of current between D and C.

To measure Rx the position of C is adjusted to a minimum as indicated by the null detector G. The position of C will change rapidly resulting variation in L_1 and L_2 automatically till the balance point is reached; where no current is detected. At equilibrium or balanced condition;

$$\frac{R}{R_{CB}} = \frac{R_X}{R_{AC}}$$

$$Rx = \frac{R \times R_{AC}}{R_{CB}} = R\frac{AC}{CB}$$

Hence, the specific conductance, $\kappa = \dfrac{1}{R} \times \dfrac{CB}{AC}$

If the length of AB is 100cm and of BC is x; then $\kappa = \dfrac{1}{R} \times \dfrac{x}{100-x}$

9.2   CONDUCTOMETRY

To understand electrochemistry, we need to understand following five important and interrelated concepts:

- The potential of electrode determines the form of analyte present at the surface of the electrode;
- The concentration of analyte at the surface of electrode may not be equal to its concentration in bulk solution;
- The analyte may participate in other reactions, in addition to an oxidation–reduction reaction;
- Current is a measure of the rate of oxidation or reduction of the analyte; and
- Simultaneous control of current and potential may not be possible always.

The conductometric titration is based on the principle that during the titration, one of the ions is replaced by the other and these two ions will always differ in their ionic conductivity. As a result, during the course of titration the conductivity of the solution will vary. By plotting the change in conductance against the volume of titrant added, the graph obtained can locate the equivalence point.

9.3   CONDUCTIVITY CELL

Measurement of conductivity

Conductivity is measured by applying an alternating electrical current (I) to two electrodes immersed in a solution and measuring the resulting voltage (V). During this process, the cations migrate to the negative electrode, the anions to the positive electrode as shown in the fig 9.2 and the solution acts as an electrical conductor.

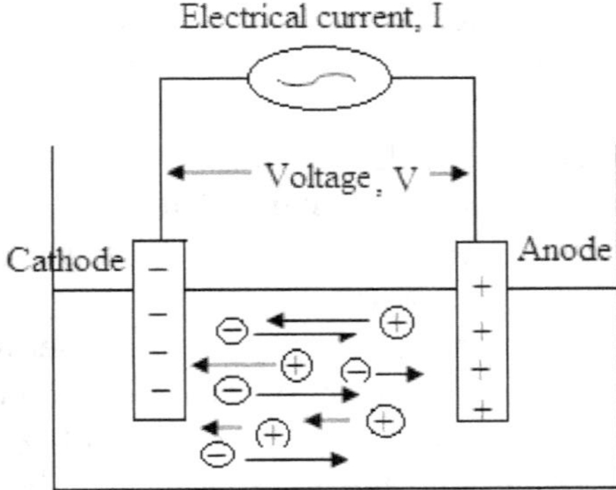

Figure 9.2 Migration of ions in solution

The cell contains two parallel sheets of platinum, fixed in position, sealed into the sides of the measuring cell. The distance between the two electrodes is constant during the determination. For a given cell with fixed electrodes the ratio of L/A (cm) is a constant which is known as cell constant. It is determined for each cell using solutions of known conductivity. The cell must be dipped in thermostatically controlled water bath or the instrumental should possess a temperature calibration device.

Conductivity = cell constant × conductance

The current source is to be adjusted so that the measured potential (V) becomes equal to the reference potential (Er) (approximately ± 200 mV). The fig 9.3 shows the schematic diagram of a simple conductivity meter.

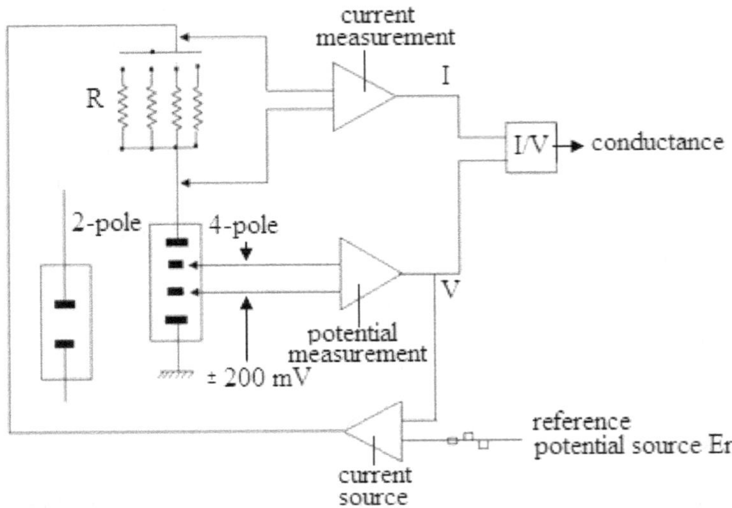

Figure 9.3 Schematic diagram of simple conductivity meter

There are various types of conductometric cells. The fig.9.4 shows few examples. Any kind of cell can be used for conductometric analysis; however, the cell must have following facilities:

- ➤ Stirring facility – the content of the cell must be stirred, preferably by mechanical means such mechanical stirrer or swirling by hand.
- ➤ Inlet for reagent addition – the cell must have a suitable provision for periodical addition of reagent whenever required.
- ➤ Resistance – the cell must be made of Pyrex or any other resistant glass.
- ➤ Area of electrode – the area of the electrode should be around 1sq.cm.
- ➤ Construction of the electrodes – the electrodes should be welded to thick platinum wires which are fused into glass tubes in which the platinum wires make contact with mercury.
- ➤ Electrodes – the ends of the copper leads that dip into mercury should be pre-amalgamated.
- ➤ Distance between the electrodes – depending on the solution being titrated (change in conductance of the solution) the distance between the electrodes varies. For low-conductance solutions the electrodes should be large and kept close together. For getting satisfactory results in many cases the electrodes are kept 2 cm apart. For precipitation titrations the electrodes must be of vertical type.
- ➤ Polarization effect – to reduce polarization effect the platinum electrodes should be platinized.

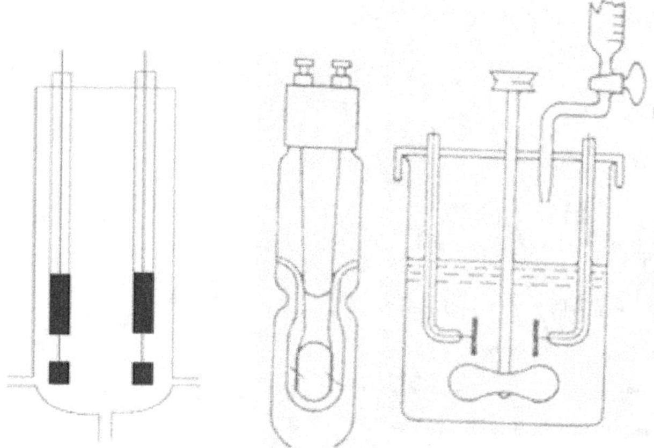

Figure 9.4 Schematic diagram of some conductometric cells

2-pole cell

When a traditional 2-pole cell is used, an alternating current is applied between the 2 poles and the resulting voltage is measured. It is used to measure the solution resistance (Rsol) only. However, the resistance caused by polarization of the electrodes (Rel) and the field effect may interfere with the measurement; hence both 'Rsol' and 'Rel' are also measured. Non-platinized 2-pole cells are suitable for measuring the conductivity ranging from 0.1μS/cm to 1 mS/cm. When platinized this type of pole can measure conductivity up to 5 mS/cm.

3-pole cell

The 3-pole cell is not popular one; because it has been replaced by the 4-pole cell. This type of pole, whether platinized or non-platinized, could measure the conductivity ranging from 0.1μS/cm to 5 mS/cm.

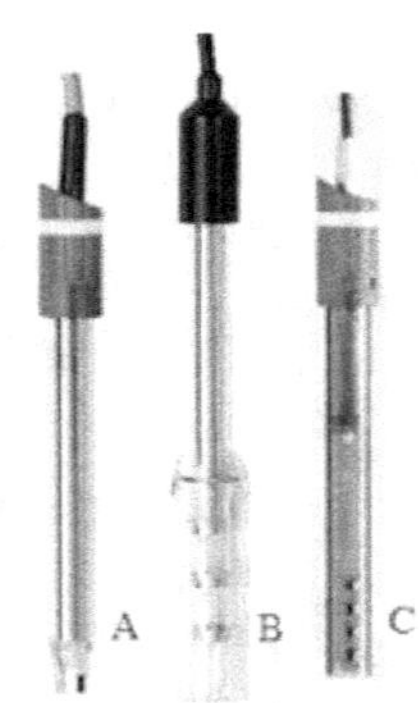

Figure 9.5 Diagram of (A) 2-pole cell, (B) 3-pole cell and (C) 4-pole cell

4-pole cell

In a 4-pole cell, a constant potential difference is maintained between the inner rings (2 and 3) by applying the current to the outer rings (1 and 4). Since the voltage measurement takes place with a negligible current, these two electrodes are not polarized ($R_2 = R_3 = 0$). Thus, the conductivity will be directly proportional to the applied current. The geometry of 4-pole cells with an outer tube is such that it minimizes the beaker field effect; since the measurement volume is well defined within the tube. Therefore, the position of the conductivity cell in the measuring vessel or the sample volume has no influence on the measurement. Non-platinized 4-pole cells are can measure the conductivity ranging from 0.1μS/cm to about 90 mS/cm. When platinized this type of pole can measure conductivity up to 1000 mS/cm. Conductivity values of some samples at 25°C are given in table 9.2 below.

Table 9.2: Conductivity values of some samples at 25°C

Sample	Conductivity
Pure water	0.055 μS/cm
Deionized water	1 μS/cm
Rainwater	50 μS/cm
Drinking water	500 μS/cm
Industrial wastewater	5 mS/cm
Seawater	50 mS/cm
1 mol/l NaCl	85 mS/cm
1 mol/l HCl	332 mS/cm

Platinized cells

To minimize polarization effects and to avoid error on the measurement the cell poles (plates or rings) are covered with a layer of platinum black. Thus, the surface of the pole is increased; the current density is decreased; as a result, the polarization effect is reduced. The platinum black must not be damaged or scratched, because this will modify the surface of the poles and therefore the cell constant.

However, one minor limitation of platinized cells is that the cell constant tends to drift faster than that of non-platinized cells.

It is therefore necessary to use platinized cells only in non-viscous samples, and to perform frequent calibrations.

Flow-through cell

These type of conductivity cells are designed to measure the flow in small volumes of sample. The measurements can be done in a closed liquid system protected from air. However, when the measurement is done in pure water, a flow cell must be used. Contact with air must be avoided; because the carbon dioxide in the air forms hydrogen carbonate ions in water and leads to a change in the conductivity. Generally, a circulation cell is used in two ways:

➢ Circulation: during the measurement the solution flows continuously.
➢ Pipette: an amount of solution is drawn into the cell. This technique is ideal for small sample volumes.

Selection of the right conductivity cell

Cell type	Advantages	Disadvantages
2-pole cell	Easier to maintain	Field effects - cell must be positioned in the centre of the measuring vessel
	Use with sample changer (no carryover)	Only cells with no bridge between the plates
	Economical	Polarization in high conductivity samples
	Recommended for viscous media or samples with suspension	Calibrate using a standard with a value close to measuring value Measurement accurate over 2 decades
4-pole cell	Linear over a very large conductivity range	Unsuitable for micro samples; depth of immersion 3 to 4 cm
	Calibration and measurement in different ranges	Unsuitable for use with a sample changer
	Flow-through or immersion type cells	
	Ideal for high conductivity measurements	
	Can be used for low conductivity measurements if cell capacitance compensated	

9.4 CONDUCTOMETRIC TITRATIONS

- **Determination of the strength of a solution of hydrochloric acid by a standard solution of sodium hydroxide.**

Materials required

1. HCl solution of unknown strength is provided.
2. 0.1N NaOH solution is provided.
3. Calibration of the instrument at room temperature.

Procedure

➢ Rinse the conductivity cell a number of times with conductivity water or double distilled water.

➢ Pipette out 20 mL of HCl in a beaker and dip the conductivity cell in it, so that the cell should dip completely in solution.

➢ Note the temperature of the sample solution and accordingly set the temperature control or keep the cell in a thermostat at room temperature.

➢ Add small amount of NaOH solution (few drops) from burette, stir it and measure the conductance after each addition.

➢ Take at least five readings beyond the end point.

Observation and Calculation

Volume of HCl taken (V_1)	Volume of NaOH added (V_2)	Conductance
20 mL		

Plot a graph between conductance and volume of titrant (NaOH solution). Two intersecting lines will be obtained and the points of intersection of these lines represent the equivalent point.

Let, V_2 be the volume of NaOH at the equivalent point (from graph) and the strength of acid is S_1 and strength of NaOH solution is $S_2 = 0.1(N)$.

Then, $20ml \times S_1 = V_2 \times S_2$

$$S_1 = \frac{S_2 \times V_2}{20mL} N = x\,N$$

Hence, the strength of the hydrochloric acid is x N.

- **Conductometric Titration of Hydrochloric Acid and Acetic Acid with Sodium Hydroxide**

Procedure

➢ Dry the potassium hydrogen phthalate in an oven at 110°C for at least 2 hours.

➢ Remove the dried material from the oven and keep it in a desiccator to cool to room temperature.

➢ Add about 6 mL of 50% sodium hydroxide solution to a 1 L volumetric flask.

- ➤ Dilute the solution to near the mark with distilled water. The resulting solution becomes 0.1 M sodium hydroxide.
- ➤ Weigh accurately 0.8 g of potassium hydrogen phthalate into each of three 250 mL Erlenmeyer flasks, previously marked.
- ➤ Add 30 mL of distilled water and two drops of phenolphthalein solution to each of the flasks.
- ➤ Rinse and fill a 50 mL clean burette with the sodium hydroxide solution. Titrate potassium hydrogen phthalate solution present in each Erlenmeyer flask. The color of the end point changes from colorless to light pink. Note three titer values.
- ➤ Mix 35 mL of an acetic acid solution and 35 mL of a hydrochloric acid solution. Mark the sample numbers.
- ➤ Add 10 mL of the hydrochloric acid solution to the 250 mL beaker through a pipette. Add about 140 mL of distilled water and put a glass rod to stir the solution in beaker. Use a clamp to suspend the electrodes in the solution. The platinum electrodes must be completely immersed into the solution; but the electrodes should not interfere with operation of the stirring rod. Adjust the stirring rate to yield a smoothly stirred solution.
- ➤ Refill the burette with sodium hydroxide solution. Measure the initial conductance of the stirred solution. Add 1 mL of the sodium hydroxide solution to the stirred solution. measure and record the conductance of the solution and also the total volume (to the nearest 0.01 mL) of the added titrant solution after each addition. Continue the titration until the end point has been reached by 100%, i.e., until a total volume that is twice the endpoint volume has been added.
- ➤ Similarly dilute and titrate twice taking 10 mL portions of the hydrochloric acid solution each time and titrate thrice taking 10 mL of the acetic acid solution each time.

Calculations

- ➤ Calculate the strength of potassium hydrogen phthalate solution and by using that calculate the strength of sodium hydroxide solution. The molecular weight of potassium hydrogen phthalate is 204.23. Use the average strength of the sodium hydroxide solution.
- ➤ Plot the graph of conductance (y axis) vs. volume of sodium hydroxide solution added (x axis). Draw a straight line through each of the two, linear portions in each titration curve. Determine the endpoint volume of each titration from the intersection of the two straight lines.
- ➤ Use the endpoint volumes and the mean sodium hydroxide concentration to calculate three values of the concentration of the original hydrochloric acid solution and three values of the concentration of the original acetic acid solution.
- ➤ Determine the mean hydrochloric acid concentration and the standard deviation of the results. Determine the mean acetic acid concentration and the standard deviation of the results.

9.5 APPLICATIONS

- **Conductivity measurements**

  Conductivity is measured simply to detect whether the ions are presence in solution. It is, therefore, a non-specific measurement. For example, conductivity measurement is done for monitoring purity of water – drinking water and process water. It is a rapid and method of determining the ionic strength of a solution.

  The conductivity κ, is calculated using the conductance G and the cell constant K as follows:

  $$\kappa = G \times K \ (S/cm)$$

- **Titration of strong acid with strong base**

  As shown the fig. 9.4 the conductivity graph falls down sharply during the first part of the titration (before equivalence) and goes up sharply after equivalence point. This is because the hydrogen ions having strong mobility of 350 are rapidly neutralized. As a result, the conductance decreases sharply. After equivalence, when slight excess of base is added the conductance goes up sharply due to high mobility (198) of hydroxyl ions.

  This method is suitable or recommended when the solution is dark and no indicator is found suitable, or the concentration is very low so that acid-base titration could not be conducted with greater accuracy. However, when the dilute solution is titrated, it must not contain any dissolved carbon dioxide. Presence of carbon dioxide produces error in the titration.

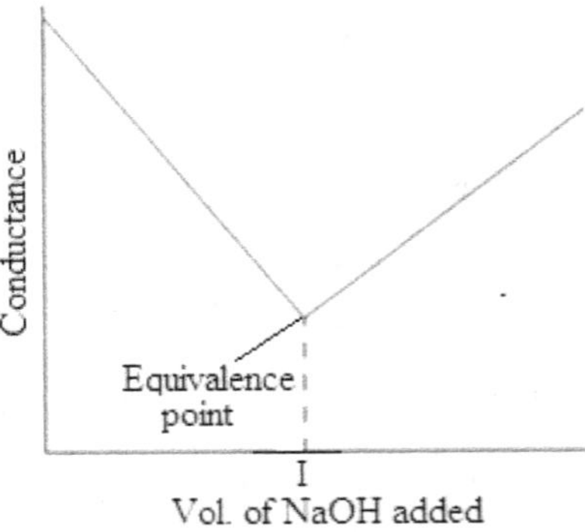

Figure 9.6 Conductometric titration of strong acid with strong base

- **Titration of strong acid with weak base**

  In this method the conductance falls down sharply in the first part of titration. Once the equivalence point is reached the curve becomes almost flat even after addition of slight excess of ammonia, as shown in Fig.9.5. For example, in titration of sulphuric acid with ammonia, ammonia in water does not ionize appreciably in presence of ammonium sulphate.

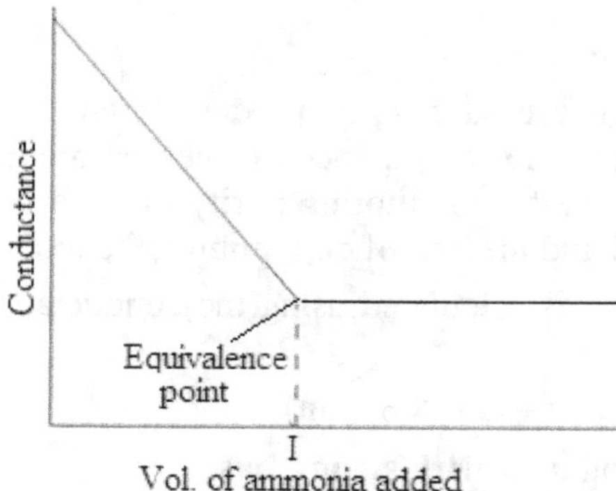

Figure 9.7 Conductometric titration of strong acid with weak base

- **Titration of weak acid with strong base**

  When a weak acid is titrated with a strong base, the shape of the curve depends on;
  - Concentration of the acid, and
  - Dissociation constant of the acid being titrated.

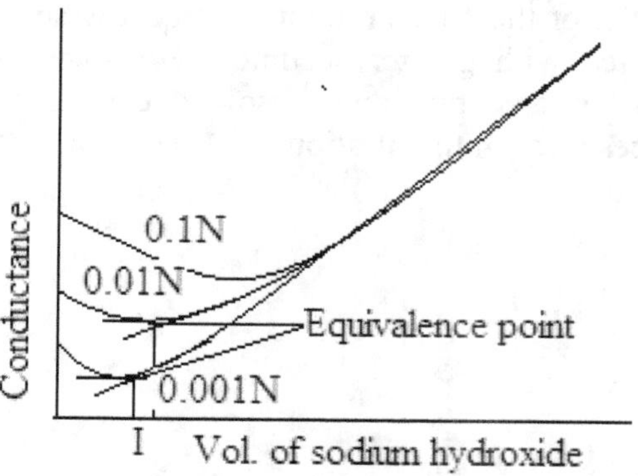

Figure 9.8 Conductometric titration of acetic acid with sodium hydroxide

For example, acetic acid is titrated with sodium hydroxide. The dissociation constant of acetic acid is 1.8×10^{-5}. During the first part of titration sodium acetate formed hinders the ionization of acetic acid remaining in the solution. As a result, the conductance does not decrease sharply as in earlier cases. Hence, the fall of conductance will be hindered as shown in the fig.9.6. Near the equivalence the weak acid say acetic acid starts ionizing; this results in slight increase in conductance and rounding at equivalence point. But, after attainment of equivalence point addition of slight amount of sodium hydroxide in excess, the conductance will increase sharply.

- **Titration of weak acid with weak base**

  When very dilute solution of acetic acid such as 0.003N is titrated with dilute solution of ammonia such as 0.1, the change of conductance is similar to that in titration of weak acid with strong base. However, the decrease in conductance is less as shown in the fig.9.7. Almost near to the equivalence hindrance caused by ammonium acetate is reduced and the weak acid say 0.003N acetic acid starts ionizing; this results in slight increase in conductance and rounding at equivalence point. Once equivalence point reached the conductance increases sharply on addition of slight excess of the base. The increase in conductance up to a certain point; thereafter it does not increase on further addition of the base. The curve becomes flat. The equivalence point is not sharp as in the titration of titration of weak acid with strong base. The equivalence point can be found out after extrapolation as indicated in the graph.

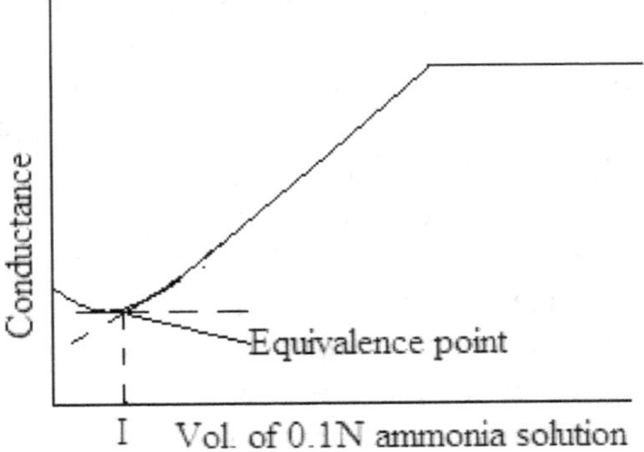

Figure 9.9 Conductometric titration of 0.003N acetic acid with 0.1 N ammonia

- **Titration of mixture of strong and weak acids with strong base**

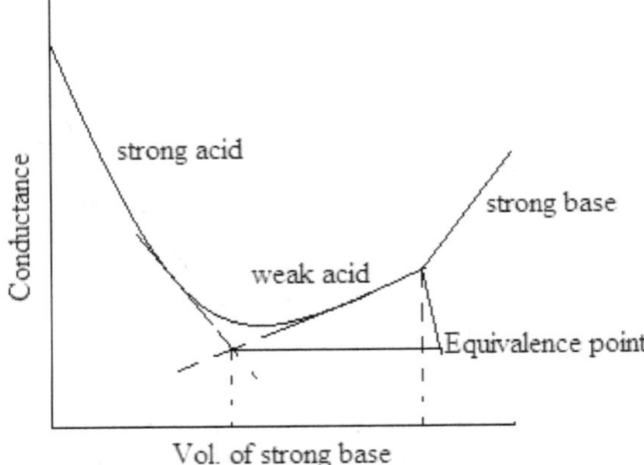

Figure 9.10 Conductometric titration curve of mixture of strong acid and weak acid with strong base

When a strong base is added to a mixture of a strong acid and a weak acid such as hydrochloric acid and acetic acid, the decreases until the strong acid is neutralized. Thereafter the weak acid is converted into its salt and conductance increases. A typical graph of this type of titration is shown in the fig.9.8. The graph shows three straight lines indicating that –

1. The weak acid dissociates increasing which results rounding off at the first end point.
2. The salt of weak acid hydrolyzes and second rounding off takes place at the second end point.

The end points can be located by extrapolating the three straight lines of the graph obtained.

- **Displacement or replacement titration**

In this type of titration, a salt of weak acid is titrated with a strong acid or titration of a salt of weak base is titrated with a strong base. When a salt of weak acid is titrated with a strong acid, the anion of the stronger acid replaces the anion of the weak acid. Similarly, the cation of the weak base is replaced by that of the stringer base. For example, if 1N hydrochloric acid is added to 0.1N sodium acetate. At the beginning the chloride ion replaces the acetate ion. The conductivity increases due to the higher mobility of chloride ion than that of the acetate ion. When the replacement of acetate is about to complete, sodium acetate concentration in the solution becomes high and it suppress the ionization of acetic acid produced through replacement of it by chloride ion. Near the equivalence point acetic acid ionizes sufficiently and changes the conductivity of the solution. Thus, due to the increase of conductivity the curve is rounded off. After attainment of equivalence, if slight excess of hydrochloric acid is present in the solution ionization of acetic acid is again suppressed.

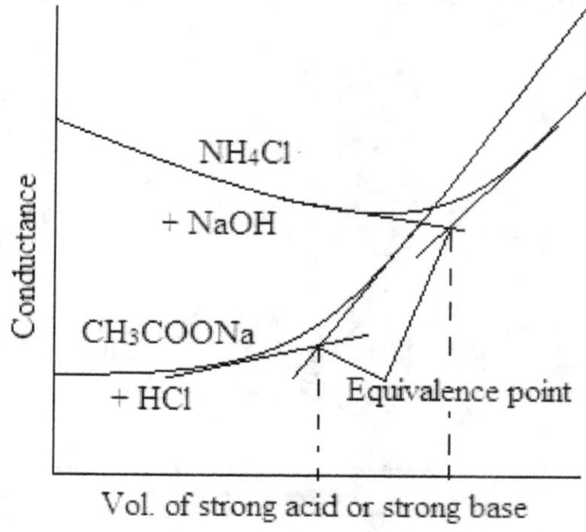

Figure 9.11 Conductometric displacement of replacement titration

- **Precipitation and complex formation reactions**

  Conductometric titration can be applied to some precipitation and complex formation reactions, provided that such reactions produce sparingly soluble precipitates or complexes. The angle between two sides of the curve should be as small as possible. If the angle is large a small error can result large deviation in the final result. Hence, applicability and accuracy of the titration depend on the following factors:

  ➢ The mobility of the ion that replaces the reacting ion should be smaller.

  ➢ If the mobility of the reacting anion is larger than that of cation to be determined, the angle between two sides would be more acute. Similarly, if the mobility of the reacting cation is larger than that of anion to be determined, the angle between two sides would be more acute.

  ➢ The salts which would be completely ionized in the solution should be titrated. The reagents to be used in the reaction should also be ionizable.

  ➢ Solubility of the precipitate should be less than 5%. In some cases, alcohol is added to reduce the solubility.

  ➢ The rate of precipitation should not be slow and the precipitate formed should not be microcrystalline. Seeding or addition of alcohol up to 30 – 40% is recommended.

  ➢ The precipitate should not have marked adsorptive properties. So that its composition remains constant. Otherwise there shall be error in the determination.

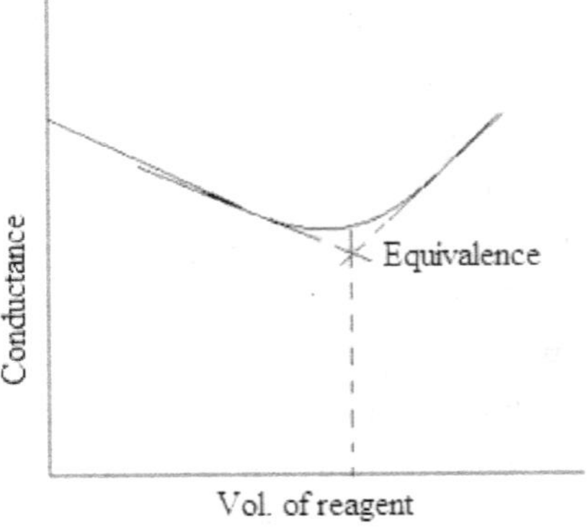

Figure 9.12 Conductometric precipitation and complex formation reactions

- **Resistivity measurements**

  Measurement of resistivity can be used as a reliable method for determination of quality of water for its ionic strength; particularly for ultrapure water (UPW). Sometimes the resistivity value is preferred to a conductivity value; for example, checking of water for its contamination in organic solvents.

The resistivity of a solution is calculated on the basis of the conductance, G compensated for the cable resistance, cable capacitance and cell constant of the conductivity cell used. The resistivity, ρ is calculated as follows:

$$\text{v} \quad \rho = \frac{1}{\kappa} \, \Omega.\text{cm}^{-1}$$

- **TDS measurements**

In the pulp and paper industry the total organic and inorganic dissolved solids in water can be accurately and easily determined by measuring TDS. TDS (Total Dissolved Solids) corresponds to the total weight of cations, anions and the undissociated dissolved species in one litre of water. The standard method to determine TDS is to evaporate a measured volume of sample water to dryness at 180°C, and carefully weigh the amount of dry solids left. The precision of the standard method depends on the nature of the dissolved species. However, by use of conductivity meter the TDS can be accurately determined.

- **Concentration measurements**

For measurement of concentration, the first step is to know the conductivity of the solution as a function of the concentration of the species of interest. This information can be available from published data (conductivity vs. concentration curves for electrolytes) or from laboratory measurements.

In a solution the charge of the ions facilitates the conductance of electrical current and the conductivity of the solution is greatly (but not totally) proportional to its ionic concentration. Since conductivity is a non-specific technique, concentration can be calculated by using conductivity measurements and it is valid for samples containing only the species of interest.

- **Salinity measurements**

Salinity refers to the weight of dissolved salts in seawater or in other water. The salinity is calculated from an empirical relationship between the conductivity and the salinity of a seawater sample. Oceanographic Tables and Standards provided by the UNESCO/SCOR/ICES/IAPSO are used for the calculation.

Salinity measurements are performed with no direct temperature correction. The calculation is valid for salinity values in the range 2 to 42 at a sample temperature of −2 to +35°C.

A. MULTIPLE CHOICE QUESTIONS

1. Alternative name of conductometry is
   - (a) Electrochemical method
   - (b) Electro gravimetric method
   - (c) Conductimetric method
   - (d) None of the above

2. Electrochemical method is based on measuring
   - (a) Electrolytic conductance
   - (b) Resistance
   - (c) Absorbance
   - (d) None of the above

3. The flow of electricity in a solution depends on
   - (a) Concentration
   - (b) Mobility of ions
   - (c) Valence of ions
   - (d) All of the above

4. Which one of the following statements is true?
   - (a) Aweak electrolyte dissociates completely into ions in its solutions
   - (b) A strong electrolyte dissociates completely into ions in its solutions
   - (c) Weak electrolyte does not dissociate even to only small extents
   - (d) None of the above

5. Which one of the following statements is true?
   - (a) If the temperature is increased by 1°C the conductance increases by 2 %.
   - (b) If the temperature is increased by 2°C the conductance increases by 1 %.
   - (c) If the temperature is increased by 0.1°C the conductance increases by 2 %.
   - (d) None of the above

6. Which one of the following statements is correct?
   - (a) The cell constant (K) is the ratio of the width of the cell to the area (a) of the electrodes.
   - (b) The cell constant (K) is the ratio of the area (a) of the electrodes to the distance (d) between the electrodes.
   - (c) The cell constant (K) is the ratio of the distance (d) between the electrodes to the area (a) of the electrodes.
   - (d) None of the above

7. Which one of the following statements is correct?
   - (a) Equivalent conductance (Λ) is defined as the conductance of one gram equivalent of a solute when placed between two electrodes spaced one centimeter apart.
   - (b) Equivalent conductance (Λ) is defined as the conductance of one gram of a solute when placed between two electrodes spaced one centimeter apart.
   - (c) Equivalent conductance (Λ) is defined as the conductance of one gram of a solute when presentin the solution.
   - (d) Equivalent conductance (Λ) is defined as the conductance of one gram equivalent of a solute when presentin the solution.

8. Which one of the following statements is correct?
   - (a) In conductometry current is a measure of the rate of oxidation of the analyte
   - (b) In conductometry current is a measure of the rate of reduction of the analyte
   - (c) In conductometry current is a measure of the rate of oxidation and reductionof the analyte
   - (d) None of the above

9.   The potential of electrode indicates
     (a)   the form of analyte present at the surface of the electrode;
     (b)   the form of analyte present in the solution;
     (c)   the amount of analyte present at the surface of the electrode;
     (d)   the amount of analyte present in the solution;

10. Conductivity is measured by applying an alternating electrical current
     (a)   To one of the electrodes immersed in a solution and measuring the resulting voltage.
     (b)   To two electrodes immersed in a solution and measuring the resistance
     (c)   To two electrodes immersed in a solution and measuring the resulting voltage
     (d)   To two electrodes and measuring the resulting voltage

11. Which one of the following statements is correct?
     (a)   The content of the cell must not be stirred
     (b)   The content of the cell must be stirred
     (c)   The cell must be made of any glass.
     (d)   The area of the electrode should be fixed.

12. Which one of the following statements is correct?
     (a)   To reduce polarization effect the platinum electrodes should be platinized.
     (b)   To reduce polarization effect the platinum electrodes should be used.
     (c)   To reduce polarization effect any electrodes should be used.
     (d)   To increase polarization effect the platinum electrodes should be used.

13. Which one of the following statements is correct?
     (a)   The mobility of ions carrying the electric current towards the electrodes varies with the size of the ion.
     (b)   The mobility of ions carrying the electric current towards the electrodes varies with their molecular weight
     (c)   The velocity or mobility of ions carrying the electric current towards the electrodes varies with the number of charges the ion possesses
     (d)   All of the above

14. Which one of the following statements is correct?
     (a)   Conductometry can be used in weak acid-weak base titration
     (b)   Conductometry can be used in weak acid-strong base titration
     (c)   Conductometry can be used in strong-strong base titration
     (d)   All of the above

15. Conductometry can be used for
     (a)   Resistivity measurements   (b)   TDS measurement
     (c)   Concentration measurement   (d)   All of the above

16. Which one of the following statements is correct?
    (a) 4-pole cell is ideal for high conductivity measurements
    (b) 4-pole cell is easier to maintain
    (c) 4-pole cell is economical
    (d) 4-pole cell is recommended for viscous media or samples with suspension

B. SHORT QUESTIONS

1. Define Ohm's law and resistance.
2. What are equivalent conductance and equivalent ionic conductance?
3. How does the conductivity of a solution vary?
4. What is the application of Wheatstone Bridge?
5. What is platinized cell?
6. Mention the applications of Conductometry.

C. LONG QUESTIONS

1. Explain the factors influencing the conductance of the solution
2. Describe the method of measurement of conductivity.
3. Write down the principle of conductometric analysis.
4. How does the conductivity cell works?
5. Write down how the strength of a solution of hydrochloric acid can be determined by a standard solution of sodium hydroxide.
6. How can you perform conductometric titration of Hydrochloric Acid and Acetic Acid with Sodium Hydroxide?
7. Explain with the help of a graph the conductometric determination of a weak acid and strong base.
8. Explain with the help of a graph the conductometric determination of a weak acid and weak base.
9. Discuss the applications of conductometry.

CHAPTER 10

Potentiometry

INTRODUCTION

There are various indicators which are used to detect endpoint of titrations. The endpoints are detected visually by observing the color change of the indicator. But there are some substances such as colored substances or very dilute solutions which cannot be titrated by using an indicator or the colorimetric titration does not produce accurate result. These substances can be easily estimated by using physico-chemical method such as potentiometric titration. If this method is used; a single operation can determine two compounds accurately in a mixture. For example, a mixture of chloride and iodide can be titrated with standard solution of silver nitrate using silver election. The first inflexion is for iodide and second inflexion is for chloride. The concept of potentiometric titration is same as that of ordinary titration.

The potential of a metal electrode in a solution containing the ions of the electrode material at 25°C is given by;

$$E_{25}^{o} = E^{o} + \frac{0.0591}{n} \log C_{M}^{n+} \quad .....(10.1)$$

Where, E^{o} is the standard potential of the metal, n is the valency of the ions and C_{M}^{n+} is the ionic (activity). If C_{M}^{n+} is written in the exponential form, that is $-\log [M^{n+}] = pM^{n+}$, then the eqn.1 can be written as;

$$E_{25}^{o} = E^{o} - \frac{0.0591}{n} pM^{n+} \quad .....(10.2)$$

In case of hydrogen electrode, the eqn.2 is expressed as;

$$E_{25}° = E_H^O - 0.0591pH \qquad\qquad .....(10.3)$$

Where, E_H^O is the standard potential of the normal hydrogen electrode. In case of an oxidation-reduction electrode the eqn.3 can be expressed as;

$$E_{25}° = E° + \frac{0.0591}{n} \log \frac{[Ox]}{[Red]}$$

Where, $E°$ is the standard reduction potential, n is the number of electrons gained by the oxidant during its reduction, [Ox] and [Red] are the concentrations (activities) of oxidant and reductant respectively.

The main objective of potentiometric titration is to find out the value of E. this is used to measure either the value of $\frac{[Ox]}{[Red]}$ of a solution or change in $\frac{[Ox]}{[Red]}$ during titration.

In eqn.3 $E°$ is the hydrogen electrode potential in a solution containing hydrogen ions. If the activity of H^+ ions is in equilibrium with hydrogen gas at 1 atm, then $E°$ is considered as zero at all temperatures. Under these circumstances the eqn.3 becomes

$$E = - 0.0591pH \text{ (at } 25°C)$$

Since, here the term pH refers to the activity of H^+ ions; the term pH can be defined as;

$$pH = -\log aH^+$$

Where aH^+ is the activity of H^+ ions. The definition of pH (Sorensen) has been modified by both US National Bureau Standard (NBS) and the British Standards 1647 for 1950.

If the pH of two solutions (S, standard and U, unknown) are measured at the same temperature using same reference electrode, and at same hydrogen pressure, the difference between the pH can be calculated as;

$$pH(U) - pH(S) = \frac{E_U - E_S}{2.303RT/F}$$

Where, E_A is the emf of the cell,

$$H_2, Pt \left| Solution\ U \right| 3.5M\ KCl \left| Reference\ electrode \right.$$

E_S is the emf of the cell,

$$H_2, Pt \left| Solution\ A \right| 3.5M\ KCl \left| Reference\ electrode \right.$$

R is the universal gas constant, T is the temperature in absolute scale, and F is the faraday. At 25°C the value of 2.303RT/F is 0.05916, when f = 96493 coulombs.

According to the British Standards 0.05M potassium hydrogen phthalate is considered as reference standard solution, pH of this solution is 4.000 at 15°C. The change in pH due to change in temperature can be calculated by using following equation;

$$pH = 4.000 + \frac{1}{2}\left(\frac{t-15}{100}\right)^2$$

Where, 't' is the temperature other than 15°C.

A typical apparatus required for potentiometric titration is shown in figure 10.1.

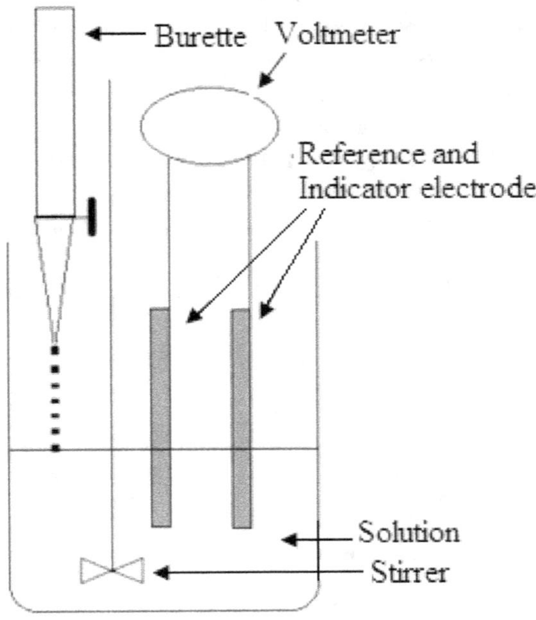

Figure 10.1 Typical apparatus for potentiometric titration

10.1 ELECTROCHEMICAL CELL

Zinc can ionize faster than copper and loses electrons. A spontaneous reaction takes place if zinc and copper rods (electrodes) dipped in an electrolyte solution, say copper sulphate are connected with a wire externally. Zinc ions (Zn^{2+}) go into solution leaving electrons in zinc electrode (anode) and the electrons move to the copper electrode (cathode) through the wire. Hence, the copper ions of the solution move towards copper electrode, gain electrons and deposit on the copper electrode. Two electrodes have two half-reactions – anode reaction (oxidation):

$$Zn = Zn^{2+} + 2e,$$

E_{left}, and E_{right} cathode reaction (reduction): $Cu^{2+} + 2e = Cu$

$$E_{cell} = E_{left} + E_{right}$$

Individual electrode potential is the difference in potentials of each electrode and its surrounding solution. Thus, two half-cell reactions can be written as;

$$Zn\left|Zn^{2+}\ (c_{Zn2+})\right\|Cu^{2+}(c_{Cu2+})\left|Cu\right.$$

Where single vertical line represents the junction between two phases of a half-cell and double vertical line represents the liquid junction; in other words, between two half-cells. A redox reaction involves transfer of electrons from one chemical species to another. The energy from a redox reaction can be used to do work by constructing an electrochemical cell. In an electrochemical cell, the oxidation process and the reduction process are separated into two *half-cells*. These half-cells are connected by an external wire. The half-cell with the oxidation process is loses the negative charge (e– loss) while the half-cell with the reduction process gains the negative charge (e– gain). To keep electrical neutrality in both half-cells, a salt bridge (or semipermeable membrane) must connect the two half-cells so that the ions move between two solutions. Thus, the salt bridge completes the electrical circuit between the half cells. The transfer of electrons through the external wire develops a current that can do work. The voltage difference between the two half-cells works as driving force movement of electrons through the wire. This voltage difference is called the *cell potential (E_{cell})* and is measured in volts.

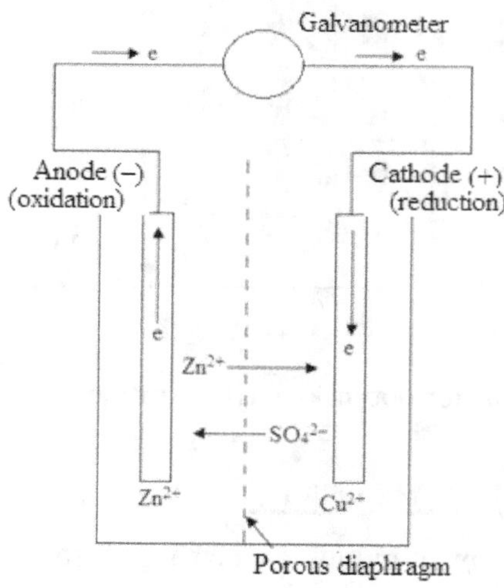

Figure 10.2 Schematic diagram of a simple electrochemical cell (Daniel cell)

The cell potential (E_{cell}) is directly related to the magnitude of the equilibrium constant for the overall oxidation-reduction reaction occurring in the cell. A reaction that more strongly favors product formation (larger K_{eq}) will have a higher cell potential (larger E_{cell}) than a reaction which moderately favors product formation.

In a potentiometric measurement system there are (1) two electrodes – one is reference and the other one is indicator electrode, (2) potentiometer and (3) a solution of analyte.

10.2 CONSTRUCTION AND WORKING OF REFERENCE ELECTRODE

The potential difference between an electrode and a solution can be determined when there is another electrode and a solution of accurately known potential difference. If the two electrodes are combined, it forms a voltaic cell and the emf of the cell can be directly measured. The emf of the cell is the arithmetical sum or difference of the electrode potentials. The value depends on the sign of the potentials. It has been mentioned earlier that out of two electrodes one is primary standard or reference and other one is unknown. Thus, the value of unknown potential can be easily calculated. Usually standard hydrogen electrode is used as reference electrode.

10.2.1 Standard Hydrogen Electrode

Construction: This consists of a piece of platinum foil coated with platinum black electrolytically. The electrode is immersed in a solution of hydrochloric acid containing hydrogen ions of unit activity. Hydrochloric acid of 1.8M produces hydrogen ions of unit activity at 25°C. The schematic diagram of standard hydrogen electrode is shown in Fig 10.3. As shown in the figure through the side tube, A hydrogen gas is passed over the platinum foil at one atmospheric pressure. Through the small holes B the gas escapes in the surrounding glass tube C. The level of the liquid inside the tube may fluctuate due to frequent bubbling. A portion of the platinum foil is exposed to the solution and hydrogen. To avoid interruption of the electric current the lower portion of the foil is continuously dipped into the solution. Inside the tube C there is a tube D which contains mercury. The mercury connects the platinum foil and the external circuit. The platinum foil is coated with platinum black because the platinum black can adsorb large quantity of hydrogen and it allows conversion of hydrogen gas to hydrogen ions and hydrogen ions to hydrogen gas freely. Thus, it behaves in such a way that the electrode is made up of hydrogen only. For this reason, it is called hydrogen electrode. Under standard conditions that is passing hydrogen gas at 1 atm and the solution would have hydrogen ions of unit activity, the hydrogen electrode will have a definite potential. Conventionally the potential of a standard hydrogen electrode is considered to be zero at all temperatures. The standard electrode potential can be measured by connecting this hydrogen electrode with a metal electrode through a salt bridge such as potassium chloride. The metal electrode means a piece of metal in contact with a solution containing its ions of unit activity. Figure 10.3 depicts a schematic diagram of a Hydrogen electrode.

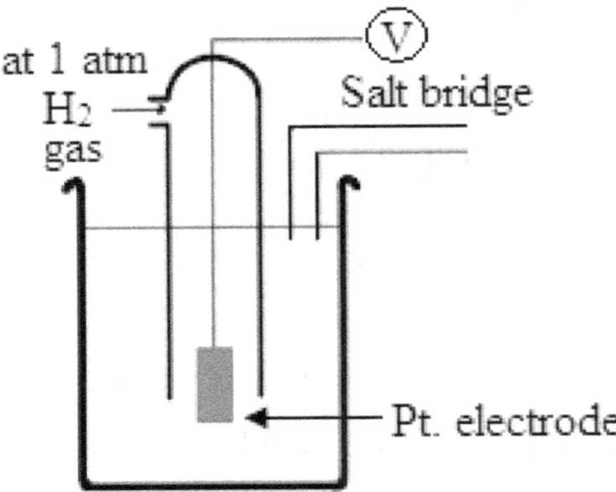

Figure 10.3 Schematic diagram of Hydrogen electrode

The cell is schematically written as;

$$\text{Pt, } H_2 \Big| H^+ (a = 1) \Big\| M^{n+} (a = 1) \Big| M$$

The single vertical line in the expression shows metal–electrode boundary at which potential difference is measured and the double vertical line indicates a liquid junction at which the potential is eliminated by a salt bridge.

Working

For routine work supply of hydrogen gas is made by using a hydrogen cylinder. Hydrogen gas can be steadily obtained by opening the valve of the cylinder in such a way that the pressure of the gas released is 1 atm. The gas released is purified by passing it through 0.2N potassium permanganate, alkaline Pyrogallol solution (2g of Pyrogallol mixed with 35mL of 4N sodium hydroxide), 0.1N sulphuric acid, and finally washed by passing through distilled water. The purified gas is then passed into the electrode. All these solutions are kept in all glass bottles. The hydrogen electrode is immersed in a solution whose pH is to be determined. The half-cell is coupled with a normal hydrogen electrode through a saturated solution of potassium chloride to eliminate the potential at liquid-junction. The emf of the cell is measured by using a potentiometer. The half-cell reactions are expressed as;

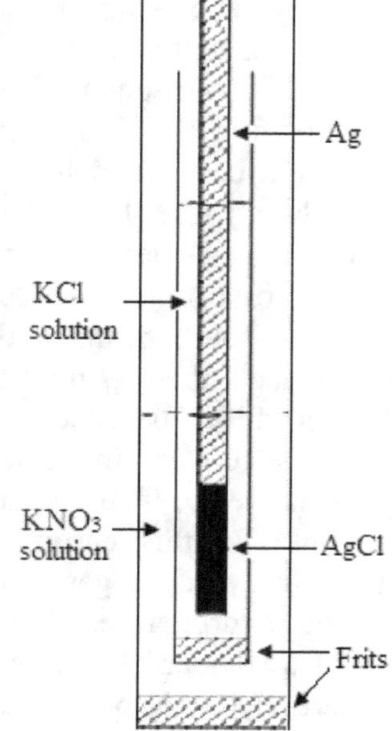

Figure 10.4 Schematic diagram of Silver-Silver chloride electrode

$$\text{Pt} \Big| \underset{a=1}{H_2, H^+} \Big\| \underset{a=x}{H_2, H^+} \Big| \text{Pt}$$

The emf of the cell is calculated by;

$$E = \frac{0.0591}{n} \log \frac{c_2}{c_1} = \frac{0.0591}{1} \log \frac{1}{[H^+]}$$
$$= 0.0591 \text{ pH}$$

Thus, $\text{pH} = \dfrac{0.0591}{E}$

Hydrogen electrode cannot be used in solution containing oxidizing agent such as permanganate, nitrate, ceric, ferric ions and other substances such as unsaturated organic compounds, or in presence of sulphides, compounds of arsenic, etc. These substances destroy the catalytic property of platinum black.

10.2.2 Silver Chloride Electrode

This is another important electrode and is used as a reference half-cell. It is difficult to prepare. It contains a silver wire or a platinum wire coated with silver. Coating is done electrolytically by plating a thin layer of silver chloride. The electrode is dipped into the solution of potassium chloride of known concentration. At 25°C the potentials of saturated solution of silver-silver chloride electrode and 0.1M solution are 0.199 volts and 0.290 volts respectively with respect to normal or standard hydrogen electrode. Fig 10.4 represents schematic diagram of a silver-silver chloride electrode.

The silver-silver chloride electrode is represented as;

$$Ag \left| AgCl \right| Cl^- \ (c, \text{ moles per lt})$$

and the electrode process is

$$Ag = Ag^+ + e^-$$
$$\underline{Ag^+ + Cl^- = AgCl}$$

Overall
$$Ag + Cl^- = AgCl + e^- \ (c, \text{ moles/lt})$$

10.2.3 Calomel Electrode

This is also called Mercury-mercurous chloride electrode. There are various forms of calomel electrode. The electrode 0.1N, 1N potassium chloride, but saturated solution is widely used; particularly in routine analysis.

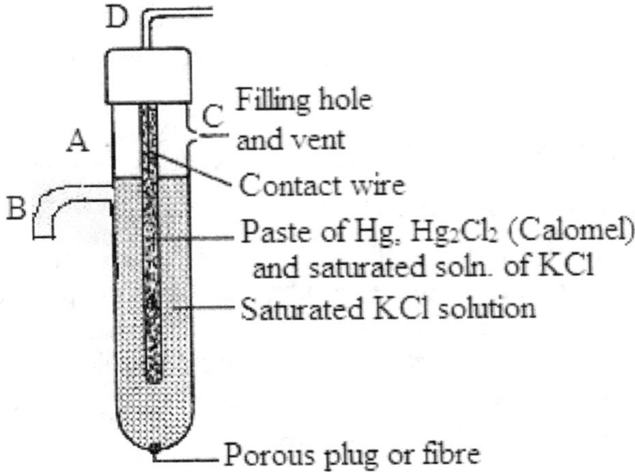

Figure 10.5 Schematic diagram of Calomel electrode

It consists of a relatively wide glass tube, A one end of which is round, and the other end is open. The tube is joined with two narrow tubes, B and C on two sides. The tube, B is inverted closed ended U-tube as shown in Fig 10.5 and tube; C is open ended bent tube.

The tube, C is closed with a screw clip. There is one narrow, closed ended tube, D in which a platinum wire is placed. The tube, D contains little amount of pure mercury into which an amalgamated copper wire is dipped. The other end of the tube is sealed, and the platinum is extended for electrical connection. The tube, A is filled with pure mercury up to a depth of 0.5 – 1 cm. The mercury layer is covered with a layer of calomel paste. Calomel paste is prepared by rubbing pure calomel, mercury, and saturated solution of potassium chloride in a glass mortar. The supernatant liquid is poured off and the process is repeated twice with fresh saturated solution of potassium chloride and the paste is poured over the mercury layer into in to the tube, A. Then the tube D is inserted in to the tube A through a rubber bung in such a way that the platinum wire dips in to the mercury layer. The rubber bung is rightly placed in to the mouth of the tube A. The tube A is then filled with saturated solution of potassium chloride presaturated with calomel by shaking with calomel. The saturated solution of potassium chloride is inserted through the bent tube C.

Now the electrode becomes ready for use.

Working

The calomel electrode is represented by

$$Hg \mid Hg_2Cl_2 \mid Cl^- \ (c, \ moles \ per \ lt)$$

The electrode reaction is

$$Hg = Hg^+ + e^-$$
$$Hg^+ + Cl^- = \tfrac{1}{2} Hg_2Cl_2$$

Overall
$$\overline{Hg + Cl^- = \tfrac{1}{2} Hg_2Cl_2 + e^- \ (c, \ moles/lt)}$$

10.3   CONSTRUCTION AND WORKING OF INDICATOR ELECTRODES

Calomel electrode and silver-silver chloride electrode are most frequently used as reference electrode. Reference electrodes produce an constant potential which does not change with change in concentration of solution. Hence, these electrodes are used with another electrode called *indicator electrode*. Such set of electrodes can measure the potential of a solution even when very small and negligible amount of current flows.

There are two types of indicator electrodes – metal and membrane indicator electrodes.

10.3.1 Metal Indicator Electrodes

These electrodes produce an electric potential in response to a redox reaction at the metal surface. The measurements are done using a reference electrode which has a known, stable potential. Generally, Pt or Au are used for making the metal indicator electrode because these are inert; that is these do not react. The metal indicator electrodes may be or may not be specific to the metal ion to be analyzed in an electrochemical measurement. These are of two types – first type responds directly to changing activity of electrode ion; this type is not selective for a specific analyte.

$$E_{cell} = E_{indicator} - E_{ref}$$

Electrodes of the first type are used where the electrode potential is directly related to the concentration of the metal ion being analyzed,

$$Cu^{2+}, \text{ with a } Cu(s) \text{ electrode; } Cu^{2+} + 2e^- \leftrightarrow Cu(s)$$

This type of indicator electrode consists of a pure metal of the analyte which is to be or being analyzed. There are a limited number of metals which are suitable for such reactions such as Ag, Bi, Cd, Cu, Hg, Pb, Sn, Ti & Zn.

The potential in a redox reaction for such cells can be reduced to a simple equation containing a single constant which depends on the concentration of the metal ion.

For example, in case of copper indicator electrode

$$Cu^{2+} + 2e^- \leftrightarrow Cu(s)$$

$$E_{cell} = E_{ind} - E_{ref}$$

$$E_{ind} = E^o - \frac{0.0591}{n} \log \frac{1}{[Cu^{2+}]}$$

$$E_{cell} = E^o - \frac{0.0591}{n} \log \frac{1}{[Cu^{2+}]} - E_{ref}$$

Since E^o, E_{ref} are constant, the above equation can be written as

$$E_{cell} = K + \frac{0.0591}{n} \log [Cu^{2+}]$$

Where, K represents all the constants. The value of K can be determined by calibrating the instrument using known concentration of the metal ion, Cu^{2+}. When the value of K is known, unknown solution can be measured, and cell potential can converted in to the concentration.

Electrodes of the second type are used where the metal ions are in equilibrium with the analyte being measured; this equilibrium influences the availability of the metal ion to interact with the electrode.

$$Cu^{2+} + 2I^- \leftrightarrow CuI_2(s) \text{ with the above electrode system}$$

The electrodes usually categorized as first type can also be used to determine the concentration of other species in the solution, if the metal ions interact with these species.

These electrodes are termed categorized as second type electrodes, provided there is equilibrium between the metal ion and the analyte. Then the potential for the cell can be expressed in terms of that analyte. The S.C.E. and Ag/AgCl reference electrodes are electrodes of the second type.

Thus, $\qquad\qquad E_{cell} = E_{ind} - E_{ref}$

Let us consider the example: $Cu^{2+} + 2I^- \leftrightarrow CuI_2(s)$

$$K_{sp} = [Cu^{2+}] [I^-]^2$$

So,
$$[Cu^{2+}] = \frac{K_{sp}}{[I^-]^2}$$

Now,
$$E_{ind} = Eo - \frac{0.0591}{n} \log \frac{1}{[Cu^{2+}]}$$

$$= \frac{0.0591}{n} \log \frac{1}{\frac{K_{sp}}{[I^-]^2}}$$

$$= \frac{0.0591}{n} \log \frac{[I^-]^2}{K_{sp}}$$

Since, E_{ref}, $E°$, and K_{sp} are constant, the above equation can be written as;

$$K = E° - E_{ref} + \frac{0.0591}{n} \log (K_{sp}) \; \left[\log \frac{[I^-]^2}{K_{sp}} = \log [I^-]^2 - \log K_{sp} \right]$$

Thus,
$$E_{cell} = K - \frac{0.0591}{n} \log [I^-]^2$$

There are several ways that a second type metal indicator electrode can be used to analyze or measure an interacting ion. However, in each case the original concentration of the metal ion is to be known before measuring the unknown concentration. These electrodes can be used to analyze the analyte by titration, or to analyze the solutions of the analyte.

10.3.2 Glass Electrode

The glass electrode is widely used, and it can respond to hydrogen ions. Hard glasses such as Pyrex are not pH responsive; hence not suitable. Special soft-glass of soda-lime type such as Corning 015 glass is pH responsive. It contains 72% of SiO_2, 22% of Na_2O, and 6% of CaO. This type of glass has low melting point, relatively high electrical conductivity and high hygroscopicity.

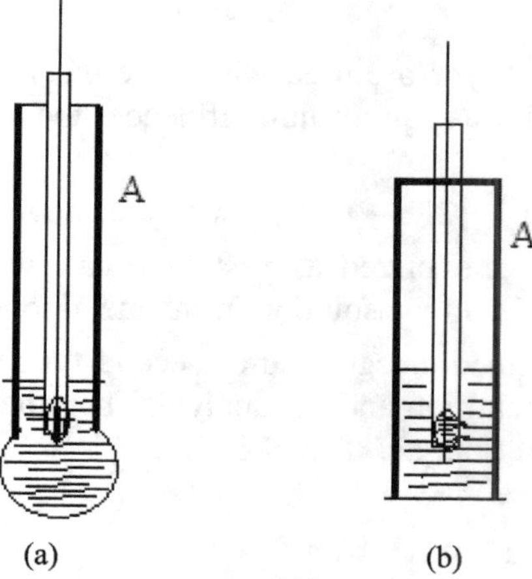

Figure 10.6 Schematic diagram of Glass electrode

The Fig 10.6 shows two simple types of glass electrodes. The Fig 10.6*a* shows that the tube A made of special glass is blown at its lower end to make an extremely thin walled bulb. The Fig 10.6b shows that the lower end of the tube is sealed by a pH responsive thin special-glass membrane. Most of the glass electrodes commonly used are made of two glasses – pH responsive relatively soft glass and hard glass. The bulb (working part of the electrode) and the membrane are made of pH-responsive special glass. These potions are sealed or fused with the stem of the electrode made of high-resistant hard glass. The stem part of the electrode resists strongly the ion-transfer. This may result error in the determination when the electrode is dipped in solution at different depth. By making the bulb or membrane pH-responsive, the cause of error is eliminated. If the working part of the electrode (bulb or membrane) is immersed in the solution the electrode will work. The stem part of the electrode is made in such a way that the electrode is protected from mechanical damage.

The electrical contact with the membrane is ensured by –

- ➢ Filling the bulb with dilute hydrochloric acid or a buffer solution containing sodium chloride and potassium chloride,

- ➢ Immersing a reference electrode (calomel or silver-silver chloride) in the bulb containing the electrolyte solution as mentioned.

The external connection with the electrode is provided by extending the wire of the reference electrode through the molded cap at the top of the stem.

The arrangement of the cell is thus expressed as;

$$\text{Ag} \,\big|\, \text{AgCl}_{(s)}, \text{HCl} \,\big|\, \text{Glass} \,\big|\, \text{Test solution} \,\big\|\, \text{KCl}_{(satd.\ Or\ 3.5M)} \,\big|\, \text{Hg}_2\text{Cl}_2 \,\big|\, \text{Hg}$$

Glass exhibits resistance to emf. Due to this resistance (1 – 100megohms) the emf of the cell is measured by using a valve potentiometer or valve voltmeter. At 25°C the emf of the cell is given by;

$$E = K + 0.0591 pH$$

Where, K is the constant for glass material. Its value depends on the composition of the glass. The above expression holds over the pH range of 1 – 10.

The exact mechanism of glass electrode is not known. It is suggested that the glass acts as semipermeable membrane. It permits the transfer or passage of hydrogen ions probably in hydrated form. When electric current is passed through the glass membrane the H^+ ions pass through the glass membrane as per the Faraday's law. For this reason, the glass must be in contact with water. The electrode does not function if it is dry or immersed in dehydrating liquid such as concentrated sulphuric acid or alcohol. It starts working after immersing in water for overnight or 10 – 12 hrs.

If the electrode is made of Corning 015 or similar glass, and if the pH of the solution is more than 10, the electrode gives lower value. That is *alkaline error* will occur; because, the membrane permits the passage of other ions along with H^+ ions. The error increases with increase in concentration of alkali metals in the solution. For measurement of these solutions special glass electrodes have been developed. Similarly, if the pH of solution is less than zero, the *acid error* will take place. The acid error is of opposite sign. For example, for pH = –1, the error would be +0.3. Acid error is not as important as alkaline error. The glass electrodes can be used when –

1. Oxidizing or reducing agents are present in solution,
2. The solution is viscous,
3. The solution contains proteins and similar substances,
4. The volume of solution is less.

Note:

1. The electrode should be standardized at least once in a day using two buffer solutions of known pH.
2. It must be calibrated before measurement of pH of test solution, and preferably after measurement.
3. Both glass and reference electrodes should be thoroughly washed with distilled water after measurement of test solutions.
4. Before measurement of test solutions, the electrodes should be rinsed thrice with portions of test solution.
5. The glass electrode should not be allowed to dry, unless it is stored for long period.
6. Before use of a dry electrode, it must be immersed in distilled water at least for 10 – 12 hrs.

10.4 METHODS TO DETERMINE END POINT OF POTENTIOMETRIC TITRATION

In potentiometric titration the equivalence point or end point can be determined by locating the point in the curve where the potential changes suddenly. The plot of emf reading against the volume of titrating solution (titrant) is drawn. The plot may be drawn as done in case of normal acid-base titration, or by plotting the derivatives against the volume of titrant. Accordingly, three types of curves may be obtained.

1. *Normal curve* similar to neutralization curve is obtained when the emf (E) values are plotted as ordinates against the volumes of titrant (V) used as abscissa. The curve obtained is sigmoidal as shown in Fig 10.7. The point in the graph where the value of slope is maximum would be the equivalence or end point of the titration. The value of V at the endpoint is the volume of titrant required for attaining the equivalence. Usually this procedure does not produce accurate results; because it requires drawing best fit curve and identifying the point of maximum slope. These depend on the individual judgement and may from person to person. For this reason, derivative of E and V values are used to draw the curve.

2. *First derivative* curve is constructed by plotting the values of $\Delta E/\Delta V$ as ordinates against the volumes of titrant (V) required. $\Delta E/\Delta V$ is called first derivative. The pattern of curve would be obtained is shown in Fig 10.8. It shows that the plot ascends up to a certain point; thereafter it falls down sharply. The point of inflexion (peak point) if is very sharp, a perpendicular line is drawn on the abscissa to know the volume of titrant required for attainment of equivalence point. If the point of inflexion is not sharp; the personal judgement would be required to determine the end point.

3. Since the first derivative curve is not always capable of providing accuracy of the result, it would be better to construct the *second derivative* curve. This method is the so called 'analytical method' of locating the equivalence or end point of a potentiometric titration. In this method the values of $\Delta^2 E/\Delta V^2$ (second derivative) are plotted as ordinates and the volumes of titrant (V) as abscissa. The type of curve obtained is shown in Fig 10.9. The second derivative, $\Delta^2 E/\Delta V^2$ of the curve is zero at the point where slope of the normal curve (Fig 10.7) is maximum.

To facilitate the calculation or for convenience of determination, equal volumes of titrant should be added near to the equivalence point. Of course, it is not essential for determination of the end point.

Example 1: Results of a potentiometric titration is given below. Draw the normal curve, first derivative curve, and calculate the volume of titrant required for equivalence.

Volume of titrant consumed V(mL)	Potential E (mV)	First Derivative $(\Delta E/\Delta V)$	Second Derivative $(\Delta^2 E/\Delta V^2)$	Volume of titrant consumed V (mL)	Potential E (mV)	First Derivative $(\Delta E/\Delta V)$	Second Derivative $(\Delta^2 E/\Delta V^2)$
2	-250	0.5	0	8.2	-190	260	-31500
4	-249	1	0	8.3	-164	190	-24000
5	-248	1	0	8.4	-145	110	-5700
6	-247	2	12	8.5	-134	80	1700
6.5	-246	4	48	8.6	-126	45	-1125
7	-244	20	0	8.8	-117	30	-500
7.2	-240	20	225	9	-111	20	0
7.4	-236	25	600	9.2	-107	13.34	-77.78
7.6	-231	35	1275	9.5	-103	6	0
7.8	-224	50	-475	10	-100	3	-5
8	-214	90	14400	11	-97	2	9021
8.1	-205	150	45100	12	-95		

Solution: As per the curve 10.7 and 10.8 the equivalence point is 21.05mL

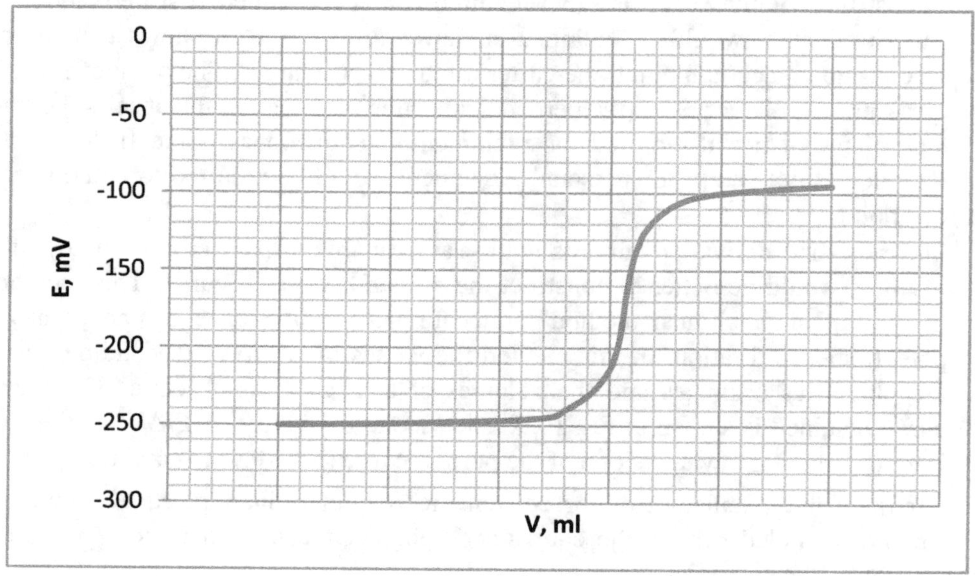

Figure 10.7 Plot of emf values vs. volume of titrant consumed (Normal Curve)

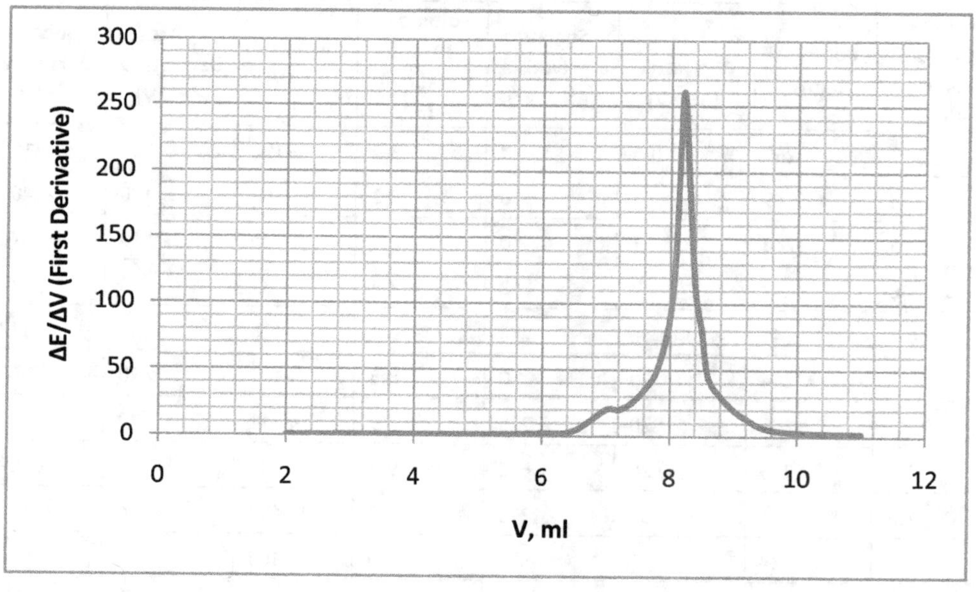

Figure 10.8 Plot of first derivative vs. volume of titrant consumed

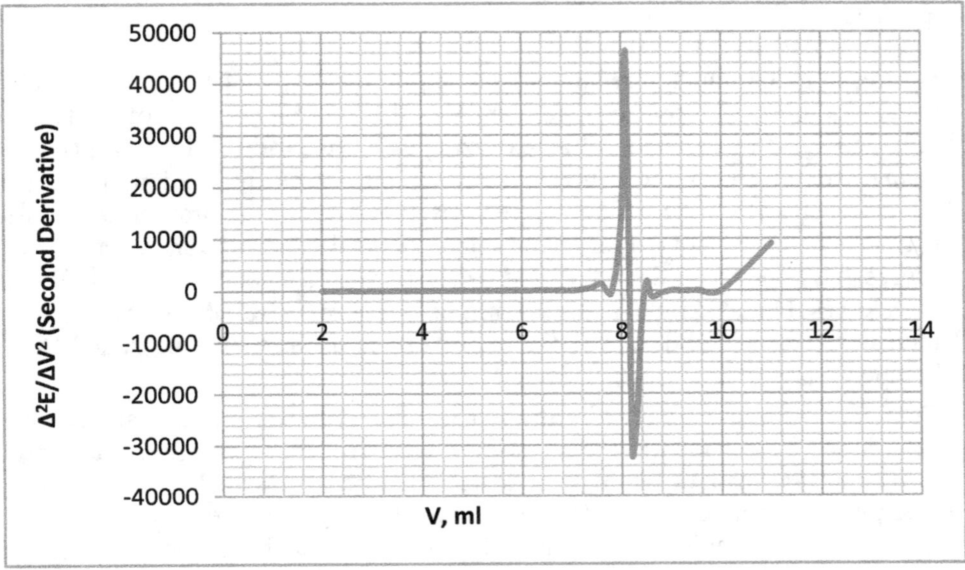

Figure 10.9 Plot of second derivative vs. volume of titrant consumed

10.5 APPLICATIONS

Potentiometric method can be used for analysis of different substances including some drug substances and chemical of different nature. Some are given here.

1. *Neutralization titrations:* In this type of potentiometric titration any one out of hydrogen, glass, antimony, or quinhydrone electrodes can be used as indicator electrode and usually calomel electrode is used as reference electrode. The accuracy of this potentiometric titration greatly depends on the concentration and strength of acid and alkali used. Satisfactory results can be obtained if

   Either acid or base is very weak, $K < 10^{-8}$ and the solution is dilute.

   Both acid and alkali are weak. In this case about 1% accuracy may be obtained with 0.1N solution.

   The potentiometric method can be used to analyze mixture of acids having great difference in their strengths; such as mixture of acetic acid and hydrochloric acid. The first break indicates the neutralization of strong acid such as hydrochloric acid, while the second break indicates the complete neutralization of weaker acid such as acetic acid.

2. *Oxidation-reduction titration:* Such titration can be done potentiometrically, but the success of this titration depends on the ratio of concentrations of oxidized and reduced forms of certain ion species. For example,

   Oxidized form + n electron $\leftrightarrow$ reduced form

   The potential E gained by the indicator electrode at 25°C is calculated by

$$E = E^\circ + \frac{0.0591}{n} \log \frac{[Ox]}{[Red]}$$

Where, E° is the standard reduction potential of the system. Thus, the ratio of these concentrations will influence the potential of the electrode. In case of oxidation of a reducing agent or reduction of an oxidizing agent, the ratio and the emf (potential) changes rapidly near the equivalence point. This type of titrations can be done potentiometrically. For example, the reaction of ferrous iron with potassium permanganate, or potassium dichromate, or with ceric sulphate can be done successfully and the end point would be characterized by sudden change of emf. In such cases the electrode made of bright platinum wire or foil is suitable for indicator electrode and the solution of oxidizing agent should be added from the burette.

3. *Precipitation titration:* In this titration ion concentration at equivalence point is determined by calculating the solubility product of the sparingly soluble product formed during the titration. If a suitable reagent is added to a solution, the precipitation of an ion I from the solution may take place. The concentration of I in the solution will rapidly and clearly change in the vicinity of the end point. If the indicator electrode is responsive to the concentration of I, the potential of the indicator electrode will change. The change in emf (potential) can be recorded in potentiometric titration. Usually a saturated calomel electrode and an electrode which will readily come into equilibrium with one of the ions of the precipitate are used. Hydrogen electrode is less commonly used in place of calomel electrode. For example, a silver electrode is used in the titration of silver ions with a halogen such as chloride, bromide, or iodide. The electrode may be made of silver wire, or a platinum wire or a foil which may be plated with silver and sealed within a glass tube. For analysis of a halide the salt bridge used should be a saturated solution of potassium nitrate. If silver nitrate is titrated with thiocyanate excellent result could be attained. The solution is to be stirred mechanically to attain equilibrium in solubility.

4. *Complexometric titration:* Potentiometric titration can be used to analyze metals such as copper, chromium, calcium, magnesium, aluminium, nickel, cobalt, mercury, zinc, bismuth, lead, thorium, etc. In this titration the indicator electrode used is mercury ∣ mercury-EDTA complex electrode. A mercury electrode shows change in potential when kept in contact with a solution containing metal ion (Mn+) to be titrated and a small amount of HgY-EDTA complex added to the solution. the half-cell equation can be written as;

$$Hg \mid Hg^{2+}, HgY^{2-}, MY^{(n-4)+}, M^{n+}$$

At equilibrium the potential can be calculated by,

$$E = E^{\circ\prime}_{Hg^{2+},Hg} + \frac{RT}{2F} \ln\frac{[HgY^{2-}]}{[MY^{(n-4)+}]} \times \frac{K_{MY}}{K_{HgY}} + \frac{RT}{2F} \ln [M^{n+}]$$

Where, K_{MY} and K_{HgY} are the stability (or formation) constants of the metal-EDTA and mercury-EDTA complexes respectively.

5. *Assay of drug substances:* Certain drugs such as tinidazole, captopril, sulpha drugs, Ziprasidone hydrochloride, hydrochloride salt of chlorpromazine, promethazine, imiprazine, clomipramine, opipramol, amitryptiline, etc.

A. MULTIPLE CHOICE QUESTIONS

1. Potentiometric titration is suitable for
   (a) Colored substances difficult to be titrated by ordinary titrations
   (b) Very dilute solutions which cannot be titrated by using an indicator
   (c) Substances not suitable for colorimetric titration which does not produce accurate result.
   (d) All of the above

2. Potentiometric titration is suitable for
   (a) Determination of the components in a mixture
   (b) Determination of a single component
   (c) Titration using indicator
   (d) None of the above

3. The main objective of potentiometric titration is
   (a) To measure E_H^o
   (b) To measure $\dfrac{[Ox]}{[Red]}$
   (c) To measure $\dfrac{[Red]}{[Ox]}$
   (d) To measure pH

4. Potentiometric titration using hydrogen electrode measures
   (a) $E_{25}^o = E^o - \dfrac{0.0591}{n} pM^{n+}$
   (b) $E_{25}^o = E^o + \dfrac{0.0591}{n} \log \dfrac{[Ox]}{[Red]}$
   (c) $E_{25}^o = E^o - \dfrac{0.0591}{n} pM^n$
   (d) $E_{25}^o = E_H^o - 0.0591 pH$

5. The change in pH due to change in temperature can be calculated by using following equation
   (a) $pH = 4.000 + \dfrac{1}{2}\left(\dfrac{t-15}{100}\right)^2$
   (b) $pH = 3.99 + \dfrac{1}{2}\left(\dfrac{t-15}{100}\right)^2$
   (c) $pH = 4.000 + \left(\dfrac{t-15}{100}\right)^{\frac{1}{2}}$
   (d) $pH = 4.000 + \dfrac{1}{2}\left(\dfrac{t-10}{100}\right)^2$

6. The calomel electrode reaction is expressed as
   $$\text{Pt, } H_2 \,\big|\, H^+ (a = 1) \,\big\|\, M^{n-} (a = 1) \,\big|\, M$$
   (a) $Ag + Cl^- = AgCl + e^-$ (c, moles/lt)
   (b) $Hg + Cl^- = \dfrac{1}{2}Hg_2Cl_2 + e^-$
   (c) moles/lt)
   (d) None of the above

7. Which one of the following statements is correct?
   (a) The electrode should be standardized at least once in a day using two buffer solutions of known pH.

   (b) It must be calibrated before measurement of pH of test solution, and preferably after measurement.

   (c) Both glass and reference electrodes should be thoroughly washed with distilled water after measurement of test solutions.

   (d) All of the above

8. Which one of the following statements is correct?

   (a) Before measurement of test solutions, the electrodes should be rinsed thrice with portions of test solution.

   (b) The glass electrode should not be allowed to dry, unless it is stored for long period.

   (c) Before use of a dry electrode, it must be immersed in distilled water at least for 10 – 12 hrs.

   (d) All of the above

9. Which one of the following statements is correct?

   (a) The first derivative curve is not always capable of providing accuracy of the result,

   (b) The first derivative curve always provides accuracy of the result,

   (c) The second derivative curve should not be constructed.

   (d) None of the above

10. In potentiometric neutralization titration which one out of following can be used as indicator electrode?

   (a) Hydrogen electrode   (b) Glass electrode

   (c) Antimony electrodes   (d) All of the above

11. When complexometric titration is carried out using a potentiometer

   (a) Mercury $|$ mercury-EDTA complex electrode is used as the indicator electrode.

   (b) Silver silver chloride electrode is used as the indicator electrode.

   (c) Mercury $|$ mercury chloride electrode is used as the indicator electrode.

   (d) All of the above

12. Which of the following statements is correct?

   (a) The glass electrode does not function if it is dry

   (b) The glass electrode does not function if it is immersed in dehydrating liquid such as concentrated sulphuric acid or alcohol.

   (c) The glass electrode t starts working after immersing in water for overnight or 10 – 12 hrs.

   (d) All of the above

B. SHORT QUESTIONS

1. What is the principle of the potentiometric titration?
2. Discuss the advantages of potentiometric titration.
3. Explain Null Balance Potentiometer along with its principle and working.
4. Describe the electrode used in oxidation reduction titration.
5. What is the process of performing acid base titration by potentiometric titration?
6. What are the different variations in the potentiometric titration?

B. LONG QUESTIONS

1. Describe the potentiometric titration assemblage with the help of diagram and elucidate its operation.
2. What are the various types of electrodes used in potentiometric titration? Discuss each category with example of one electrode including its advantage and working.
3. Describe the assemblage required for the potentiometric titration of V^{2+} and MnO_4^-
4. What is the principle used in measurement of EMF by the potentiometric titration method? Illustrate with help of diagram the principle involved in the potentiometric titration.
5. Elaborate the advantage and disadvantage of potentiometric titration.

CHAPTER 11

Polarography

The polarographic method is a method of chemical analysis which is based on the interpretation of the current-voltage curves obtained and measured by an instrument called *polarograph*. Thus, *polarography* is an electroanalytical technique, a branch of voltammetry, in which a dropping mercury electrode is used as the indicator electrode. In this method a dropping mercury electrode is used as the indicator electrode. The solutions of electrooxidizable and/or electroreducible substances are electrolyzed between an indicator electrode (dropping mercury electrode [DME]) and some reference electrode (RE). The potential between these electrodes is varied and the consequent change in the flow of current is measured, Fig. 11.1. If the changes in current flow are plotted

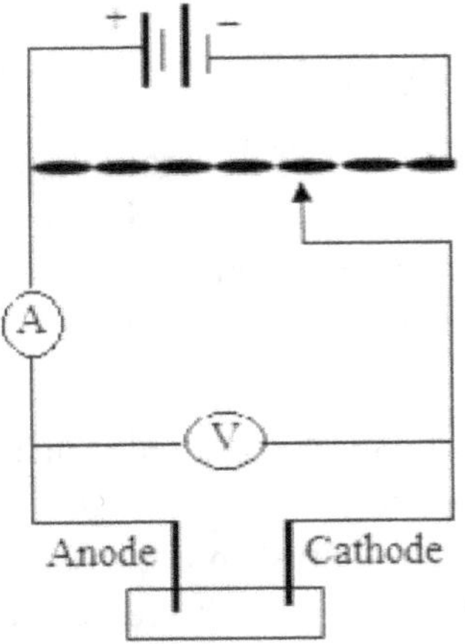

Figure 11.1 Schematic diagram of polarography

against the potential variation, an **i - E** curve known as *polarogram* is obtained. Jaroslave Heyrovsky in 1922 first discovered the use of the DME in electrolysis and received the Nobel Prize in Chemistry in 1959. This technique is used for qualitative and quantitative analysis of electro-reducible or oxidizable elements or groups. Polarograph has various applications in chemical analysis.

11.1 PRINCIPLE

The solutions containing electro reducible or electro oxidizable substances are electrolyzed using two electrodes. One of which is very small; usually mercury dropping from a fine-bore capillary. Due to smaller in size the mercury can be assumed to be completely polarized; while the other one is practically unpolarizable. From the position and magnitude of certain steps observed in these curves, both qualitative and quantitative information related to the electrolyzed material can be obtained.

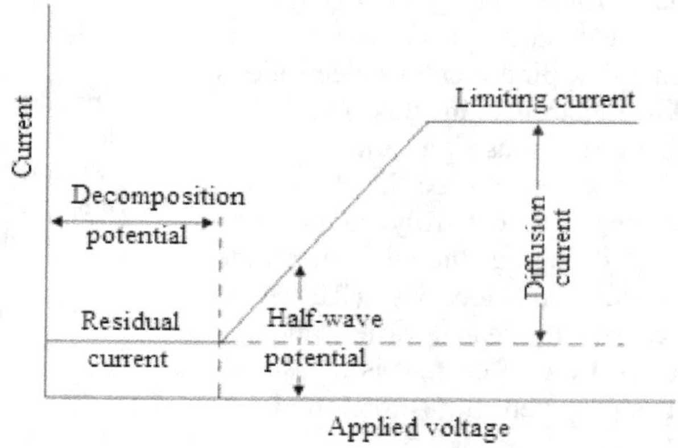

Figure 11.2 Graphical interpretation of analytical data obtained from polarographic analysis

The polarograph measures the effect of the potential of an electrode on the current that flows in the electrolysis cell. The electrode whose potential is varied is called the indicator electrode. Various materials such as mercury, platinum, gold and graphite, having varying shapes and construction may be used to prepare the voltammetric indicator electrodes.

For example, an applied negative potential (voltage) is gradually increased between a polarizable and non-polarizable electrode and the corresponding current (μA) is recorded. When the emf in terms of volts applied is plotted against the current (μA) produced, a sigmoid curve is obtained. With the help of this curve a sample can be analyzed both qualitatively and quantitatively.

The figure 10.2 explains the various stages of the polarogram and how the analytical data can be interpreted. The point of inflection in the curve is called Half-wave potential

($E^{\frac{1}{2}}$). It varies with the element or functional group. It is characteristic to the type of element or functional group being analyzed. Hence, for qualitative analysis the Half-wave potential is used.

The diffusion current (I_d) measured varies proportionally with the concentration, C of the particular substance being analyzed. Thus, I_d can be used for quantitative analysis. The position of a wave in a polarogram along the potential axis indicated the identity of the substance while the magnitude of the limiting current indicates the concentration variation of the sample. By distilling under vacuum a very pure mercury (99.99 %) patch can be obtained through distillation under vacuum. Each drop can work as a fresh electrode with a new exposed surface. The reproducibility of geometry of each drop with the laps of time is another advantage of the DME over other electrodes.

Advantages of polarographic analysis
- ➤ Both organic and inorganic substances can be analyzed,
- ➤ Useful for both qualitative and quantitative analysis,
- ➤ Can measure very low concentration up to 10^{-8}M,
- ➤ Requires very less time,
- ➤ It can analyze the concentration without separating the components of a mixture,
- ➤ Very small volume of sample up to 0.05mL can be used to measure.

11.2 ILKOVIC EQUATION

The electrical force on the reducible ions is nullified when an excess amount of the supporting electrolyte is present in solution. This happens because the ions of added salt carry practically all the current. The potential gradient is compressed or shortened to a region very nearest to the electrode surface and the electrode surface cannot attract electro-reducible ions. Under this condition the limiting current becomes diffusion current. D. Ilkovic in 1934 examined various factors that govern the diffusion current and deduced an equation which is called Ilkovic equation. It is a relation between the diffusion current (I_d) and the concentration of the substance (c) reduced or oxidized at the dropping mercury electrode. The equation can be written as;

$$I_d = 607 \times n \times D^{\frac{1}{2}} \times C \times m^{\frac{2}{3}} \times t^{\frac{1}{6}}$$

Where, I_d is the diffusion current in microamperes,

n is the number of electron equivalents per mole of electrode reaction,

D is the diffusion coefficient of the reducible (or oxidizable) substance,

C is its concentration in millimoles per liter, m is the mass flow of mercury from the dropping electrode in milligrams per second,

t is the drop-time in seconds, and

607 is a natural constant including the faraday at 25°C. It depends slightly on temperature. In this equation the quantity $knD^{\frac{1}{2}}$ is a constant particular ion being estimated. Other factors either depend on the concentration of the ion or are physical constants of the apparatus used.

11.3 CONSTRUCTION AND WORKING OF DROPPING MERCURY ELECTRODE

Dropping mercury electrode (DME) is the basic apparatus in polarography. The figure 11.3 shows the schematic diagram of the apparatus. Usually it works as a cathode. Sometimes it is called indicator electrode or micro-electrode. The pool of mercury works as anode. Its area is relatively large. Mercury does not polarize easily; hence its potential remains almost constant in a medium containing anions such as SO_4^{2-}, Cl^-, etc. which can readily form insoluble salts of mercury. Thus, it acts as a reference electrode. The exact potential of it depends on the concentration of anions of supporting electrolyte present in the solution. Hence, the polarization of the cell depends on the reaction taking place at the minute dropping mercury cathode. Two tubes – inlet, B and outlet, A are attached to the cell for removal of dissolved oxygen from the solution by passing an inert gas such as hydrogen or nitrogen before the measurement. Not during the measurement. In figure P is the potentiometer by which any e.m.f up to 3 volts can be gradually applied to the cell. S is a shunt for adjustment of the sensitivity of the galvanometer, G. This should be selected according to the nature and concentration of the substance being analyzed. Under these conditions the current – voltage curve is actually a current – cathode potential curve; but is displayed by a constant voltage corresponding to the potential of the anode. In certain cases, external anode of known potential such as a saturated calomel electrode is connected. The initial potential of the mercury cathode is uncertain and will show the potential that is applied to it from external source.

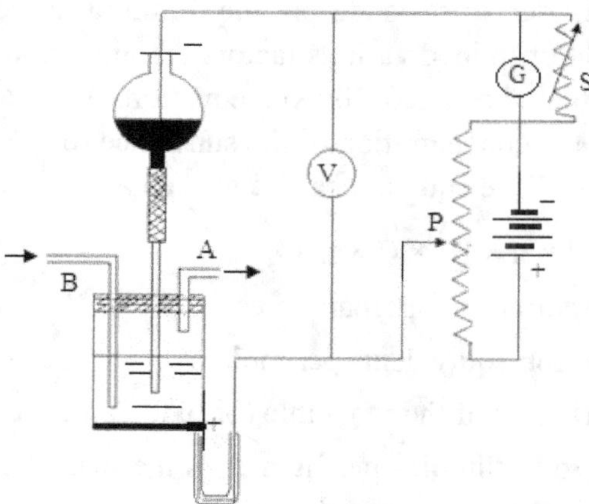

Figure 11.3 Schematic diagram of Dropping mercury electrode

It is considered to be polarized when its potential will be different from that shown in absence of electrical connection.

Construction

Dropping mercury electrode assembly designed by Heyrovsky has been given in figure 11.4. The assembly is made up of a mercury reservoir, a tube that connects the reservoir and the capillary tube, and a glass electrolysis cell. The unknown solution or the solution of analyte is placed in the cell. About 80 – 100 cm long sulphur free heavy walled rubber tube or neoprene tube is used. The inner surface of the tube needs to be steamed for 30 min and then dried by filtered air before use. A platinum wire is used for electrical connection to the mercury in the reservoir. The wire is sealed into the end of a soft-glass tube which is partly filled with mercury and held in place by the stopper of the reservoir.

The length of the effective capillary tube is about 5 – 10 cm with a internal diameter of about 0.05mm and external diameter is about 6 – 7mm. The delivery tube is cut horizontally. At a given pressure the *drop time* is directly proportional to the length of the capillary and inversely proportional to the third power of the internal radius of the capillary. The drop time is also inversely proportional to the pressure on the drop. The drop time is the time taken for fall of two successive drops. For polarographic analysis the desired drop time is about 3 – 6sec and each drop should be of 6 – 10 mg when immersed in distilled water. The position at which the dropping mercury electrode is mounted is an important factor for accuracy of the dropping.

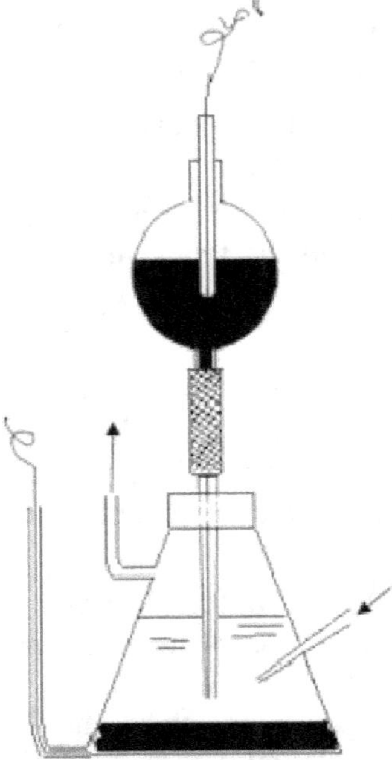

Figure 11.4 Simple assembly of Dropping mercury electrode

Note:

1. The capillary must be mounted within ±5% of the vertical.

2. No solid matter of any kind must be allowed to enter into the capillary.

3. The electrode must not be allowed to stand in a solution when mercury is not flowing.

Working

The sample solution is to be deaerated first; then the mercury pressure is to be increased to at least 10 cm above the previous equilibrium height. This is done with the tip of capillary in the air. The capillary is then inserted in to the cell and mercury level is finally adjusted to desired value. When the measurement is completed the capillary must be withdrawn from the cell and washed thoroughly with a stream of water from a wash bottle.

11.4   CONSTRUCTION AND WORKING OF ROTATING PLATINUM ELECTRODE

H.A. Laitinen and L.M. Kolthoff developed this technique or electrode in 1941. Dropping mercury electrode is not suitable or cannot be used when positive potential is about 0.4 volts because the mercury gets oxidized in this condition. Under this condition of positive potential rotating platinum electrode can work satisfactorily. The rotating platinum electrode possesses following advantages over the dropping mercury electrode;

➢ Construction of this electrode is simple.

➢ It can work successfully on the positive voltage range up to 0.9 volts; where dropping mercury electrode cannot be used.

➢ Sensitivity of the electrode or of the method is high because the value of diffusion current increases even up to 20 times in polarography due to rotation of the electrode.

Construction

The electrode consists of a glass tube of 15 – 20 cm long and 6 mm wide. A short length of platinum wire extends up to 5 – 10 mm from the wall of the glass tube as shown in Fig 11.5. The electrode is mounted in the shaft of a motor and is rotated at a constant speed of about 600 revolutions per min. A simple rotating platinum electrode assembly is shown in Fig 11.6.

The construction and dimensions of the electrode may vary from manufacturer to manufacturer. As shown in Fig 11.5, it consists of two parts – the glass well and the glass tube with a bell-shaped rotating top. The glass well is the stationary part of the electrode. It is made from 40 mm and 16 mm diameter tubing. The side arm is made from 8 *mm* tubing and has a 20 mm length of platinum wire sealed through the end.

The electrode is made from Pyrex tubing. The inside diameter of the glass well and glass tube are 28 mm and 8 mm respectively. A platinum wire is sealed in the bottom of the electrode and extends to the outer edge of the bell. To assure contact, the platinum wire is tied with household cement to the side of the bell. The portion which is in contact with the mercury is left uncovered. The glass bell should not extend to a depth of more than 3 *mm* into the mercury. This prevents excessive splashing of mercury at high speeds. The mercury bath is filled to a height of 6 to 10 mm. Corks are used for bearings. The large cork which fits into the top of the well is not tied with the glass well. To provide a smooth-finished surface the inside wall of the cork is covered and is cemented completely.

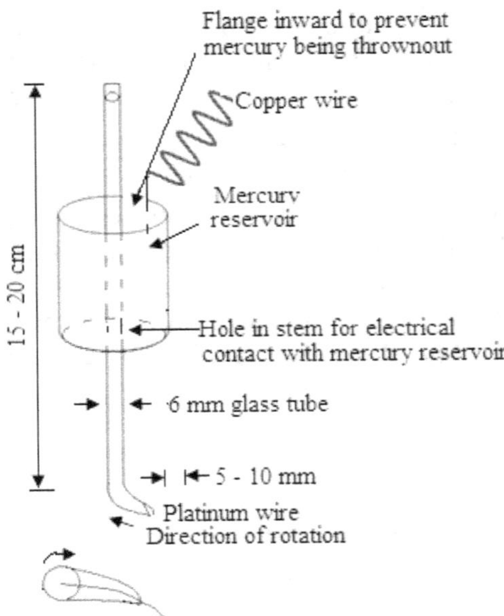

Figure 11.5 Schematic diagram of rotating platinum electrode

The inside walls of the two small corks are tied permanently with the glass well. These are also covered with cement to give a smooth surface. The upper small cork extends above the glass wall and slopes outward inside the bell to provide a run off for any mercury that splashes up. The glass electrode fits loosely into the two small corks but with a clearance of not more than 1/32 inch. This is to prevent the electrode from wobbling at high speed.

An electric power-driven variable speed laboratory stirrer is used with this electrode. The use of a small torque stirrer is advisable to prevent-applying too much strain on the electrode. It is important to note that the three corks play a leading role in the operation of this electrode. The corks should be aligned and the electrode tested by hand before attaching it to the motor.

The glass well is clamped to the stand and the stirrer is attached to the same stand. A short piece of rubber tubing connects the glass tubing of the electrode to the shaft of the motor. Minor adjustments are necessary for efficient operation of the electrode. The short tube of paper is extended from the top cork in order to stop the mercury from creeping out of the well. A glass bead near the platinum wire protects it from being broken off.

Note:

1. Once the electrode is in operating position it need not be removed except for repairs.

2. Oxidized mercury will form on the inside wall of the well and on the bell but it has not been found to interfere with the function of the electrode.

Working

This has been mentioned earlier that in amperometric titration dissolved oxygen must be removed. This is done by bubbling a purified gas such as nitrogen through the solution for about 30 min before starting the titration and for 1 min after each addition of titrant.

Supporting electrolyte such as potassium chloride and maximum suppressor such as gelatin, dyes or surfactant are added before the titration.

With stationary platinum electrode the diffusion current is attained slowly but steadily. But diffusion layer is reduced considerably. This increases the sensitivity as well as the rate of attainment of equilibrium. The potential to be applied is determined by recording the polarogram of the substance. The potential corresponding to the limiting current is then applied. At this potential all of the electro-reducible ions undergo reduction and thus, will carry the current.

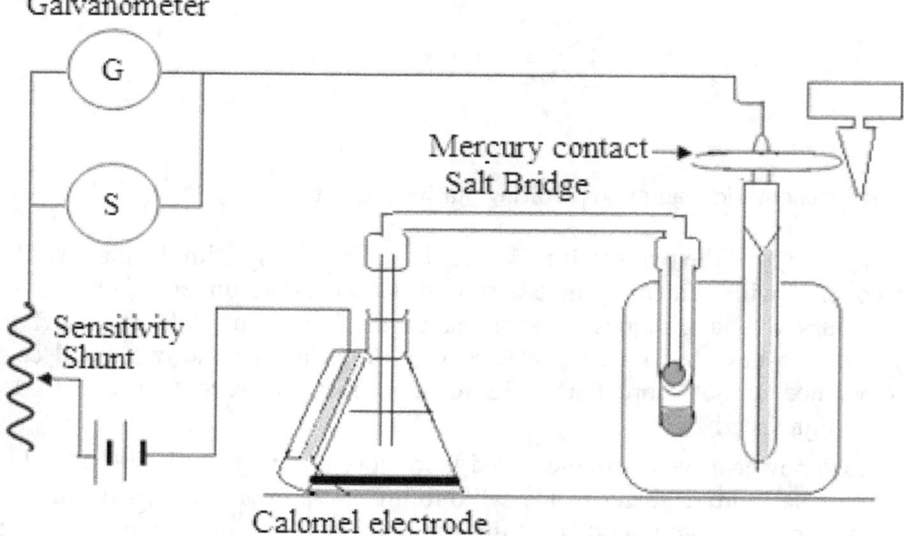

Figure 11.6 Schematic diagram of working rotating platinum electrode

11.5 APPLICATIONS

Electrochemical analysis is a powerful analytical technique and is widely utilized in Pharmaceutical industry, metal industry, and environmental applications, etc. There are several advantages of electro analysis – high sensitivity, reduction in solvent and sample consumption, rapid analysis, low operating cost and high scan rate in all cases. Some common applications are mentioned here:

- Widely applicable than Potentiometry. This method is widely used for the determination of sulphate which could not be determined accurately by potentiometric method due to lack of suitable indicator.
- Successive determination of chloride, bromine, Iodide by using rotating microelectrode.
- They are used as micro detectors in liquid chromatography.
- In bioamperometric titration this technique is widely used in Karl-fisher moisture titration.
- Other applications are determination of:

(a) Phosphate with uranyl acetate

(b) Lead with dichromate ions

(c) Sulphate with lead nitrate

(d) Cu, CO, Pt with

(e) Iodine with mercuric nitrate

A. MULTIPLE CHOICE QUESTIONS

1. Polarography is a
   (a) Chemical method of analysis
   (b) Electrochemical method of analysis
   (c) Chromatographic method of analysis
   (d) None of the analysis

2. In polarography the cell consists of
   (a) Reference electrode and dropping mercury electrode
   (b) Mercury electrode and a reference electrode
   (c) Normal electrolytic cell
   (d) None of the above

3. Polarogram is the curve obtained by
   (a) Plotting the changes in potential against the concentration
   (b) Plotting the changes in potential against the temperature variation
   (c) Plotting the changes in current flow against the potential variation
   (d) None of the above

4. Which one of the following statements is correct?
   (a) The electro-reducible substances are only analyzed by polarography
   (b) Theelectro-oxidizable substances are only analyzed by polarography
   (c) Both electro-oxidizable and electro-reducible substances are analyzed by polarography
   (d) None of the above

5. The indicator electrode of the cell used in the polarography should be
   (a) Very small in size
   (b) Of standard size
   (c) Large in size
   (d) All of the above

6. Which one of the following statements is correct?
   (a) One of the two electrodes of the cell used in polarography should be polarizable
   (b) Both the two electrodes of the cell used in polarography should be polarizable
   (c) None of the two electrodes of the cell used in polarography should be polarizable
   (d) None of the above

7. Which one of the following statements is correct?
   (a) Only organic substances can be analyzed by polarography
   (b) Only inorganic substances can be analyzed by polarography
   (c) Both organic and inorganic substances can be analyzed by polarography
   (d) None of the above

8. Which one of the following statements is correct?
   (a) Polarography can be used for only quantitative analysis
   (b) Polarography can be used for only qualitative analysis
   (c) Polarography can be used for both qualitative and quantitative analysis
   (d) None of the above

9. Which one of the following statements is correct?
   (a) Polarography can measure the concentration of solution up to 10^{-8}M
   (b) Polarography can measure the concentration of solution up to 10^{-5}M
   (c) Polarography can measure the concentration of solution up to 10^{-3}M
   (d) Polarography can measure the concentration of solution up to 10^{-1}M

10. Which one of the following statements is correct?
    (a) Polarography requires very less time,
    (b) Polarography can analyze the concentrationwithout separating the components of a mixture,
    (c) Very small volume of sample up to 0.05ml can be used to measure by polarography.
    (d) All of the above

11. In dropping mercury electrode used in polarography mercury works as
    - (a) Anode
    - (b) Cathode
    - (c) Both anode and cathode
    - (d) None of the above
12. The rotating platinum electrode can be used when
    - (a) The positive potential is very low, even less than 1 volt
    - (b) Dropping mercury electrode is not suitable
    - (c) Higher sensitivity is desired
    - (d) All of the above

B. SHORT QUESTIONS

1. What are different current possible in Polarography?
2. What is a Polalogram?
3. What do you mean by catalytic current in Polarography?
4. How can we remove migration current in Polarography?
5. What is the unique feature of polarography which separates it from other electro analytical techniques?
6. Why does an electrochemical process appear irreversible?
7. Explain the principle behind the working of an ion selective electrode.
8. A glass electrode is a specific example of an ion selective electrode. How does a glass electrode work?
9. Explain Rotating plating electrode?
10. Explain dropping mercury electrode.
11. Explain what is meant by adsorptive (or cathodic stripping voltammetry) and explain the principles behind it.

C. LONG QUESTIONS

1. Sketch a polarogram and label two important details of the polarographic wave.
2. Explain the working and instrumentation of rotating platinum electrode.
3. Explain the working and instrumentation of Dropping Mercury Electrode.
4. Describe the approaches that might be used to attach an enzyme or antibody to this electrode to produce a functional biosensor.
5. Explain the working and instrumentation of polarograph?

Appendix - I

Test Solutions

TEST SOLUTIONS (T.S.)

ACETONE, BUFFERED T.S.

Dissolve 1.7g of sodium acetate ($NaC_2H_3O_2$) and 8.4g of sodium chloride in about 20mL of water; add 13.6 mL of 0.1N hydrochloric acid and 30mL of acetone. Mix well and dilute to 100mL with water. Fill the solution in a clean reagent bottle, stopper and label properly.

ACID-FERRIC CHLORIDE T.S.

Add 7.5 mL of sulphuric acid (98%) to 90 mL of glacial acetic acid, mix thoroughly. Add 1.5 mL of *Ferric Chloride T.S.* to this mixture, mix and cool. Fill the solution in a clean reagent bottle, stopper and label properly.

ALCOHOLIC POTASSIUM HYDROXIDE T.S.

Take 10 mL of water in a 500 mL volumetric flask; add about 17.5g of potassium hydroxide (not less than 85% KOH) and dissolve. Add aldehyde free alcohol (95%) with continuous swirling sufficiently to make up the volume to 500 mL. Fill the solution in a clean reagent bottle, stopper and label properly.

ALKALINE CUPRIC TARTRATE, T.S.

See Fehling's solution

ALKALINE CUPRIC IODIDE T.S.

Take 750 mg of cupric sulphate ($CuSO_4$, $5H_2O$) in a clean 100 mL conical flask, add 10 mL of water and dissolve (solution 1). In another clean 250 mL beaker take 2.5 g of anhydrous sodium carbonate, 2.0 g of bicarbonate, and 2.5 g of potassium sodium tartrate and 45 mL of water; dissolve (solution 2). Add the solution 1 gradually with constant stirring to the solution 2 through a funnel that touches the bottom of the beaker; add

150 mg of potassium iodide (not less than 99%), 20 g of anhydrous sodium sulphate, and 7.5 mL of 0.02M solution of potassium iodate, stir the solution well and make up the volume to 100 mL with water. Fill the solution in a clean reagent bottle, stopper and label properly.

> *Note:* The volume of 0.02M potassium iodate solution to be added may vary from 5 ml to 15 ml depending on the blood sugar concentration and on the volume of blood filtrate used.

ALKALINE MERCURIC POTASSIUM IODIDE SOLUTION T.S.

See Nessler's Reagent

ALKALINE PICRATE T.S.

Mix 2 mL of trinitrophenol solution (1%) with 1mL of 5% solution of sodium hydroxide; dilute the solution to 10 mL with water. Fill the solution in a clean reagent bottle, stopper and label properly.

> *Note:* Solution should be prepared within 2 days of use

AMINONAPHTHOLSULPHONIC ACID T.S.

Weigh accurately 0.5g of sodium sulphite (Na_2SO_3), 9.43g of sodium bisulphite ($NaHSO_3$) and 70mg of 1,2,4-aminonaphtholsulphonic acid, mix the powders thoroughly. Fill the solution in a clean reagent bottle, stopper and label properly.

> *Note:* Freshly prepared solution is to be used. When required, 0.75g of this powder mixture is dissolved in 5 ml of water.

AMMONIA-AMMONIUM CHLORIDE BUFFER T.S.

Dissolve 6.75g of ammonium chloride in 30 mL of water. Add 57 mL of *Strong Ammonia water*, dilute to 100 mL with water. Fill the solution in a clean reagent bottle, stopper and label properly.

AMMONIA-CYANIDE T.S.

Dissolve 2g of potassium cyanide in 15 mL of Strong Ammonia water ($28 - 30\%$ of NH_3) and dilute to 100 mL with water. Mix well and fill the solution in a clean reagent bottle, stopper and label properly.

AMMONIA T.S.

Dilute 40 mL of Strong Ammonia water ($28 - 30\%$ of NH_3) to 100 mL with water. Mix well and preserve in tightly closed bottle in cool place, label it properly.

> *Note:* The bottle must be tightly closed. The bottle should be put in a ice bath before opening and while opening the face should be kept away from the bottle.

AMMONIA, T.S., ALCOHOLIC

It is a solution of ammonia gas in alcohol that contains $10 - 11\%$ of NH_3. The specific gravity of the solution should be 0.80. The solution should be stored in alkali resistant container in a cool place.

AMMONIA T.S., STRONG

Strong ammonia solution containing $28 - 30\%$ of ammonia calculated as NH_3.

AMMONIUM ACETATE T.S.

It is a 10% solution of ammonium acetate in water. That is dissolve 10g of ammonium acetate in water, make up the volume to 100 mL; shake well and store in bottle.

AMMONIUM CARBONATE T.S.

Dissolve 20g of ammonium carbonate in sufficient water, add 20 mL of Ammonia T.S. slowly with mild stirring and make up the volume to 100 mL. Mix thoroughly and preserve in stoppered bottle.

AMMONIUM CHLORIDE T.S. (2N)

It is a 10.5% solution of ammonium chloride in water. Fill the solution in a clean reagent bottle, stopper and label properly.

AMMONIUM CHLORIDE - AMMONIUM HYDROXIDE T.S.

Mix 50 mL of water and 50 mL of Ammonia T.S. strong well. Saturate the solution with ammonium chloride. That is, add ammonium chloride to ammonia-water mixture, shake well for at least 30 min until some amount remains undissolved. Fill the solution in a clean reagent bottle, stopper and label properly.

AMMONIUM MOLYBDATE T.S.

Powder about 7g of molybdic acid in a dry mortar pestle, take 6.5g of the fine powder of molybdic acid, and dissolve in a mixture of 14 mL of water and 14.5 mL of Ammonia T.S. strong. Cool the solution. Add 32 mL of nitric acid to 40 mL of water in another clean beaker; cool the mixture well. Add the cooled solution of molybdic acid slowly to well cooled nitric acid solution with constant stirring.

Allow the solution to stand for 48 hrs and filter through asbestos. Store the solution in a clean amber-glass bottle and keep it in dark.

> *Note:* The solution should be freshly prepared. If there is precipitation, use the clear supernatant solution.

> **Test:** Add 2 ml of sodium phosphate T.S. to 5 ml of this solution (Ammonium Molybdate T.S.); a yellow color precipitate is obtained immediately or after slight warming.

AMMONIUM OXALATE T.S. (0.5N)

It is 3.5% solution of ammonium oxalate [(NH$_4$)$_2$C$_2$H$_4$, H$_2$O] in water. Fill the solution in a clean reagent bottle, stopper and label properly.

AMMONIUM PHOSPHATE, DIBASIC T.S. / AMMONIUM PHOSPHATE T.S.

It is 13% solution of ammonium phosphate [(NH$_4$)$_2$HPO$_4$] in water. Fill the solution in a clean reagent bottle, stopper and label properly. The approximate strength of the solution is 1N.

AMMONIUM SULPHIDE T.S.

Saturate 60 mL of Ammonia T.S. with hydrogen sulphide (H$_2$S). Add 40 mL of Ammonia T.S., mix well and transfer the solution into a dark amber color bottle. Keep the bottle in dark and cold place.

> **Note:** The solution should not be turbid either by addition of Magnesium Sulphate T.S. or by Calcium Chloride T.S.
>
> The solution should not be used if precipitate of sulphur is found.

AMMONIUM THIOCYANATE T.S. (1N)

It is 8% solution of ammonium thiocyanate (NH$_4$SCN) in water. Fill the solution in a clean reagent bottle, stopper and label properly.

ANTHRONE T.S.

Add 65 mL of sulphuric acid to 35 mL of water, mix. Dissolve 35 mg of anthrone to this hot solution of sulphuric acid. Cool the solution immediately in an ice bath to bring the solution to room temperature. Filter the solution through glass wool. Allow the solution to room temperature for 30 min before use.

> **Note:** The solution should not be prepared before 12 hr of use.

ANTIMONY TRICHLORIDE T.S.

It is 20% solution of antimony trichloride in water. The solution should be filtered if necessary. Fill the solution in a clean reagent bottle, stopper and label properly.

BARIUM CHLORIDE T.S.

It contains 12g of barium chloride ($BaCl_2$, $2H_2O$) in 100mL of solution prepared with water. Fill the solution in a clean reagent bottle, stopper and label properly.

BARIUM HYDROXIDE T.S.

It is a saturated solution of barium hydroxide [$(BaOH)_2$, $8H_2O$] in recently boiled water. Freshly prepared solution should be used. Fill the solution in a clean reagent bottle, stopper and label properly.

BARIUM NITRATE T.S.

It contains 6.5g of barium nitrate in 100mL of solution prepared with water. Fill the solution in a clean reagent bottle, stopper and label properly.

β-NAPHTHOL T.S.

Dissolve 1g of β-Naphthol in 1% solution of sodium hydroxide to make 100 mL solution. Fill the solution in a clean reagent bottle, stopper and label properly.

BROMINE WATER (BROMINE T.S.)

It is a saturated solution of bromine in water. Take 2 – 3 mL of bromine in 100 mL of cold water contained in a glass stoppered conical flask.

> *Note:* Preserve the solution in a cool and dark place. Fill the solution in a clean reagent bottle, stopper and label properly.

BROMOCRESOL GREEN T.S.

Take 50 mg of bromocresol green in a 100 mL stoppered cylinder, dissolve in *alcohol* and make up the volume with alcohol. If required, filter the solution; fill in stoppered bottle.

> *Note:* For pH determination, the solution is prepared by dissolving 50 mg of Bromocresol green in 1.4 ml of 0.05N sodium hydroxide solution and then the volume is made up to 100 ml with freshly boiled and cooled distilled water.

BROMOPHENOL BLUE T.S.

Dissolve 100 mg of bromophenol blue in 100 mL of *diluted alcohol*. If required filter the solution and then preserve in reagent bottle.

> *Note:* For pH determination, the solution is prepared by dissolving 50 mg of Bromophenol blue in 1.5 ml of 0.05N sodium hydroxide solution and then the volume is made up to 100 ml with freshly boiled and cooled distilled water.

BROMOTHYMOL BLUE T.S.

Dissolve 100 mg of bromothymol blue in 100 mL of *diluted alcohol*. If required filter the solution and then preserve in reagent bottle with proper label.

> ***Note:*** For pH determination, the solution is prepared by dissolving 50 mg of Bromothymol blue in 1.6 ml of 0.05N sodium hydroxide solution and then makes up the volume to 100 ml with freshly prepared distilled water.

CALCIUM CHLORIDE T.S.

It is a 7.5% solution of calcium chloride ($CaCl_2$, $2H_2O$) in water. Fill the solution in a clean reagent bottle, stopper and label properly.

CALCIUM HYDROXIDE T.S.

The solubility of calcium hydroxide in water depends on temperature. Take about 0.3g of calcium hydroxide and add to 100 mL of cold water, shake vigorously for one hour. Keep the mixture undisturbed and allow the undissolved calcium hydroxide to settle completely. Decant the clear supernatant liquid carefully and store the solution at cool place. If necessary filter the solution before use. Fill the solution in a clean reagent bottle, stopper and label properly.

CALCIUM SULPHATE T.S.

It is a saturated solution of calcium sulphate ($CaSO_4$, $2H_2O$) in water. Take 100 mL of water in a stopper conical flask, add some calcium sulphate; stopper the flask and put it in a shaker. Shake for 1hr; if there is no undissolved calcium sulphate, add some more and repeat the process until there is some amount of calcium sulphate remains undissolved. Filter the solution and fill in a clean reagent bottle, stopper and label properly.

CERIC AMMONIUM NITRATE T.S.

Dissolve 12.50g of ceric ammonium nitrate [$Ce(NO_3)_4.2NH_4.NO_3$, $2H_2O$] in 20 mL of 0.25 N Nitric acid. Fill the solution in a clean reagent bottle, stopper and label properly.

> ***Note:*** The solution can be preserved only for 2 days.

CHLORAL HYDRATE T. S.

Mix 15 mL of water and 10 mL of glycerin. To the solution add 50g of chloral hydrate and dissolve. Fill the solution in a clean reagent bottle, stopper and label properly.

CHLORINE T.S. (CHLORINE WATER)

It is a saturated solution of chlorine in water. The solution is prepared by passing chlorine gas prepared by any chemical reaction through water. The solution should be completely filled in an dark amber color bottle in cool place.

> *Note:* Even on proper storage it deteriorates; hence the solution should be freshly prepared and if full concentration is required.

CHROMOTROPIC ACID T.S.

Add 75 mL of concentrated sulphuric acid very slowly to 33.3 mL of ice cooled water. It is better that during mixing, the conical flask should be place in an ice bath. After each addition the solution should be gently agitate and cool. Once the solution becomes cool, add the next portion of sulphuric acid. In 100 mL of 75% solution of sulphuric acid, thus prepared, dissolve 50 mg of chromotropic acid ($C_{10}H_8O_8S_2$, $2H_2O$) or its sodium salt.

> *Note: Never add water to concentrated sulphuric acid to water.* While sulphuric acid is added to water, the volume of the mixture reduces. Hence, excess of water is taken. If 33.3 ml of water is mixed with 75 ml of concentrated sulphuric acid it will produce 100 ml. keep the conical flask immersed into the ice bath during mixing.

COBALT-URANYL ACETATE T.S.

Mix 6 mL of glacial acetic acid with sufficient water to make 100 mL of solution (6%v/v solution of glacial acetic acid). To this solution add 8 g of uranyl acetate [$UO_2(C_2H_3O_2)_2$, $2H_2O$], warm and dissolve. Similarly prepare another 100 mL of 6%v/v solution of glacial acetic acid and dissolve 40g of cobaltous acetate [$Co(C_2H_3O_2)_2$, $4H_2O$] by warming, if necessary. Mix the two solutions while warm; cool the solution to $20^{\circ}C$ and keep it for at least 2 hrs to settle the precipitate, if any. If precipitation takes place, filter the solution and store in tightly closed glass bottle and label properly.

COBALTOUS CHLORIDE T.S.

Dissolve 2 g of cobaltous chloride ($CoCl2$, $6H2O$) in 1 mL of hydrochloric acid and dilute to 100 mL with eater. Store in a reagent bottle. This is approximately 0.16N solution.

CONGO RED T.S.

Take a 50 mL measuring cylinder. Pour 5 mL of alcohol and 45 mL of water in it. Transfer the mixture into a 100 mL conical flask. Dissolve 250 mg of Congo red in the mixture of solvent. Fill in a glass bottle, stopper and label properly.

CRESOL RED T.S.

Triturate 40 mg of cresol red in a mortar pestle with 10.50 mL of 0.01N sodium hydroxide until a complete solution is obtained. Dilute the solution to 100 mL with water, mix well and keep it in a stoppered glass bottle, label properly.

CRESOL RED-THYMOL BLUE T.S.

Add 15 mL of thymol blue T.S. to 5 mL of cresol red T.S.; mix well, fill the solution in a stoppered glass bottle (reagent bottle), label properly.

CUPRIC OXIDE, AMMONIATED T.S.

See Schweitzer's Reagent

CUPRIC SULPHATE T.S.

Dissolve 12.5 g of cupric sulphate ($CuSO_4$, $5H_2O$) in sufficient water to make 100 mL of solution. mix thoroughly and preserve in a stoppered glass bottle. The strength of this solution is approximately 1 N. fill the solution in a clean reagent bottle, stopper and label properly.

CUPRIC TARTRATE T.S., ALKALINE

See Fehling's solution

CRYSTAL VIOLET T.S.

See Methylrosaniline Chloride, T.S.

DELAFIELD'S HEMATOXYLIN T.S.

Solution A: Prepare 200 mL of saturated solution of ammonium alum. Dissolve 2 g of hematoxylin in 12.5 mL of alcohol. Add this solution to solution A and mix. Keep the solution in a flask stoppered with a pledget of purified cotton; expose it to light and air. After 4 days, filter the solution.

Solution B: Mix 50 mL of glycerin and 50 mL of methanol in a clean beaker; add the solution to solution A and mix thoroughly. Keep the solution in warm place (at about 40°C), exposed to light and air until the solution becomes dark. Fill the solution in tightly closed bottle with proper label.

> *Note:* Dilute the solution with equal volume of water before use for staining endocrine tissue.

DENIGES' REAGENT

See Mercuric Sulphate, T.S.

DIAZOBENZENESULPHONIC ACID T.S.

Dry about 2 g of sulphinilic acid at 105°C for 3 hrs. Weigh accurately 1.57g, take into a clean beaker. Add 80 mL of water and 10 mL of dilute hydrochloric acid; heat on a boiling water bath until a solution is produced. Cool to 15°C; add slowly 6.5 mL of 10% solution of sodium nitrite with constant stirring. Dilute the solution to 100 mL with water. Fill the solution in a clean reagent bottle, stopper and label properly.

> *Note:* During cooling to 15°C some of the sulphinilic acid may precipitate which would redissolve subsequently.

DICHLOROFLUORESCEIN T.S.

Weigh 100 mg of Dichlorofluorescein and take into a clean 100mL beaker; add 60 mL of alcohol and shake well to dissolve. Add 2.5 mL of 0.1N sodium hydroxide; mix well and dilute to 100 mL with water. mix and transfer into a clean reagent bottle; stopper and label properly.

Þ-DIMETHYLAMINOBENZALDEHYDE T.S.

Carefully mix 65 mL of sulphuric acid with 35 mL of cold water in a clean beaker; dissolve 125 mg of

Þ-dimethylaminobenzaldehyde. Add 0.05 mL of Ferric chloride T.S. and mix well.

Fill the solution in a clean and dry reagent bottle, stopper and label properly.

> *Note:* Use the solution within 7 days.

DIPHENYLAMINE T.S.

Take about 90 mL of sulphuric acid in a clean and dry beaker; add 1.0 g of Diphenylamine, stir with a glass rod to dissolve. Make up the volume to 100 mL with sulphuric acid. Mix well; transfer the solution into a clean and dry reagent bottle; stopper and label properly.

> *Note:* The solution prepared should be colorless.

EOSIN Y T.S.

Dissolve 50 mg of eosin Y in 10 mL of water. Preserve the solution in 25 mL of reagent bottle, stopper and label properly.

> *Note:* The solution is used as absorption indicator.

ERIOCHROME BLACK T.S.

Take about 40 mL of methanol in a clean and dry 50 mL cylinder; add 200 mg of Eriochrome black T and 2 g of hydroxylamine hydrochloride. Stir to dissolve. Make up the volume up to 50 mL with methanol. Transfer the solution into a clean and dry 100 mL reagent bottle, stopper tightly and label properly.

FEHLING'S SOLUTION T.S.

Solution A (Cupric sulphate solution): take 17.33 g of small fresh crystals of cupric sulphate ($CuSO_4$, $5H_2O$) which is free from efflorescence and deliquescence in a 250 mL volumetric flask, dissolve in water and make up the volume, mix well and stopper the flask, label properly.

Solution B (Alkaline Tartrate solution): take 86.5 g of crystalline potassium sodium tartrate ($KNaC_4H_4O_6$, $4H_2O$) and 25 g of sodium hydroxide; dissolve in 200 mL of water in a conical flask. Make up the volume up to 250 mL with water, mix well and preserve in a stoppered flask with a proper label.

> *Note:* When required, mix equal volumes of the two solutions A and B and use.

FERRIC AMMONIUM SULPHATE T.S.

Take about 80 mL of water in a 100 mL measuring cylinder; add 8 g of Ferric Ammonium Sulphate [$FeNH_4(SO_4)_2$, $12H_2O$] and dissolve. Make up the volume to 100 mL with water; mix well. Transfer the solution into a clean reagent bottle, stopper and label properly.

FERRIC CHLORIDE T.S.

Take about 80 mL of water in a 100 mL measuring cylinder; add 9 g of Ferric Chloride ($FeCl_3$, $6H_2O$) and dissolve. Make up the volume to 100 mL with water; mix well. Transfer the solution into a clean reagent bottle, stopper and label properly.

> *Note:* The strength of the solution is about 1N.

FERROUS SULPHATE T.S.

Take about 90 mL of freshly boiled and cooled distilled water in a 100 mL volumetric flask; add 8 g of crystals of Ferrous Sulphate ($FeSO_4$, $7H_2O$) and dissolve. Make up the volume to 100 mL with sulphuric acid; mix well. Transfer the solution into a clean reagent bottle, stopper and label properly. Standardize the solution with 0.1N potassium permanganate.

> *Note:* The strength of the solution should be measured frequently; it is about 0.25N.

FERROUS SULPHATE T.S., ACIDIC

Take about 80 mL of freshly boiled and cooled distilled water in a 100 mL measuring cylinder; add 7 g of crystals of Ferrous Sulphate ($FeSO_4$, $7H_2O$) and dissolve. Make up the volume to 100 mL with water; mix well. Transfer the solution into a clean reagent bottle, stopper and label properly.

> *Note:* The solution should be freshly prepared and used.

FORMALDEHYDE T.S.

Formaldehyde solution contains not less than 37% of formaldehyde. The solution also contains methanol to prevent polymerization. It is Formaldehyde solution I.P. fill the solution in a clean reagent bottle, stopper and label properly.

FUCHSIN-PYROGALLOL T.S.

Boil about 100 mL of water for 15 min and cool; when the water is warm to 50 mL of this water dissolve 100 mg of basic fuchsin. Allow to cool completely. Add 2 mL of saturated solution of sodium bisulphite.

Mix well and keep it for 3 hrs. Add 0.9 mL of hydrochloric acid, mix and keep it for overnight. Add 100 mg of Pyrogallol stir until it dissolves. Dilute the solution with water to 100 mL, fill in an amber-glass bottle, stopper and label properly.

Note: Preserve the solution in a refrigerator.

FUCHSIN-SULPHUROUS ACID T.S.

Take 60 mL of freshly boiled hot water, add 100 mg of basic fuchsin and dissolve. Allow the solution to cool to room temperature. Dissolve separately 1 g of anhydrous sodium sulphite in 10 mL of water. Add this solution to the solution of fuchsin, mix well. Add 1 mL of hydrochloric acid, mix and dilute to 100 mL with water, mix well. Fill the solution in an amber-glass bottle, stopper and label properly.

Note: This solution should freshly prepared and used.

GASTRIC FLUID SIMULATED T.S.

In 7.0 mL of hydrochloric acid dissolve 2.0 g of sodium chloride and 3.2 g of pepsin. Dilute the solution to 1000 mL with water.

Note: The pH of the solution would be 1.2

GELATIN T.S.

Take 170 g of acid-treated gelatin (Type A) and dissolve in about 450 mL of water. Mix well and dilute to 500 mL with water. Heat the solution in an autoclave at 115oC for 30 min. take out the solution from the autoclave, cool and add 5 g of phenol and 500 mL of water. Mix well. Fill the solution in a 1 lt bottle, tightly stopper, label properly.

Note: Store the solution in a refrigerator. The solution is used in determination of Corticotrophin injection.

GOLD CHLORIDE, T.S.

Take 35 mL of water and dissolve 1 g of gold chloride ($HAuCl_4$, $3H_2O$). Fill the solution in a 1 tightly stopper reagent bottle and label properly.

Note: Strength of this solution is 0.2N.

HYDROGEN PEROXIDE, T.S.

It is Hydrogen Peroxide solution, I.P. It should contain 2.5 to 3.5%w/v of H_2O_2 and a suitable preservative not more than 0.05%. Preserve the solution in an air tight reagent bottle with proper label.

HYDROGEN SULPHIDE, T.S.

It is a saturated solution of hydrogen sulphide in cold water. The hydrogen sulphide gas is prepared in Kip's apparatus. Pass the gas through cold water.

> If the solution is to be stored; it is to be stored in small, amber-glass bottle, filled nearly to the top. The filled and sealed bottle is stored in dark and cold place.

HYDROXYLAMINE HYDROCHLORIDE, T.S.

Take 63 mL of alcohol (95%) in a 100 mL clean and dry measuring cylinder, pour into a clean and dry 250 mL conical flask. Measure 37 mL of water, add to alcohol, and mix well to prepare 60% alcohol. Measure 95mL of 60% alcohol in to another conical flask, add 3.5 g of Hydroxylamine Hydrochloride and dissolve. To this add 0.5 mL of 0.1% solution of bromophenol blue solution and then, add drop wise 0.5N alcoholic potassium hydroxide until greenish color is obtained. Transfer the solution into the 100 mL measuring cylinder and make up the volume to 100 mL with prepared 60% alcohol. Fill the solution in a clean and dry reagent bottle, stopper tightly and label properly.

INDIGO CARMINE, T.S./SODIUM INDIGOTINDINSULPHONATE, T.S.

Dissolve a quantity of Sodium Indigotindinsulphonate equivalent to 180 mg of $C_{16}H_8N_2O_2(SO_3Na)_2$, in about 95 mL of water. Make up the volume to 100 mL with water, mix well. Fill the solution in a clean and dry reagent bottle, stopper tightly and label properly.

> *Note:* Use the solution within 60 days from its preparation.

INDOPHENOL-ACETATE, T.S.

Solution A: Pipette out 24 mL of standard dichlorophenol-indophenol solution and transfer into a clean 100 mL volumetric flask, dilute the solution to 100 mL with water, mix well.

Solution B: Dissolve 2.732g of anhydrous sodium acetate in sufficient water to make 100 mL.

In a 250 mL clean beaker take solution A; to this Add solution B, mix well. Adjust the pH of the final solution to 7 with o.5N acetic acid. Fill the solution in a clean and dry reagent bottle, stopper tightly and label properly.

> *Note:* Store the solution in a refrigerator and use it within 2 weeks. The solution is used for the assay of Corticotropin injection.

INTESTINAL FLUID, SIMULATED, T.S.

Take about 250 mL of water 1000 mL clean beaker, add 6.8 g of monobasic potassium phosphate and dissolve. Add 190 mL of 0.2N sodium hydroxide and 400 mL of water, stir with a clean glass rod to mix. Add 10 g of pancreatin, mix well. Adjust the pH of the solution to 7.5 ± 0.1 with 0.2N sodium hydroxide. Transfer the solution into a clean 1000 mL measuring cylinder and make up the volume to 1000 mL with water. Mix well and store in a 1 lt reagent bottle, stopper tightly and label.

> *Note:* Freshly prepared solution should be used in dissolution test.

IODINE, T.S.

Take 3.6 g of potassium iodide into a 250 mL clean glass stopper conical flask; dissolve in 50 mL of water. To this solution add 1.4 g of iodine and stopper the flask, swirl the flask until iodine is complete dissolved. Add 2 drops of hydrochloric acid, mix thoroughly. Transfer the solution to a 100 mL measuring cylinder. Wash the flask with aliquots of water, add the washings to main solution; make up the volume to 100 mL with water.

> *Note:* Strength of this solution is 0.1N iodine.

IODINE MONOCHLORIDE, T.S.

In a glass stopper conical flask take 75 mL of water; dissolve 10 g of potassium iodide and 6.44 g of potassium iodate in it. Add 75 mL of hydrochloric acid and 5 mL of chloroform. The chloroform layer at the bottom shall be colored depending on the amount of iodine liberated/present free. Adjust the color of chloroform layer to faint brown by gradual addition of 0.01M potassium iodide or potassium iodate solution.

If much of iodine is liberated stronger solution of potassium iodate can be initially used and finally with 0.01M solution. Fill the solution in amber-glass bottle, stopper tightly and label properly.

> *Note:* Store the solution in dark place.

IODINE AND POTASSIUM IODIDE, T.S.

Take 25 mL of water in a 50 mL of glass stopper cylinder or flask; add 1.5 g of potassium iodide and 500 mg of iodine. Stopper the flask and swirl till a complete solution is made. Transfer the solution into an amber-glass clean bottle, stopper tightly and label properly.

> *Note:* Store the solution in dark place.

IODOBROMIDE, T.S.

Take a clean and dry stoppered conical flask; measure 100 mL of glacial acetic acid using a clean and dry measuring cylinder. Add 1.32 g of iodine to the acetic acid, stopper the flask. Swirl and heat over a boiling water bath to dissolve iodine. While putting over the water bath, open the stopper and loosely put it over the mouth of the flask. After complete dissolution of iodine, cool the solution to room temperature and titrate 10 mL of the solution with 0.1N sodium thiosulphate. Determine the amount of iodine present in 10 mL of the solution and then calculate the amount of iodine present in 90 mL of the solution.

Add a quantity of bromine equivalent to that of the iodine present, mix thoroughly. Transfer the solution into an amber-glass clean bottle, stopper tightly and label properly.

> *Note:* Store the solution in dark place.

LEAD ACETATE, T.S.

Take 90 mL of freshly boiled and cooled distilled water in a clean conical flask; add 9.5 g of transparent, clear crystals of lead acetate [$Pb(C_2H_3O_2)_2, 3H_2O$] and dissolve. Transfer the solution into a 100 mL measuring cylinder. Make up the volume to 100 mL with freshly boiled and cooled distilled water. Fill the solution in a clean well stoppered reagent bottle and label properly.

> *Note:* Approximate strength of the solution is 0.5N.

LEAD SUBACETATE, T.S.

Take 14 g of lead monoxide into a clean glass mortar pestle; add 10 mL of freshly boiled and cooled distilled water. Triturate to a smooth paste. Transfer the paste into a clean stoppered conical flask. Rinse the mortar pestle with 10 mL of freshly boiled and cooled distilled water, add to the flask. In another flask dissolve 22 g of lead acetate in 70 mL of freshly boiled and cooled distilled water. Add this solution to lead oxide mixture. Stopper the flask and shake vigorously for 5 min. Allow to stand the mixture for 7 days with occasional shaking. Filter the mixture; rinse the precipitate with freshly boiled and cooled distilled water and make up the volume to 100 mL. Fill the filtrate into a well stoppered reagent bottle, stopper firmLy and label properly.

LEAD SUBACETATE, T.S., DILUTED

Take about 95 mL of freshly boiled and cooled distilled water into a 100 mL measuring cylinder, add 3.25 mL of lead Subacetate, T.S. and make up the volume to 100 mL with freshly boiled and cooled distilled water. Transfer the solution into a clean, well stoppered regent bottle; stopper tightly and label properly.

LOCKE-RINGER'S T.S.

See Locke-Ringer's solution

LOCKE-RINGER'S SOLUTION

Dissolve the following substances in sufficient freshly boiled and cooled distilled water to make 100 mL of the solution.

Sodium chloride	900 mg
Potassium chloride	42 mg
Calcium chloride	24 mg
Magnesium chloride	20 mg
Sodium bicarbonate	50 mg
Dextrose	50 mg

Note: This solution should be freshly prepared every day.

MAGNESIA MIXTURE, T.S.

Take 65 mL of water in a well stoppered conical flask, add 5.5 g of magnesium chloride ($MgCl_2$, $6H_2O$) and 7 g of ammonium chloride; dissolve. Add 35 mL of ammonia, T.S. and mix well. Stopper the flask tightly and keep for 4 days. Filter the solution through Whatmann 42 filter paper. Transfer the filtrate in a clean well stoppered reagent bottle, stopper tightly and label properly.

Note: If the solution becomes turbid, filter it before use.

MAGNESIUM SULPHATE, T.S.

Dissolve 12 g of clear crystals of magnesium sulphate ($MgSO_4$, $7H_2O$) in sufficient water to make 100 mL of solution. Fill the solution in a clean reagent bottle, stopper tightly and label properly. Crystals should not undergo efflorescence.

Note: The approximate strength of the solution would be 1N.

MALLORY'S STAIN

Take 40 of water in a conical flask add to it 250 mg of water-soluble aniline blue, 1 g of orange G and 1 g of oxalic acid; dissolve. Transfer the solution into a 50 mL measuring cylinder and rinse the flask with aliquot of water and make up the volume with washing. Transfer the solution into a well stoppered reagent bottle, stopper firmly and label properly.

MAYER'S REAGENT

Dissolve 5 g of potassium iodide in 10 mL of water in a small conical flask. In another flask dissolve 1.358 g of mercuric chloride in about 40 mL of water. Mix the two solutions and make up the volume with water. Transfer the solution into a well stoppered reagent bottle, stopper firmly and label properly.

MERCURIC-POTASSIUM IODIDE, T.S.

See Mayer's Reagent

MERCURIC ACETATE, T.S.

Take 40 mL of glacial acetic acid in a clean and dry conical flask, add 3.0 g of mercuric acetate and dissolve. Transfer the solution into a clean and dry 50 mL measuring cylinder; make up the volume with glacial acetic acid. Fill the solution into a well stoppered amber-glass reagent bottle, stopper firmly and label properly.

> *Note:* Store the solution away from sunlight and keep it tightly closed after use.

MERCURIC BROMIDE, T.S., ALCOHOLIC

Take 50 mL of alcohol in a clean and dry stoppered conical flask; add 2.5g of mercuric bromide and dissolve by warming over boiling water bath; cool to room temperature. Transfer the solution into a clean and dry 50 mL measuring cylinder; if necessary add alcohol to make up the volume to 50 mL. Transfer the solution into a well stoppered amber-glass reagent bottle, stopper firmly and label properly.

> *Note:* Exposure to heat for longer time causes the loss of alcohol. Approximate strength of the solution would be 0.3N.

MERCURIC CHLORIDE, T.S.

Dissolve 3.25g of mercuric chloride in sufficient water to make 50 mL of solution. Store the solution in a clean reagent bottle, stopper tightly and label properly. Approximate strength of the solution would be 0.5N.

MERCURIC IODIDE, T.S.

Take 7g of mercuric iodide in a beaker; add very slowly 50 mL of 10% potassium iodide solution with continuous stirring until mercuric iodide is almost dissolved. Filter the solution and fill it in a clean amber-glass reagent bottle, stopper tightly and label properly.

MERCURIC NITRATE, T.S.

Take 15 mL of water, add and mix 32 mL of nitric acid in a conical flask. Add 40g of mercuric oxide (red or yellow), stopper and shake until mercuric oxide is dissolved. Fill the solution in a clean amber-glass reagent bottle, stopper tightly and label properly.

> *Note:* Approximate strength of the solution would be 4N. The solution must be kept away from light.

MERCURIC-POTASSIUM IODIDE, T.S.

In about 60 mL of water dissolve 1.358g of mercuric chloride. Transfer the solution into a 100 mL measuring cylinder. In another flask take 5g of potassium iodide in 10 mL of water. Add this solution to mercuric chloride solution. Make up the volume to 100 mL with water. Fill the solution in a clean amber-glass reagent bottle, stopper tightly and label properly.

MERCURIC POTASSIUM IODIDE SOLUTION, T.S., ALKALINE

See Nessler's Reagent

MERCURIC SULPHATE, T.S.

Take 40 mL of water in a 250 mL beaker, add 5g of mercuric oxide (yellow) and stir continuously. Add gradually 20 mL of sulphuric acid with continuous stirring; add another 40 mL of water, mix well; cool to room temperature. Make up the volume to 100 mL with water. Fill the solution in a clean amber-glass reagent bottle, stopper tightly and label properly.

MERCUROUS NITRATE, T.S.

Take 90 mL of water; add 10 mL of diluted nitric acid (10.5% solution). Mix well and add 15g of mercurous nitrate, stir to dissolve. Transfer the solution into an amber-glass reagent bottle containing a small globule of mercury. Stopper the bottle tightly and label properly.

> **Note:** Keep the solution in dark. Approximate strength of the solution would be 0.5N.

METAPHYLENEDIAMINE HYDROCHLORIDE, T.S.

Dissolve 500mg of Metaphylenediamine Hydrochloride in 100mL of water. Fill the solution in a reagent bottle, stopper and label properly. The solution should be colorless at time of use. If required heat the solution with activated charcoal. Then filter and use.

METAPHOSPHORIC-ACETIC ACID, T.S.

Dissolve 7.5g of Metaphosphoric acid in 20mL of glacial acetic acid; add sufficient water to make 250 mL solution. Store the solution in reagent bottle in a cool place.

> **Note:** Use the solution within 2 days of preparation.

METHYL ORANGE, T.S.

Dissolve 50mg of methyl orange in 50 mL of water. If required filter the solution and store in a reagent bottle; stopper and label properly.

METHYL RED, T.S.

Dissolve 50mg of methyl red in 50 mL of alcohol. Filter if required; store in a reagent bottle; stopper and label properly.

> *Note:* For determination of pH the solution is prepared by dissolving 50 mg of methyl red in 3.7ml of 0.05N sodium hydroxide; dilute the solution to 50 ml with water. Store the solution in a reagent bottle; stopper and label properly.

METHYLROSANILINE CHLORIDE, T.S.

Dissolve 100mg of methylrosaniline chloride in 10 mL of glacial acetic acid. Store in a suitable small reagent bottle, stopper and label properly.

METHYLTHIONINE PERCHLORATE, T.S.

Take 200 mL of 0.1% solution of potassium perchlorate in a beaker; add dropwise 1% solution of methylene blue with constant stirring until a slight turbidity results permanently. Stop stirring. Allow the solution to stand until the precipitate settles down. Decant the supernatant liquid into a reagent bottle. Stopper the bottle and label properly.

> *Note:* Use only the clear solution.

MILLON'S REAGENT

In an Erlenmeyer flask take 2 mL of mercury, add 20 mL of nitric acid; shake under a fuming chamber until the mercury is broken into fine globules; after 12 min add 35 mL of water and mix. If precipitates or crystals appear; add dilute nitric acid gradually until the precipitates or crystals get dissolved. Add 10% sodium hydroxide solution dropwise with constant stirring until curdy precipitate does not redissolve and form suspension. Add 5 mL of dilute nitric acid, mix well. Transfer the solution in a clean reagent bottle, stopper and label properly.

> **Note:**
> 1. Nitric acid used should be freed from oxides by blowing air through the acid until the acid becomes colorless.
> 2. Dilute nitric acid shall be prepared by diluting 10.5 ml of nitric acid to 100ml with water.
> 3. The solution should be freshly prepared and used.

METHYL VIOLET, T.S.

See Methylrosaniline Chloride, T.S.

NAPHTHOL GREEN, T.S.

Dissolve 50 mg of Naphthol green B in sufficient water to produce 100mL. Transfer the solution in a clean reagent bottle, stopper and label properly.

NESSLER'S REAGENT

Take 5g of potassium iodide and dissolve in 5 mL of water. To this solution add slowly with continuous stirring the saturated solution of mercuric chloride until a slight red color precipitate remains undissolved. Dissolve 15g of potassium hydroxide in 30 mL of water, cool in ice-bath; when the solution is ice-cooled, add this solution to the main mixture with gentle stirring.

Then add 0.5 mL of saturated solution of mercuric chloride. Dilute the solution to 100 mL with water. Allow the precipitate to settle solution, take out the supernatant clear solution. preserve the solution in a clean amber-glass tightly closed reagent bottle with a proper label.

> ***Test:*** Add 2 ml of the Nessler's reagent to 100 ml of a 1 in 300 000 solution of ammonium chloride in ammonia free water. A yellowish brown color will be produced immediately.

NINHYDRIN T.S.

Dissolve 200mg of triketohydrindene hydrate in water to make 10mL. label the solution properly.

> ***Note:*** The solution should be freshly prepared and used.

Þ-NITROANILINE, T.S.

Take 175 mg of Þ-Nitroaniline in a 25 mL stoppered measuring cylinder, add 0.75mL of hydrochloric acid and mix well. Dilute the volume to 25 mL, stopper and shake to mix thoroughly. Allow the solution to settle. Pipette out 5mL of clear supernatant liquid into a 100 mL volumetric flask; place the flask in an ice bath; after 5 min add 0.5mL of hydrochloric acid while the flask is in ice bath. Then add 1mL of 1% sodium nitrite solution dropwise and swirl the flask occasionally. Remove the flask from ice bah and dilute the content to 100 mL with water. Mix thoroughly and preserve in a clean amber-glass reagent bottle, stopper and label properly.

ORTHOPHENANTHROLINE, T.S.

Take 20 mL of water in a 25mL stoppered measuring cylinder, add 0.296g of clear crystals of ferrous sulphate ($FeSO_4$, $7H_2O$); dissolve. Add 300mg of Orthophenanthroline and dissolve. Transfer the solution into well stoppered small reagent bottle, stopper tightly and label properly.

OXALIC ACID, T.S.

Take 6.3 g of oxalic acid ($C_2H_2O_4$, $2H_2O$) in a 100mL stoppered measuring cylinder, dissolve in water and dilute to 100mL with water. stopper the cylinder, shake and transfer into a reagent bottle, stopper and label properly.

PHENOL RED, T.S.

Dissolve 50 mg of Phenolsulphonphthalein in 50 mL of alcohol (95%); filter if necessary, transfer the filtrate into a clean and dry reagent bottle, stopper tightly and label properly.

Note: For pH determination; dissolve 50 mg of Phenolsulphonphthalein in 2.85 ml of 0.05N sodium hydroxide and dilute to 100 ml with water. Fill the solution in well closed reagent bottle.

PHENOLSULPHONPHTHALEIN, T.S.

See Phenol Red, T.S.

PHENOLDISULPHONIC ACID, T.S.

In a 100mL flask take 2.5g of phenol; dissolve in 15mL of sulphuric acid. Add 7.5mL of fuming sulphuric acid, stir well, and heat at 100°C for 2hrs. While it is in fluid state transfer the material into a glass stoppered bottle. Before use, place the flask over a boiling water bath until the product is liquefied.

PHENOLPHTHALEIN, T.S.

Take 1g of phenolphthalein in a clean and dry 100mL measuring cylinder, dissolve in alcohol (95%) and make up the volume to 100mL with alcohol. Transfer the solution into a clean and dry reagent bottle, stoppered tightly and label properly.

PHENYLHYDRAZINE ACETATE, T.S.

Take 5mL of glacial acetic acid in a clean 100mL measuring cylinder, add and dissolve 10mL of phenylhydrazine acetate; dilute the solution to 100mL with water. Transfer the solution into a reagent bottle, stoppered tightly and label properly.

PHENYLHYDRAZINE-SULPHURIC ACID, T.S.

Mix 60 mL of sulphuric acid with 60mL of ice-cooled water, mix well. Take 65mg of phenylhydrazine hydrochloride in a 250mL clean conical flask; add about 90mL of water-sulphuric acid mixture. Transfer the solution into a 100mL measuring cylinder and make up the volume to 100mL with water-sulphuric acid mixture. Transfer the solution into a clean reagent bottle, stopper tightly and label properly.

PHOSPHOTUNGSTIC ACID, T.S.

Take 1g of phosphotungstic acid ($24WO_3.2H_3PO_4$, $48H_2O$) in a 100mL of measuring cylinder, dissolve in water and make up the volume up to 100mL with water. Transfer the solution into a clean reagent bottle, stopper tightly and label properly.

PICRIC ACID, T.S.

See Trinitrophenol T.S.

PLATINIC CHLORIDE, T.S.

Take 2.6g of platinic chloride (H_2PtCl_6, $6H_2O$) in a 50mL stoppered measuring cylinder, dissolve in sufficient water to make 20mL. the strength of this solution is almost 0.5N. Transfer the solution into a clean reagent bottle, stopper tightly and label properly.

POTASSIUM ACETATE, T.S.

Take 10g of potassium acetate in a clean 100mL measuring cylinder, add water to dissolve. Make up the volume of the solution to 100mL with water. Transfer the solution into a clean reagent bottle, stopper tightly and label properly. The approximate strength of the solution would be 1N.

POTASSIUM CHROMATE, T.S.

Take 10g of potassium chromate in a clean 100mL measuring cylinder, add water to dissolve. Make up the volume of the solution to 100mL with water. Transfer the solution into a clean reagent bottle, stopper tightly and label properly.

POTASSIUM DICHROMATE, T.S.

Take 7.5g of potassium dichromate in a clean 100mL measuring cylinder, add water to dissolve. Make up the volume of the solution to 100mL with water. Transfer the solution into a clean reagent bottle, stopper tightly and label properly.

POTASSIUM FERRICYANIDE, T.S.

Dissolve 1g of potassium ferricyanide in 10mL of water. Approximate strength of the solution would be 1N.

> **Note:** The solution should be freshly prepared.

POTASSIUM FERROCYANIDE T.S.

Dissolve 1g of potassium ferrocyanide in 10mL of water. Approximate strength of the solution would be 1N.

> **Note:** The solution should be freshly prepared.

POTASSIUM HYDROXIDE T.S.

Take 6.5g of potassium hydroxide in a 100mL measuring cylinder, add water to dissolve. Make up the volume to 100mL with water. Transfer the solution into a clean reagent bottle, mix well, stopper and label properly. Approximate strength of the solution would be 1N.

POTASSIUM HYDROXIDE T.S., ALCOHOLIC

Take 3.5g of potassium hydroxide in a 100mL measuring cylinder, add 2mL of water to dissolve. Make up the volume to 100mL with aldehyde-free alcohol (95%). Transfer the solution into a clean reagent bottle, mix well, stopper and label properly. Approximate strength of the solution would be 0.5N.

POTASSIUM IODIDE T.S.

Take 16.5g of potassium iodide in a 100mL measuring cylinder, add water to dissolve. Make up the volume to 100mL with water. Transfer the solution into a clean amber-glass reagent bottle, mix well, stopper and label properly. Approximate strength of the solution would be 1N.

POTASSIUM PERMANGANATE T.S.

Dissolve about 0.33g of potassium permanganate in 100mL of water in a stoppered flask; boil the solution for 15 min and keep it standing for at least 2 days. Filter the solution through asbestos and preserve in an amber-glass reagent bottle, stopper and label properly. Approximate strength of the solution would be 0.1N.

QUINALDINE RED T.S.

Take 100mg of Quinaldine red in a 100mL clean and dry measuring cylinder, add and dissolve in glacial acetic acid. Make up the volume with glacial acetic acid. Transfer the solution into a clean amber-glass reagent bottle, mix well, stopper and label properly.

SALINE T.S.

Dissolve 0.9g of sodium chloride in 100mL of water. Transfer the solution into a clean amber-glass reagent bottle, mix well, stopper and label properly.

SCHWEITZER'S REAGENT

Take 10g of cupric sulphate ($CuSO_4$, $5H_2O$) and dissolve in 100 mL of water, add sufficient sodium hydroxide solution (20%) so that copper hydroxide is precipitated. Filter the precipitate and wash with cold water to make the precipitate free from sulphate. Dissolve the wet precipitate in the minimum quantity of ammonia T.S.

SILVER-AMMONIUM NITRATE T.S.

Take 1g of silver nitrate in a conical flask; dissolve in 20mL of water. Add Ammonia T.S. dropwise with constant stirring. When the precipitate being formed is almost but not completely dissolved, stop adding Ammonia T.S. Filter the solution through Whatmann No 1 filter paper into a clean, amber-glass reagent bottle. Stopper firmly and label properly.

SILVER NITRATE T.S.

Dissolve 1.75g of silver nitrate in sufficient water to make 100ml. Transfer the solution into a clean amber-glass reagent bottle, mix well, stopper and label properly.

SODIUM ACETATE T.S.

Dissolve 13.6g of sodium acetate in sufficient water to make 100mL solution. Transfer the solution into a clean reagent bottle, mix well, stopper and label properly.

SODIUM BISULPHITE T.S.

Dissolve 5g of sodium bisulphite in 15mL of water, label properly.

> *Note:* The solution should be freshly prepared.

SODIUM BITARTRATE T.S.

Dissolve 1g of sodium bitartrate in 10mL of water. Approximate strength of the solution would be 1N, label properly.

> *Note:* The solution should be freshly prepared.

SODIUM CARBONATE T.S.

Dissolve 10.5g of anhydrous sodium carbonate in sufficient water to make 100mL. Transfer the solution into a clean reagent bottle, mix well, stopper and label properly. Approximate strength of the solution would be 2N.

SODIUM COBALTINITRITE T.S.

Dissolve 5g of sodium cobaltinitrite in 50mL of water, filter if required. Transfer the solution into a clean small reagent bottle, mix well, stopper and label properly.

SODIUM HYDROSULPHITE T.S., ALKALINE

Solution A: In a small clean reagent bottle (25mL capacity) take 5g of potassium hydroxide in 7mL of water, stopper and label properly.

Solution B: In another clean reagent bottle take 5g of sodium hydrosulphite and dissolve in 25mL of water, stopper and label properly.

Mix 2mL of solution A and 12.5mL of solution B to prepare the test solution.

> *Note:* The solution should be freshly prepared.

SODIUM HYDROXIDE T.S.

Take 4.3g of sodium hydroxide flakes or beads into a 100mL clean measuring cylinder, dissolve in water and make up the volume to 100mL with water. Transfer the solution into a clean reagent bottle, mix well, stopper and label properly. Approximate strength of the solution would be 1N.

SODIUM HYPOBROMITE T.S.

Dissolve 20g of sodium hydroxide in 75mL of water in a stoppered flask. Add 5mL of bromine, stopper the flask and swirl to make the solution. When the solution is made, make up the volume to 100mL with water.

Note: The solution should be freshly prepared.

SODIUM IODOHYDROXYQUINOLINE SULPHONATE T.S.

Dissolve 3.52g of Iodohydroxyquinoline sulphonic acid in 80mL of water; add 2.6mL of 4N sodium hydroxide. Add sufficient water to make 100mL with water, mix and filter. Transfer the solution into a clean reagent bottle, mix well, stopper and label properly.

SODIUM NITROFERRICYANIDE T.S.

Dissolve 0.5g of sodium nitroferricyanide in water to make 10mL of solution. Label the solution properly.

Note: The solution should be freshly prepared.

SODIUM PHOSPHATE T.S.

Dissolve 12g of clear crystals of sodium phosphate in sufficient water to make 100mL of solution. Transfer the solution into a clean reagent bottle, mix well, stopper and label properly. Approximate strength of the solution would be 1N.

SODIUM SULPHIDE T.S.

Take about 9mL of water, add and dissolve 1g of sodium sulphide. Make up the volume to 10mL with water.

Note: The solution should be freshly prepared.

STANNOUS CHLORIDE T.S.

Mix 9.8mL of water, add 0.2mL of hydrochloric acid, add and dissolve 1.5g of stannous chloride. Transfer the solution into a clean reagent bottle, put a small portion of tin, mix well, stopper and label properly.

Note: The solution should be freshly prepared.

STANNOUS CHLORIDE T.S., ACID

Dissolve 1.6g of stannous chloride in 100mL of hydrochloric acid. Transfer the solution into a clean reagent bottle, mix well, stopper and label properly.

Note: The solution should be used within 3 months from the date of preparation.

STARCH IODIDE PASTE T.S.

Prepare a solution of 0.75g of potassium iodides in 5mL of water. Prepare separately a solution of 2g of zinc chloride in 10mL of water. Heat 100mL of water to boiling, add potassium iodide solution; add zinc chloride solution and allow the solution to boil. Add a smooth suspension of 5g of potato starch in 30mL of cold water gradually with constant stirring. Boil the suspension for 2 min, cool to room temperature. Transfer the paste in a clean reagent bottle, stopper tightly and label properly. Store the paste in a cold place.

> *Note:* Efficacy of the starch iodide paste – dip a glass rod in a mixture of solution of 0.1ml of 0.1M sodium nitrite, 50ml of water and 1ml of hydrochloric acid. Streak the rod on a smear of the paste. A definite blue color streak would be produced.

STARCH-POTASSIUM IODIDE T.S.

Take 100mL of freshly prepared starch T.S., add and dissolve 500mg of potassium iodide. Label the solution properly.

> *Note:* The solution should be freshly prepared and used.

STARCH T.S.

Triturate 500mg of arrowroot starch in 5mL of cold water; add the slurry slowly into 100mL of boiling water with constant stirring. Boil the mixture until a translucent fluid is obtained. Allow the fluid to cool and settle. Decant the clear liquid and use.

> *Note:* The solution should be freshly prepared and used.

SULPHINILIC-A-NAPHTHYLAMINE T.S.

Solution A: Dissolve 100mg of sulphinilic acid in 30mL of acetic acid. Solution B: Dissolve 20mg of Naphthylamine hydrochloride in 30mL of acetic acid. Mix the two solutions and transfer it into a clean and dry reagent bottle, stopper tightly and label properly.

> *Note:* The solution may develop a pink color which may be removed by treating with zinc.

SULPHURIC ACID T.S.

Add an amount of sulphuric acid of known concentration to water to make a solution of concentration of $95.0\pm0.5\%$ w/v of H_2SO_4. Preserve the solution in tightly closed reagent bottle with proper label.

TANNIC ACID T.S.

Dissolve 1g of tannic acid in 1mL of alcohol, dilute to 10mL with water. label the properly.

> *Note:* The solution should be freshly prepared and used.

TETRAMETHYLAMMONIUM HYDROXIDE T.S.

Prepare 10% aqueous solution of Tetramethylammonium hydroxide in water. Transfer the solution in a clean reagent bottle, stopper and label properly.

THYMOL BLUE T.S.

In a clean and dry 50mL measuring cylinder take 50mg of thymol blue and dissolve in alcohol (95%), make up the volume to 50mL with alcohol. if required filter the solution and fill in a clean and dry reagent bottle, stopper tightly and label properly.

> *Note:* For pH determination – dissolve 50mg of thymol blue in 2.15ml of 0.05N sodium hydroxide and dilute to 100ml with freshly boiled and cooled water.

THYMOLPHTHALEIN T.S.

In a clean and dry 50mL measuring cylinder take 50mg of thymolphthalein and dissolve in alcohol (95%), make up the volume to 50mL with alcohol. if required filter the solution and fill in a clean and dry reagent bottle, stopper tightly and label properly.

TRIKETOHYDRINDENE HYDRATE T.S.

See Ninhydrin T.S.

TRINITROPHENOL T.S.

Dry about 1.5g of trinitrophenol at 105oC for 3hrs, cool in a desiccator. Take 1g of anhydrous trinitrophenol in a stoppered conical flask, add 100mL of hot water, stopper the flask and shake to dissolve. Cool the solution to room temperature, filter if necessary. Transfer the solution into a clean reagent bottle, stopper and label properly.

VALSER'S REAGENT T.S.

See Mercuric Iodide, T.S.

APPENDIX - II

Volumetric Solutions

The solutions used in volumetric analysis are called volumetric analysis. Their concentrations or strengths must be determined accurately, and methods used to determine their strength must be accurate and reproducible. Hence the methods of preparation and standardization of various volumetric solutions are given here. However, there may be different methods with obviously different accuracy. For the purpose of knowledge and practice the methods most commonly used and accepted are given here.

ACETIC ACID (1N)

Chemical formula: $C_2H_4O_2$ **Mol. wt: 60.05**   **Eq. wt.: 60.05**

For preparing its 1N solution 60.05g of acetic acid should be present in 1000mL.

It is very convenient to transfer a liquid by volume in place of by weight. Its specific gravity or density is 1.045.

Hence, 60.05g /1.045g/mL = 57.46mL or 58mL of glacial acetic acid should be dilute to 1000mL with freshly boiled and cooled distilled water to prepare its 1N solution.

Acetic Acid (xN): Dilute $58x$ ml of glacial acetic acid to 1000ml with freshly boiled and cooled water. Standardize with sodium hydroxide xN.

Method: Take a clean 1000mL volumetric flask. Measure 58mL of glacial acetic acid by a 100mL cylinder, transfer into the flask. Rinse the cylinder thrice with freshly boiled and cooled distilled water. Add the washings to the flask. Make up the volume with freshly boiled and cooled distilled water, stopper the flask and mix thoroughly. Transfer the solution into a suitable clean container. Label properly.

Standardization: Take clean 250mL of conical flask, 25mL volumetric pipette and one 50mL burette. Rinse the burette with standard 1N sodium hydroxide solution thrice; then fill the burette with sodium hydroxide solution above the zero mark. Open stop cock and drain some solution to fill and remove air entrapped. Set the volume at the mark zero.

Pipette out accurately 25mL of acetic acid solution and take it into the conical flask, add 25mL of freshly boiled and cooled water and 5-6 drops of phenolphthalein T.S.

Titrate the solution with sodium hydroxide until a faint pink color persists. Note the volume of titer value. Repeat the titration twice more and record the titer values. The titer values should be precise. Use the average titer value for calculation.

Calculation:

Say, strength (S_1) of sodium hydroxide solution is 0.1004N,

Average titer value (V_1) = 25.07mL

Volume of acetic acid taken (V_2) = 25.00mL

Then strength of acetic acid $(S_2) = \dfrac{S_1 \times V_1}{V_2} = \dfrac{0.1004N \times 25.07mL}{25.00mL} = 0.10068N$ or **0.1007N**

AMMONIUM THIOCYANATE (1N)

Chemical formula: NH_4SCN Mol. wt: 76.12   Eq. wt.: 76.12

1N solution of ammonium thiocyanate should contain 76.12g in 1000mL. Weigh 76.12g of ammonium thiocyanate, transfer into a clean 1000mL volumetric flask, add sufficient water to dissolve. Mix well, make up the volume to 1000mL with water, stopper and mix thoroughly. Transfer the solution into a clean container. Label properly.

Standardization:

Standardize the solution with 1N silver nitrate. Take a clean 50mL burette, rinse with ammonium thiocyanate solution. Fill the burette with ammonium thiocyanate solution; adjust the meniscus at zero mark. Pipette 25mL of 1N silver nitrate solution accurately and transfer into a clean 250mL conical flask. Add 50mL of water measured through 50mL cylinder; add 2mL of nitric acid and 2mL of ferric ammonium sulphate T.S. Titrate 1N silver nitrate solution with ammonium thiocyanate solution until a red-brown color is obtained. Record the titer value. Repeat the titration twice; take the average titer value for calculation.

Calculation:

Say, the strength of silver nitrate solution is 0.1005N

The average titer value = 25.00mL

Volume of silver nitrate solution taken = 25.00mL

The strength of ammonium thiocyanate solution $= \dfrac{25.00mL \times 0.1005N}{25.00mL} = 0.1005N$

BROMINE 0.1N

Chemical formula: Br   Mol. Wt.: 79.92   Eq. wt.: 79.92

1N solution of bromine should contain 7.992g of bromine in 1000mL.

In a 1000mL clean volumetric flask take 3g of potassium bromate and 15g of potassium bromide into the flask. Add sufficient water to dissolve; make up the volume and mix well. Transfer the solution into a clean amber-glass suitable container, stopper tightly.

> Bromine xN: Dissolve $3x$g of potassium bromate and $15x$g of potassium bromide in sufficient water to make 1000ml.

Standardization:

Pipette out accurately 25.00mL into 500mL iodine flask, measure 5mL of hydrochloric acid in a 10mL measuring cylinder and add; stopper and shake gently. Add 5mL of potassium iodide T.S.; stopper the flask again and shake well, allow it to stand for 5min. take a clean 50mL burette, rinse thrice with standard 0.1N sodium thiosulphate. Fill the burette with standard 0.1N sodium thiosulphate, adjust the meniscus to zero. Titrate the liberated iodine with 0.1N sodium thiosulphate. When the color of the solution is slightly brown, use starch T.S. as indicator. A deep blue color is obtained. Continue titration dropwise until the blue color disappears. Note the titer value. Repeat the titration twice more. Take the average value for calculation.

Calculation:

Calculate the strength of bromine solution as explained earlier.

CERIC SULPHATE 0.1N

Chemical formula: $Ce(SO_4)_2$ Mol. Wt.: 332.26   Eq. wt.: 332.26

1000mL of 0.1N solution contains 33.26g of ceric sulphate.

Take about 500mL of water in a clean 1000mL volumetric flask, add and dissolve 42g of ceric sulphate, if necessary, heat to dissolve completely. Once ceric sulphate is completely dissolved, cool the solution to room temperature and make up the volume with water; stopper the flask and shake well. Transfer the solution into a suitable amber-glass bottle. Standardize the solution as mentioned below.

Standardization:

Weigh accurately 180mg of clean, rust free iron wire; place the iron into a 250mL stoppered flask. Add 50mL of diluted sulphuric acid; stopper the flask and place it over a boiling water bath with frequent swirling until dissolved completely. Cool the solution; pass it through a freshly prepared reductor. Rinse the reductor with 2×50mL of dilute sulphuric acid. Add the washings to the main solution; add 2 drops of orthophenanthroline T.S. and titrate with the ceric sulphate solution from a burette until red color turns into pale blue. Calculate the normality of the ceric sulphate solution. 1 mL of 0.1N ceric sulphate is equivalent to 5.585mg of iron.

Standard Dichlorophenol-Indophenol solution

Dissolve 53 mg sodium bicarbonate in 50 mL of distilled water taken in a 250 mL clean volumetric flask. Weigh 62.5 mg of 2,6-dichlorophenol-indophenol sodium stored in a desiccator over soda lime and transfer into the sodium bicarbonate solution. Stopper and shake the volumetric flask. Add sufficient water to make 250 mL, mix well.

Weigh accurately 50 mg of ascorbic acid U.S.P. of known potency. Transfer it into a 50 mL volumetric flask; dissolve in sufficient metaphosphoric-acetic acids T.S. to make

50 mL. Take 2 mL of ascorbic acid solution into a 50 mL Erlenmeyer flask containing 5 mL of metaphosphoric-acetic acids T.S. and titrate immediately with 2,6-dichlorophenol-indophenol sodium solution until a distinct rose-pink color is produced and persists for at least 5 seconds. Carry out a blank titration using 7 mL of metaphosphoric-acetic acids T.S. Calculate the strength of the 2,6-dichlorophenol-indophenol sodium solution based on its equivalent weight.

Disodium Ethylenediamine tetra-acetate, 0.05M

Chemical formula: $C_{10}H_{14}N_2Na_2O_8, 2H_2O$	**Mol. Wt. 372.25**	**Eq. wt.: 372.25**

Dissolve 9.3g of disodium ethylenediamine tetra-acetate in sufficient water to make 500 mL. *Standardization*

Weigh accurately 200 mg of dried calcium carbonate; transfer it to a 250 mL conical flask. Add 50 mL of water and sufficient dilute hydrochloric acid to dissolve the carbonate completely. Dilute the solution to 150 mL with sufficient water. Add 15 mL of sodium hydroxide T.S., 40 mg of murexide indicator, and 3 mL of naphthol green T.S. Then titrate the solution with disodium ethylenediamine tetra-acetate solution from a burette until a deep blue color appears. Note the titer value. Repeat the titration twice and take average of the three titer values. Carry out a blank determination and subtract from the average titer value. Calculate the strength of the 0.05M disodium ethylenediamine tetra-acetate solution.

1 mL of 0.05M disodium ethylenediamine tetra-acetate solution is equivalent to 100.1 mg of $CaCO_3$.

FERRIC AMMONIUM SULPHATE, 0.1N

Chemical formula: $FeNH_4(SO_4)_2, 12H_2O$	**Mol. Wt.: 482.21**	**Eq. wt.: 482.2**

Dissolve 25g of ferric ammonium sulphate in a mixture of 150 mL of water and 3 mL of sulphuric acid, dilute with sufficient water to make 500 mL. Mix well.

Standardization

Pipette out accurately 40.00 mL of the ferric ammonium sulphate solution, transfer to a 250 mL glass stoppered conical flask. Add 5 mL of hydrochloric acid, mix. Add 3g of potassium iodide dissolved in 10 mL of water, stopper immediately and allow to stand for 10 min. Then titrate the liberated iodine with 0.1N sodium thiosulphate solution from a burette until a light brown color appears. Add 3 mL of starch T.S., a blue color is produced. Titrate the solution until a single drop of 0.1N sodium thiosulphate solution changes the blue color to colorless. Note the titer value. Repeat the titration twice and take average of the three titer values. Carry out a blank determination and subtract from the average titer value. Calculate the strength of the ferric ammonium sulphate solution by using the equation, $S \times V = S_1 \times V_1$. Where S is the strength of ferric ammonium sulphate solution, V is 40.00 mL, V_1 is the titer value, and S_1 is the strength of 0.1N sodium thiosulphate solution.

FERROUS AMMONIUM SULPHATE, 0.1N

Chemical formula: $Fe(NH_4)_2(SO_4)_2, 6H_2O$ Mol. Wt.: 392.16   Eq. wt.: 392.2

Dissolve 20g of ferrous ammonium sulphate in a cooled mixture of 100 mL of water and 20 mL of sulphuric acid. Dilute the solution with sufficient water to make 500 mL. Mix well.

Standardization

Pipette out accurately 25.00 mL of the ferrous ammonium sulphate solution, transfer to a 250 mL conical flask. Add 2 drops of orthophenanthroline T.S. and titrate with 0.1N ceric sulphate from a burette until the red color is changed to pale blue color. Note the titer value. Repeat the titration twice and take average of the three titer values. Carry out a blank determination and subtract from the average titer value. Calculate the strength of the ferrous ammonium sulphate solution by using the equation, $S \times V = S_1 \times V_1$. Where S is the strength of ferric ammonium sulphate solution, V is 40.00 mL, V_1 is the titer value, and S_1 is the strength of 0.1N ceric sulphate solution.

HYDROCHLORIC ACID, 0.1N

Chemical formula: HCl   Mol. Wt.: 36.46   Eq. wt.: 36.46

Dilute 48 mL of hydrochloric acid with sufficient water to make 500 mL. Mix well.

Standardization

Dry about 5g of anhydrous sodium carbonate (primary standard) at 270°C for 1 hr., allow to cool the material in a desiccator. Weigh accurately 1.5g of anhydrous sodium carbonate, transfer it into a clean 250 mL conical flask, add 100 mL of water and dissolve. Add 2 drops of methyl red and titrate with hydrochloric acid slowly from a burette with constant stirring until a faint pink color appears. Heat the solution to boiling and continue titration dropwise until the pink color does not disappear on boiling. Note the titer value. Repeat the titration twice and take average of the three titer values. Calculate the strength of the hydrochloric acid solution. 1 mL of 0.1N hydrochloric acid is equivalent to 0.05299g of anhydrous sodium carbonate.

IODINE, 0.1N

Chemical formula: I   Mol. Wt.: 126.91   Eq. wt.: 126.9

Dissolve 7g of iodine in a solution of 18g of potassium iodide in 50 mL of water. Add 1 drop of hydrochloric acid and dilute with sufficient water to make 500 mL. Mix well.

Standardization

Weigh accurately about 150 mg of arsenic trioxide; transfer it into a 250 mL conical flask. Add 20 mL of 1N sodium hydroxide, dissolve by warming if required. Add 40 mL of water, mix and add 2 drops of methyl orange T.S., add 1N hydrochloric acid with constant stirring until a faint pink color appears. Add 2g of sodium bicarbonate, 50 mL of water and 3 mL of starch T.S., stir to dissolve sodium bicarbonate. Titrate the solution with iodine from a burette with constant swirling until a permanent blue color appears. Note the titer value and repeat the titration twice more. Take the average of three titer value for calculation of the strength of iodine solution.

1 mL of 0.1N iodine solution is equivalent to 4.946mg of arsenic trioxide.

Note: Preserve the iodine solution in an amber color bottle, stopper the bottle tightly. Keep it away from light.

OXALIC ACID, 0.1N

Chemical formula: $H_2C_2O_4, 2H_2O$	**Mol. Wt.: 126.07**	**Eq. wt.: 63.04**

Dissolve 6.45g of oxalic acid in sufficient water to make 1000mL.

Standardization

Pipette out accurately 25.00 mL of oxalic acid solution and take in a 250 mL conical flask. Add 7 mL of sulphuric acid; heat to about 70°C and titrate slowly with 0.1N potassium permanganate solution from a burette with constant stirring until the faint pink color that persists for at least 15 sec appears. The temperature of the solution should not be less than 60°C at the end of the titration. Note the titer value and repeat the titration twice more. Take the average of three titer values and calculate strength of the oxalic acid solution.

Note: Preserve oxalic acid solution in a amber color bottle, tightly stoppered and away from light.

PERCHLORIC ACID, 0.1N

Chemical formula: $HClO_4$	**Mol. Wt.: 100.46**	**Eq. wt.: 100.46**

Measure 4.25mL of perchloric acid using a dry 10 mL measuring cylinder, mix with 250 mL of glacial acetic acid in a clean and dry 500 mL volumetric flask. Add 15 mL of acetic anhydride and mix. Cool the mixture and dilute to 500 mL with glacial acetic acid, mix well. Allow to stand for 24 hrs. Determine the water content by titrimetric method. The water content should be less than 0.05%. If required more of acetic anhydride is to be added.

Standardization

Dry about 1 g of potassium hydrogen phthalate at 105°C for 2 hrs., cool it in a desiccator. Weigh accurately 700mg of dried potassium hydrogen phthalate and transfer it into a 250 mL clean and dry conical flask. Add 50 mL of glacial acetic acid and dissolve. Add 2 drops of methylrosaniline chloride T.S. and titrate with perchloric acid filled in a dry burette until the violet color of the solution changes to emerald-green. Note the titer value. Repeat the titration twice and make the average. Carry out a blank titration, deduct the blank titer value from the average titer value and calculate the strength of the perchloric acid solution.

1 mL of 0.1N perchloric acid is equivalent to 0.02042g of potassium hydrogen phthalate.

POTASSIUM BROMATE, 0.1N

Chemical formula: $KBrO_3$ Mol. Wt.: 167.02   Eq. wt.: 27.84

Dissolve 1.4g of potassium bromate in sufficient water to make 500 mL. Mix well.

Standardization

Pipette out exactly 40.00 mL of potassium bromate solution and take in a 250 mL iodine flask. Add 3 g of potassium iodide and 3 mL of hydrochloric acid, stopper immediately. Allow to stand for 5 min. Titrate the liberated iodine with 0.1N sodium thiosulphate solution from a burette until light brown is produced. Add 2 mL of starch T.S. as indicator. A blue color is produced. Continue titration by adding 0.1N sodium thiosulphate solution dropwise until the solution becomes colorless. Note the titer value and repeat the titration twice more and take the average titer value. Carry out a blank titration, deduct the blank titer value from the average titer value and calculate the strength of the potassium bromate solution using normality of 0.1N sodium thiosulphate.

POTASSIUM DICHROMATE, 0.1N

Chemical formula: $K2Cr_2O_7$ Mol. Wt.: 294.22   Eq. wt.: 49.04

Dissolve 2.5g of potassium dichromate in sufficient water to make 500 mL, mix well.

Standardization

Pipette out exactly 25.00 mL of potassium dichromate and take it into a 500l stopper conical flask. Add 2g of potassium iodide (iodate free), 200 mL of water, 5mL of hydrochloric acid, stopper immediately and keep it for 10 min in a dark place. Titrate the liberated iodine with 0.1N sodium thiosulphate from a burette. Use starch T.S. as indicator and continue titration until the blue color disappears with a single drop of 0.1N sodium thiosulphate. Note the titer value and repeat the titration twice more and take the average titer value. Carry out a blank titration, deduct the blank titer value from the average titer value and calculate the strength of the potassium dichromate solution using normality of 0.1N sodium thiosulphate.

POTASSIUM FERRICYANIDE, 0.05M

Chemical formula: $K_3Fe\,(CN)_6$ Mol. Wt.: 329.26

Dissolve 8.5g of potassium ferricyanide in sufficient water to make 500mL of solution.

Standardization

Pipette out exactly 50.00mL of potassium ferricyanide solution in a 500mL stoppered conical flask. Add 50mL of water, 10mL of potassium iodide T.S., 10mL of dilute hydrochloric acid, and keep it stoppered for 2min. Add 15mL of 10% zinc sulphate solution and titrate the liberated iodine with 0.1N sodium thiosulphate from a burette. Use starch T.S. as indicator and continue titration until the blue color disappears with a single drop of 0.1N sodium thiosulphate. Note the titer value and repeat the titration twice more and take the average titer value. Carry out a blank titration, deduct the blank titer value from the average titer value and calculate the strength of the potassium dichromate solution using normality of 0.1N sodium thiosulphate.

1mL of 0.1N sodium thiosulphate is equivalent to 2mL of 0.05M potassium ferricyanide.

POTASSIUM HYDROXIDE, 0.1N

Chemical formula: KOH	**Mol. Wt. 56.11**	**Eq. Wt. 56.11g**

Purity of potassium hydroxide is less (85%) and also it is hygroscopic. Hence, to make its deci-normal solution 7.0g of potassium hydroxide should be taken in place of 5.6g per litre of solution.

Dissolve 7g of potassium hydroxide in about 900mL of water; add dropwise freshly prepared saturated solution of barium hydroxide until no more precipitate is formed. Shake the solution vigorously and keep it in a stoppered flask overnight. Either decant the clear supernatant solution or filter through Whatmann No 42 filter paper. Make up the volume to 1000mL with sufficient water, mix well.

Standardization

Dry about 1 g of potassium hydrogen phthalate at 105°C for 2 hrs., cool it in a desiccator. Weigh accurately 500mg of dried potassium hydrogen phthalate and transfer it into a 250 mL conical flask. Add 75 mL of water and dissolve. Add 2 drops of phenolphthalein T.S. and titrate with 0.1N potassium hydroxide solution from a burette until a permanent pink color appears. Note the titer value. Repeat the titration twice and make the average. Carry out a blank titration, deduct the blank titer value from the average titer value and calculate the strength of the potassium hydroxide solution.

1 mL of 0.1N potassium hydroxide is equivalent to 0.02042g of potassium hydrogen phthalate.

POTASSIUM HYDROXIDE, ALCOHOLIC, 0.1N

Chemical formula: KOH	**Mol. Wt. 56.11**	**Eq. wt.: 56.11**

Dissolve 3.5g of potassium hydroxide in about 5mL of water; add sufficient alcohol (aldehyde free) to make 500 mL of solution, mix well. Keep the solution for 24 hrs, decant the supernatant solution and fill in a clean stopper bottle. Shake to mix thoroughly.

Standardization

Pipette accurately 25.00mL of standard 0.1N hydrochloric acid, add 50 mL of water and 2 drops of phenolphthalein T.S. and titrate with potassium hydroxide solution from a burette until a pink color appears permanently.

Note the titer value. Repeat the titration twice and make the average. Carry out a blank titration, deduct the blank titer value from the average titer value and calculate the strength of the potassium hydroxide solution.

Note: Store the solution in a tightly closed amber color bottle, away from light.

POTASSIUM IODATE, 0.1N

Chemical formula: KIO_3	Mol. Wt. 214.01	Eq. wt.: 53.50

Anhydrous potassium iodate is a primary standard. Take about 5.350g of potassium iodate, dry at 110°C to constant weight, cool it in a desiccator. Weigh accurately about 21.4g of the dried potassium iodate, transfer into a 1000mL volumetric flask, dissolve in sufficient water to make 1000mL. Stopper the flask and shake to mix thoroughly.

Standardization

Note the actual weight of potassium iodate taken.

$$\text{The strength of } 0.1\text{M potassium iodate} = \frac{\text{Actual weight}}{\text{Theoretical weight}} = \frac{\text{Actual weight (g)}}{21.40\text{g}}$$

POTASSIUM PERMANGANATE, 0.1N

Chemical formula: $KMnO_4$;	Mol. Wt.: 158.04;	Eq. wt.: 31.61

Dissolve about 3.3g of potassium permanganate in sufficient water to make 1000mL. Boil the solution for about 15 min, stopper the flask and keep it for 2 days. Filter the solution and standardize.

Standardization

Dry about 1g of sodium oxalate at 110°C for 3 hrs or until constant weight is obtained. Cool it in a desiccator. Weigh accurately about 200mg of dried sodium oxalate in a 500 mL conical flask. Add 250 mL of water, 7 mL of sulphuric acid; heat to about 70°C. Titrate the solution with potassium permanganate solution from a burette until a pale pink color appears which persists for 15 secs. Till the end of the titration the temperature of the solution must remain within 60 – 65°C. Note the titer value. Repeat the titration twice and make the average. Carry out a blank titration, deduct the blank titer value from the average titer value and calculate the strength of the potassium permanganate solution.

1 mL of 0.1N potassium permanganate solution is equivalent to 6.700mg of dried sodium oxalate.

Note: potassium permanganate oxidizes rubber; hence preserve the solution in an amber color bottle with glass stopper. Keep it away from light.

SILVER NITRATE, 0.1N

Chemical formula: $AgNO_3$; Mol. Wt.: 169.89;   Eq. wt.: 169.9

Dissolve 8.75g of silver nitrate in water and make 500mL solution.

Standardization

Pipette accurately 25.00mL of silver nitrate solution in a beaker; add about 40mL of water. Heat the solution to about 80°C and add slowly dilute hydrochloric acid with constant stirring until no more precipitate is formed. Boil the suspension carefully, so that there is no loss of material, for about 5 min; keep it in dark till the precipitates settle and a completely clear supernatant solution is produced. Dry a G4 sintered glass crucible at 120°C for 2 hrs, cool in a desiccator and weigh (xg). Filter the precipitate through the tared crucible, wash the precipitate with wash acidified with nitric acid. Dry the crucible with precipitate at 110°C for 2 hrs or till a constant weight (x_1g) is obtained. Calculate the strength of silver nitrate solution from weight of precipitate as follows;

The precipitation reaction is: $AgNO_3 + HCl = AgCl \downarrow + HNO_3$

Thus, 169.89g of $AgNO_3 \approx 143.34$g of $AgCl$

In other words, 143.34g of $AgCl \approx 169.89$g of $AgNO_3$

Hence, 1g of $AgCl \approx \dfrac{169.89g}{143.34g} = 1.18522$g of $AgNO_3$

Say, the weight of dry precipitate of $AgCl = (x_1g - xg) = yg \approx y \times 1.18522$g of $AgNO_3$

So, a mL of silver nitrate solution $\approx \dfrac{8.75g \times a \text{ mL}}{500mL} = 0.0175a$ g of $AgNO_3$

Hence, the normality of the solution $= \dfrac{y \times 1.18522}{a}$(N)

Where, y = weight of the dried precipitate and

   a = volume of silver nitrate solution taken.

SODIUM HYDROXIDE, 0.1N

Chemical formula: NaOH,   Mol. wt.: 40.00   Eq. wt.: 40.00

Dissolve 45g of sodium hydroxide in about 900mL of water; add dropwise freshly prepared saturated solution of barium hydroxide until no more precipitate is formed. Shake the solution vigorously and keep it in a stoppered flask overnight. Either decant the clear supernatant solution or filter through Whatmann No 42-filter paper. Make up the volume to 1000mL with sufficient water, mix well.

Standardization

Dry about 1 g of potassium hydrogen phthalate at 105°C for 2 hrs., cool it in a desiccator. Weigh accurately 500mg of dried potassium hydrogen phthalate and transfer it into a 250 mL conical flask. Add 75 mL of water and dissolve. Add 2 drops of phenolphthalein T.S. and titrate with 0.1N sodium hydroxide from a burette until a permanent pink color appears. Note the titer value. Repeat the titration twice and make the average. Carry out a blank titration, deduct the blank titer value from the average titer value and calculate the strength of the sodium hydroxide solution.

1 mL of 0.1N sodium hydroxide is equivalent to 0.02042g of potassium hydrogen phthalate.

SODIUM METHOXIDE, 0.1N

Chemical formula: CH_3ONa;   Mol. Wt.: 54.03   Eq. wt.: 54.03

Take 150 mL of methanol in a 1000mL volumetric flask, cool in ice-water. Add 2.5g of freshly cut sodium metal cut in small portions, dissolve. When the metal is dissolved completely add sufficient benzene to make 1000mL. Stopper the flask and shake well to mix thoroughly. Fill the solution in a reservoir fitted to an automatic delivery burette. The solution must be protected from moisture and carbon dioxide.

Standardization

Weigh accurately about 400mg of benzoic acid (primary standard). Transfer it into a dry 250mL conical flask, add 80 mL of dimethylformamide and dissolve. Add 3 drops of 1% solution of thymol blue in dimethylformamide. Titrate the solution with sodium methoxide from the automatic burette until a blue color is produced. Note the titer value. Repeat the titration twice and make the average. Carry out a blank titration, deduct the blank titer value from the average titer value and calculate the strength of the sodium hydroxide solution.

1 mL of 0.1N sodium methoxide is equivalent to 0.01221g of benzoic acid.

SODIUM NITRITE, 0.1M

Chemical formula: $NaNO_2$;   Mol. Wt.: 69.00

Dissolve 7.5g of sodium nitrite in sufficient water to make 1000mL, mix the solution thoroughly.

Standardization

Dry about 2g of sulphanilamide at 105°C for 3 hrs, cool in a desiccator. Weigh accurately about 500mg of sulphanilamide (USP reference standard), transfer it into a beaker, add about 50 mL of water and 5mL of hydrochloric acid. Stir the mixture with a glass rod until dissolved. Cool the solution to 15°C, add about 30g of ice and titrate slowly with sodium nitrite from a burette with constant and vigorously. The end point of the titration is detected when the titrated solution is smeared on starch iodide paste T.S. or starch iodide paper using the glass rod, a blue color is produced. Note the titer value. Repeat the titration twice and make the average. Carry out a blank titration, deduct the blank titer value from the average titer value and calculate the molarity of the sodium nitrite solution.

1 mL of 0.1M sodium nitrite is equivalent to 17.22 mg of sulphanilamide of 100% purity.

SODIUM THIOSULPHATE, 0.1N

Chemical formula: $Na_2S_2O_3, 5H_2O$ Mol. Wt.: 248.19   Eq. wt.: 248.19

Dissolve about 13g of sodium thiosulphate and 100 mg of sodium carbonate in sufficient water to make 500 mL of solution. Shake well to mix.

Standardization

Pipette out accurately 25.00 mL of 0.1N potassium dichromate standard solution into an iodine flask or glass stoppered conical flask. Add 50 mL of water, 2g of potassium iodide, and 5mL of hydrochloric acid, stopper the flask. Mix well and keep it for 10 min. Dilute with 100 mL of water and titrate the liberated iodine with 0.1N sodium thiosulphate solution until yellowish green color is produced. Add 2mL of starch T.S., a blue color is produced. Continue titration dropwise until the blue color disappears with single drop of 0.1N sodium thiosulphate. Note the titer value. Repeat the titration twice and make the average. Carry out a blank titration, deduct the blank titer value from the average titer value and calculate the normality of the 0.1N sodium thiosulphate solution.

SULPHURIC ACID, 0.1N

Chemical formula: H_2SO_4 Mol. Wt.: 98.08   Eq. wt.: 49.04

Add slowly 3 mL of sulphuric acid to 510 mL of water, mix and cool to 25°C.

Standardization

Dry about 5g of anhydrous sodium carbonate (primary standard) at 270°C for 1 hr., allow to cool the material in a desiccator. Weigh accurately 1.5g of anhydrous sodium carbonate, transfer it into a clean 250 mL conical flask, add 100 mL of water and dissolve. Add 2 drops of methyl red and titrate with 0.1N sulphuric acid slowly from a burette with constant stirring until a faint pink color appears. Heat the solution to boiling and continue titration dropwise until the pink color does not disappear on boiling. Note the titer value. Repeat the titration twice and take average of the three titer values. Calculate the strength of the sulphuric acid solution. 1 mL of 0.1N sulphuric acid is equivalent to 0.05299g of anhydrous sodium carbonate of 100% purity.

Answers

CHAPTER 1

1. (a)	2. (b)	3. (d)	4. (a)	5. (b)
6. (b)	7. (a)	8. (d)	9. (a)	10. (b)
11. (c)	12. (a)	13. (b)	14. (d)	15. (d)
16. (c)	17. (a)	18. (a)	19. (b)	10. (c)

CHAPTER 2

1. (a)	2. (a)	3. (b)	4. (c)	5. (d)
6. (a)	7. (d)	8. (c)	9. (d)	10. (a)
11. (b)	12. (c)	13. (b)	14. (b)	15. (a)
16. (c)	17. (a)			

CHAPTER 3

1. (d)	2. (d)	3. (b)	4. (a)	5. (a)
6. (b)	7. (d)	8. (b)	9. (d)	10. (a)
11. (b)	12. (d)	13. (d)	14. (a)	15. (a)
16. (c)				

CHAPTER 4

1. (b)	2. (d)	3. (d)	4. (a)	5. (a)
6. (b)	7. (c)	8. (d)	9. (a)	10. (c)
11. (b)	12. (a)	13. (c)	14. (b)	15. (a)
16. (d)				

CHAPTER 5

1. (d)	2. (a)	3. (a)	4. (c)	5. (b)
6. (c)	7. (a)	8. (c)	9. (d)	10. (b)
11. (d)	12. (a)			

CHAPTER 6

1. (d)	2. (a)	3. (b)	4. (c)	5. (d)
6. (d)	7. (c)	8. (a)	9. (c)	10. (a)
11. (d)	12. (d)	13. (c)	14. (b)	15. (d)
16. (a)	17. (b)	18. (a)	19. (d)	20. (b)

CHAPTER 7

1. (b)	2. (d)	3. (a)	4. (d)	5. (c)
6. (a)	7. (d)	8. (d)	9. (a)	10. (a)
11. (d)	12. (b)	13. (a)	14. (b)	15. (c)
16. (a)				

CHAPTER 8

1. (c)	2. (a)	3. (b)	4. (b)	5. (a)
6. (d)	7. (d)	8. (a)	9. (c)	10. (b)
11. (a)	12. (c)	13. (a)	14. (d)	15. (b)
16. (a)	17. (c)			

CHAPTER 9

1. (a)	2. (a)	3. (d)	4. (b)	5. (a)
6. (c)	7. (a)	8. (c)	9. (a)	10. (c)
11. (b)	12. (a)	13. (d)	14. (d)	15. (d)
16. (a)				

CHAPTER 10

1. (d)	2. (a)	3. (b)	4. (d)	5. (a)
6. (c)	7. (d)	8. (d)	9. (a)	10. (d)
11. (a)	12. (d)			

CHAPTER 11

1. (b)	2. (a)	3. (c)	4. (c)	5. (a)
6. (a)	7. (c)	8. (c)	9. (a)	10. (d)
11. (c)	12. (d)			

Index

R

S

T

9 789389 354195